Gender Equity in the Medical Profession

Maria Irene Bellini
Belfast Health and Social Care Trust, UK

Vassilios E. Papalois
Imperial College London, UK

A volume in the Advances in Medical Education, Research, and Ethics (AMERE) Book Series

IGI Global
DISSEMINATOR OF KNOWLEDGE

Published in the United States of America by
IGI Global
Medical Information Science Reference (an imprint of IGI Global)
701 E. Chocolate Avenue
Hershey PA, USA 17033
Tel: 717-533-8845
Fax: 717-533-8661
E-mail: cust@igi-global.com
Web site: http://www.igi-global.com

Library of Congress Cataloging-in-Publication Data

Names: Bellini, Maria Irene, 1982- editor. | Papalois, Vassilios E., editor.
Title: Gender equity in the medical profession / Maria Irene Bellini and Vassilios E. Papalois, editors.
Description: Hershey, PA : Medical Information Science Reference (an imprint of IGI Global), [2020] | Includes bibliographical references.
Identifiers: LCCN 2019003626| ISBN 9781522595991 (hardcover) | ISBN 9781522596004 (ebook)
Subjects: | MESH: Health Workforce | Sexism | Women's Rights
Classification: LCC RA564.7 | NLM W 76.1 | DDC 362.1081--dc23 LC record available at https://lccn.loc.gov/2019003626

This book is published in the IGI Global book series Advances in Medical Education, Research, and Ethics (AMERE) (ISSN: 2475-6601; eISSN: 2475-661X)

British Cataloguing in Publication Data
A Cataloguing in Publication record for this book is available from the British Library.

For electronic access to this publication, please contact: eresources@igi-global.com.

Advances in Medical Education, Research, and Ethics (AMERE) Book Series

ISSN:2475-6601
EISSN:2475-661X

Mission

Humans are living longer now than ever as a result of advances in the medical field. Having the tools available to train knowledgeable and ethical future generations of doctors and medical researchers is essential to continuing to advance our understanding of the human body and develop new ways of treating and curing sickness and disease.

The **Advances in Medical Education, Research, and Ethics (AMERE)** book series highlights publications pertaining to advancements in pedagogical practice for developing future healthcare professionals, research methods, and advancements in the medical field, as well as moral behavior and practice of healthcare professionals, students, and researchers. Featuring research-based book publications that are highly relevant to the healthcare community, this series is ideally designed for library inclusion at medical universities and research institutions as well as personal use by medical professionals, researchers, and upper-level students entering the field.

Coverage

- Clinical Research
- Conflicts of Interest
- Ethics in Medicine
- Healthcare Pedagogy
- Medical Curricula
- Medical Simulation
- Patient Data
- Professional Development
- Research Methods
- Scientific Misconduct

IGI Global is currently accepting manuscripts for publication within this series. To submit a proposal for a volume in this series, please contact our Acquisition Editors at Acquisitions@igi-global.com or visit: http://www.igi-global.com/publish/.

The Advances in Medical Education, Research, and Ethics (AMERE) Book Series (ISSN 2475-6601) is published by IGI Global, 701 E. Chocolate Avenue, Hershey, PA 17033-1240, USA, www.igi-global.com. This series is composed of titles available for purchase individually; each title is edited to be contextually exclusive from any other title within the series. For pricing and ordering information please visit http://www.igi-global.com/book-series/advances-medical-education-research-ethics/132365. Postmaster: Send all address changes to above address.

Titles in this Series

For a list of additional titles in this series, please visit:
https://www.igi-global.com/book-series/advances-medical-education-research-ethics/132365

Preparing Physicians to Lead in the 21st Century
Valerie Anne Storey (University of Central Florida, USA) and Thomas Edward Beeman (University of Pennsylvania Health System, USA)
Medical Information Science Reference • © 2019 • 245pp • H/C (ISBN: 9781522575764) • US $245.00 (our price)

Optimizing Medical Education With Instructional Technology
Erdem Demiroz (Trakya University, Turkey) and Steven D. Waldman (University of Missouri – Kansas City School of Medicine, USA)
Medical Information Science Reference • © 2019 • 291pp • H/C (ISBN: 9781522562894) • US $215.00 (our price)

Exploring the Pressures of Medical Education From a Mental Health and Wellness Perspective
Christina Ramirez Smith (University of the Bahamas, Bahamas)
Medical Information Science Reference • © 2018 • 349pp • H/C (ISBN: 9781522528111) • US $225.00 (our price)

Impact of Medical Errors and Malpractice on Health Economics, Quality, and Patient Safety
Marina Riga (Health Economist-Researcher, Greece)
Medical Information Science Reference • © 2017 • 334pp • H/C (ISBN: 9781522523376) • US $200.00 (our price)

Advancing Medical Education Through Strategic Instructional Design
Jill Stefaniak (Old Dominion University, USA)
Medical Information Science Reference • © 2017 • 349pp • H/C (ISBN: 9781522520986) • US $205.00 (our price)

Organizational Culture and Ethics in Modern Medicine
Anna Rosiek (Nicolaus Copernicus University in Toruń, Collegium Medicum in Bydgoszcz, Poland) and Krzysztof Leksowski (Nicolaus Copernicus University in Toruń, Collegium Medicum in Bydgoszcz, Poland)
Medical Information Science Reference • © 2016 • 448pp • H/C (ISBN: 9781466696587) • US $225.00 (our price)

Handbook of Research on Advancing Health Education through Technology
Victor X. Wang (Florida Atlantic University, USA)
Medical Information Science Reference • © 2016 • 588pp • H/C (ISBN: 9781466694941) • US $335.00 (our price)

IGI Global
DISSEMINATOR OF KNOWLEDGE

701 East Chocolate Avenue, Hershey, PA 17033, USA
Tel: 717-533-8845 x100 • Fax: 717-533-8661
E-Mail: cust@igi-global.com • www.igi-global.com

Associate Editors

Table of Contents

Detailed Table of Contents

It comes as no surprise that to tackle gender inequality in the future of the medical profession, the experiences of those who will become it must first be reviewed. Gender inequality is rife throughout all aspects of medical student life; from the classroom to clinical placements, from other healthcare professionals and public alike, for both male and female students. This chapter will discuss these, review literature, and share experiences. Consequently, this has an impact on their career choices, attrition, and mental health. By improving experiences and encouraging diversity, the hope is to reduce the negative effects discussed within the chapter, and break the cycle of inequality.

The challenge of diversification in the medical workforce cannot be ignored. Society and societal norms have also progressed at pace and terms and attitudes that were acceptable are now outdated. Trainers must be professionalised to ensure that training of trainees remains an exemplar role. It is accepted that boys and girls learn differently but have the same potential. Equity of opportunity ensures that the modern society retains and values all genders. By exploring whether these differences continue into the post-graduate education system, the medical profession can accommodate and mitigate to ensure equity. This chapter will explore the need for professional trainers, the educational needs of the modern-day medical trainee, and the challenges that need to be accommodated to ensure that the medical workforce retains a passion long into their careers.

Female and male physicians practice medicine differently. Female physicians engage in different communication styles, allocate more time to preventative care, and show different leadership qualities. Because gender diversity is still lacking in the top academic and clinical positions, medical organizations are not fully benefiting from these strengths. This chapter will identify three barriers that prevent women from advancing to these positions: the double burden syndrome, sexism and sexual harassment, and gender bias. This chapter will take a critical look at organizational culture and propose changes that can contribute to the pursuit of gender equity.

Communication is one of the most essential skills of the medical profession, however, it is a tool through which sexism and gender discrimination are promoted and reproduced. There is often the perception in medicine and surgery that gender inequity centres on lifestyle, family responsibilities, and childcare issues.

However, this chapter highlights that deeply engrained biases in medical communication still exist, and are perpetrated by institutions and individuals, women included. Awareness of gendered language must be raised and highlighted in order to make a change. It is achievable to speak in gender-neutral ways that are inclusive and precise as to not conjure biased attitudes towards women in medicine. Social change must be pursued at the level of the institution, the cultural structure, and at the interactional level of gender.

Female representation in medicine is increasing, however women make up only a small percentage of senior roles in the NHS. Only 36% of consultants are female with wide variation between specialties ranging from 12% of surgeons to over half of paediatricians, gynaecologists, and directors of public health. Women comprise 77% of the NHS workforce and account for 44% of chief executives of all NHS Trusts and 47% of executive directors. This chapter analyses the role of women as leaders within the medical world and compares the representation of women in senior leadership roles within medicine and other parallel, male-dominated working environments. Alternative forms of leadership such as mentoring, coaching, and sponsorship are also considered.

The gender pay gap is a symptom of the pervasive inequalities inherent in modern society. Among doctors, the gap has been increasing. The Gender Pay Gap in Medicine Review is exploring the scale of the problem and the reasons behind it. Although motherhood and flexible working both contribute to the salary discrepancy, the aetiology is complex and multifactorial, with important roles played by recruitment and representation of women at senior levels, as well as gender occupational segregation. Addressing the root causes of gender inequalities and shining a light on the pay gap data are both required in order to one day close the gap.

Every person should be valued for their skills and potential, for every moment they are present. Training on Diversity and Unconscious bias is urgently needed. All staff must see themselves as role models, creating culture and reacting to another's name badge/role, with "fake it till you make it". Those with poor behaviour may lack insight. Zero tolerance involves others taking a poorly-behaving peer for 'a Vanderbilt cup of coffee'. Informal mentors should avoid gendered assumptions, e.g. all medical students need to scrub in. Leadership roles should have a clear application process. Inequality is not just a women's issue. Improvements must focus on the women themselves, the others around them, and the structures/

Despite the consistently reported gender parity among accepted applicants to US medical schools, upstream parity in surgical training, academic promotion, leadership positions, pay equity, grant funding, and efforts to promote wellness specific to the needs of women surgeons is seriously lacking. Along with these known disparities, women surgeons disproportionally suffer from gender bias, micro-aggressions, bullying, discrimination, and harassment that together create an unjust, unsafe, undignified, intolerable if not hostile work environment. This chapter will explore these issues and offer a landscape that will set the stage for future initiatives to invoke change.

The empowerment of women as a consequence of the #MeToo initiative has undoubtedly impacted perpetrators, who are now at risk. It has also enabled an agenda for change that has visibly impacted the global workforce and placed a spotlight on the concept of authentic womanhood and the need for its protection. This is a prophylactic measure for the future, so other women who dedicate their lives to the service of others might not be subject to the violation and indignity in 21st Century workforces that has characterised generations of misogyny before them This chapter seeks to illuminate the contexts, settings, and experiences of women working at the front line of medical care and their interactions with colleagues, and is balanced by an illumination of their male counterparts and their reactions to these reported perceptions.

Preface

The presence of women in the practice of medicine goes back to the ancient times. Some women were canonized in the 10th and 11th centuries for their care during the European plagues. From the 13th century to the 18th century, women who healed wounds were considered as witches and forbidden access to the medical education of the time. It was not until the end of the 19th century that women were able to have access to training in medicine. However, up to the 1970s, women comprised only a small percentage of medical students. In the last few decades, the reality has improved significantly, but unfortunately, this change is yet to be reflected within leadership positions and in the academic world. In some male-dominated specialties such as surgery, despite the number of women is increasing steadily, still less than one third are female, with discrimination within medical school, in training programs and in consultancy positions.

Although there is lots of talk about equity in the medical profession today, eradicating sexism from our culture and from the workplace is no easy task.

Why is diversity to be considered? The value of diversity and inclusion relates to disparities and marginalization in contrast with the principles of social justice and equity at the basis of every modern democracy. Equity is more than numerical parity, it is about culture and education. If diverse members interact, they provide access to greater knowledge resources and thus a better business, in healthcare as per in any other activity.

A survey conducted through the Association of Surgeons of Great Britain and Ireland (ASGBI) in 2018 showed what are the perceived barriers for the advancement of women within the surgical field, or in any other male-dominated field (Bellini et al., 2018). When these challenges were discussed at last year's ASGBI #HowIBecameAWomanInSurgery symposium, concerns were raised about how they may be significantly impacting not only the wellbeing of female surgeons (in training or not), but also the delivery of safe and high quality care (Bellini, 2019). If we want to attract, train, and retain the best talent for our patients, we need a strong and efficient diversity strategy in place. This applies for surgery and for medicine in general. In the context of this effort and in view of a better healthcare environment, we present Gender Equity in the Medical Profession: Emerging Research and Opportunities. This book aims to provide relevant theoretical frameworks and the latest research findings in this area. It is written for professionals who want to improve their understanding in how to strategically tackle gender equity at different levels of medical education (Bellini et al, 2019). This is a global commitment of networks and organizations, of teams and work groups and, finally, of individuals as diversity will benefit for all of them.

ORGANIZATION OF THE BOOK

The book is organized into 19 chapters. A brief description of each of the chapters follows:

Chapter 1: Supporting Surgeons to Have Families – Fertility, Pregnancy, Parental Leave, and Return to Work

The main perceived barrier in male-dominated professions, such as surgery, is the incongruity with motherhood. With the changing demographic of the surgical workforce, it is becoming more common to try and combine surgical training and pregnancy, or consultant posts and pregnancy. The authors provide a view from the United Kingdom in how the environment should focus on the support of fertility, pregnancy and return to work with emotional and practical support to surgeons who might otherwise experience pregnancy loss and stillbirth.

Chapter 2: Parental Leave During Surgical Training – Gender Equity, Parental Leave, Parental Policies, Childbearing, Conciliation, Surgery

To examine the work-family conciliation or more in general the work-life balance, this author from Spain proposes an up-to-date analysis on the parental leave situation during medical training as one of the main aspects of conciliation, by analysing parental leave policies and barriers faced by surgical trainees from an additional perspective compared to chapter one.

Chapter 3: Representation of Gender Equality From the Perspective of the Medical Trainee and Its Ripple Effect – Highlighting Gender Inequality in Medical Student Experiences

Incongruity with pregnancy and family is probably the main perceived barriers encountered during surgical training, although there are also other negative experiences for male and female students from the classroom to clinical placements. This chapter aims to view in detail what are the experiences and by improving these and encouraging diversity, the hope is to reduce the negative effects discussed and break the cycle of inequality.

Chapter 4: Training Martians and Venusians on Jupiter – Gender Equity in Medical Training

From the other side, what are the challenges encountered by trainers? They must be professionalised to ensure that training of trainees remains an exemplar role. It is accepted that males and females learn differently but have the same potential. Equity of opportunity ensures that the modern society retains and values both genders. This chapter explores the need for professional trainers, the educational needs of the modern-day medical trainee and the challenges that need to be accommodated to ensure that the medical workforce retains a passion long into their careers.

Chapter 5: Understanding the Value of Gender Equity in Healthcare and How to Pursue It

As previously said, females and males learn differently, but have the same potential; this applies also to the practice of medicine. The authors of this chapter analyse physicians' practice of either gender, highlighting how females engage more in communication styles, allocating more time to preventative care and showing different leadership qualities. A critical look at organizational culture and proposal of changes that could contribute to the pursuit of gender equity is presented.

Chapter 6: Sexism in Medical Communication

Continuing on the topic of communication, awareness of gendered language must be raised and highlighted in order to make a change. It is achievable to speak in gender-neutral ways that are inclusive and precise as to not conjure biased attitudes towards women in medicine. Communication is one of the most essential skills of the medical profession, however, it is a tool through which sexism and gender discrimination are promoted and reproduced. This chapter highlights that deeply engrained biases in medical communication still exist, and are perpetrated by institutions and individuals, women included.

Chapter 7: Gender Equity in Medical Leadership

Another relevant topic is the female representation in senior roles. The authors of this chapter analyse the situation in the National Health System in the United Kingdom, where only 36% of consultants are female with wide variation between specialties ranging from 12% of surgeons to over half of paediatricians, gynaecologists and directors of public health. This chapter seeks to define the role of women as leaders within the medical world and to compare the representation of women in senior leadership roles within medicine and other parallel male dominated working environments. Alternative forms of leadership such as mentoring, coaching and sponsorship are also considered._

Chapter 8: The Gender Pay Gap in Medicine – Causes and Solutions

Directly in connection with a lack of representation in senior roles, is the gender pay gap: it is a symptom of the pervasive inequalities that are inherent in modern society with a complex and multifactorial aetiology, where important roles played by recruitment and representation of women at senior levels, as well as gender occupational segregation are at the basis. Addressing the root causes of gender inequalities and shining a light on the pay gap data are both required in order to one day close the gap.

Chapter 9: Parallels Between Improving the Culture for Women in Surgery and a Surgical Approach to Improving Health for All

Every person should be valued for their skills and potential, for every moment they are present. This chapter focuses on training on diversity to avoid unconscious bias. Inequality is not just a women's issue and there are parallels with prevention in healthcare needing 3-pronged change: in individuals, society, culture and organisations.

Chapter 10: Impostor Syndrome as a Risk Factor in the Development of Psychiatric Symptoms in Female Doctors

Directly in connection with the unconscious bias, it is the Imposter Syndrome, which can have serious repercussions for women in the medical profession. As with all lesser-known clinical conditions (those not classified as disorders), Imposter Syndrome can be fairly difficult to identify; this lack of recognition and, therefore, treatment, can lead to a worse outcome and significant potential losses at both the personal and professional levels.

Chapter 11: The Imposter Phenomenon in the Medical Profession

If the previous chapter described the Imposter syndrome as a medical condition from an expert psychiatric perspective, the author of this chapter, a surgical trainee, systematically reviewed the literature and presented the evidence on imposter syndrome in the medical profession.

Chapter 12: Who Will Take Care of Me? The Future of Human Resources in Anaesthesiology, Critical Care, and Emergency Medicine in Europe

Having predominantly focused on the surgical field, that is a very predominant male-field, this chapter shifts the view to an alternative perspective: the anaesthetic field. Anaesthesiology is a challenging specialty with an expanding scope of practice, requiring highly motivated professionals, frequent long work hours, and addressing stressful situations often. To ensure quality anaesthesia provision, the wellbeing of this diverse population of anaesthesiologists should be addressed. Themes as rational and flexible work hours, adequate compensation, and promotion of a workplace culture that fosters safety, motivation to learn and equal opportunities for leadership or academia positions are examined within a European frame.

Chapter 13: Gender Equity Evaluated by Five Successful Women in Medical Profession

The last section of the book offers a zoom on some national realties for them to be generalized in the context of a global commitment. The first is from Portugal: the authors are five women with successful experiences in different medical specialties and make a reflection about gender equity in their country over a period of 45 years of democracy.

Chapter 14: Gender Equity in the Medical Profession as a Democratic Culture – The Portuguese Experience

One of the authors of the previous chapter makes a historical framework of gender equality in Portugal and brings together demographic and statistical data on education, science, women's political participation at governments, parliament and local power levels, the medical profession and medical specialties. Also, she focuses on the governmental structures to promote gender equality and the way of recruitment/appointment for public administration leaders, providing her view to achieve true gender equity in Portugal.

Chapter 15: Gender Equity in Medicine in Sweden

Keeping on describing national realties, this chapter is about gender equity in medicine in Sweden. Starting with a historical overview over women´s situation in Sweden, the author then provides an overview of Swedish women in medicine and academia throughout the Swedish system. Although there are structural mechanisms working towards this direction, there is still a long way to go to achieve true gender equity even in this very modern democracy.

Chapter 16: Women in the Medical Field in India – A Developing Economy

There is a vast difference in the status of women in the medical field in India as compared to the western world. However, much progress has been made in the past two decades, at least in the urban areas; in fact despite having so many women who are medical leaders, the situation in rural India remains desolate at present, with episode of violence against doctor and bullying, particularly towards the females. The patriarchal nature of the society, ancient customs, inability to adapt to modern times are presented in order to critically propose a way for change.

Chapter 17: Gender Equity in Surgical Academia in Kuwait and the Arabian Gulf Region

In Kuwait and Arabian Gulf region, introduction of women in medicine was later than that of the Western World. However, in the past 40 years, women have taken a huge leap in the medical field developing gender equity in medicine and the authors describe some unique challenges their region holds based on cultural and social aspects. This chapter overviews the current status of Kuwait and the Gulf region regarding gender equity and outline the history of women surgeons. They also present the evolution of medical education and the different healthcare systems and how this may relate to gender equity in academia.

Chapter 18: Gender Inequities in the US Surgical Workforce

A pioneer in Women's rights, the US, is the theme of this chapter.

From the historical perspective, moving to the present with a call to action to ensure a cultural transformation that seeks to not only successfully retain and promote the women already part of the surgical workforce but attract more talented women to come.

Chapter 19: Prophylaxis in Action #MeToo for Women of Medical and Surgical Disciplines

This final chapter offers a view for the empowerment of women as a consequence of the #MeToo initiative. The need for change that has visibly impact on the global workforce spotting a light on the concept of authentic womanhood and the need to protect this. This is a prophylactic measure for the future, so other women who dedicate their lives to the service of others might not be subject to the violation and indignity in 21st Century workforces that has characterised generations of misogyny before them.

REFERENCES

Bellini, M. (2019). *Women in surgery—if you can see it, you can be it. BMJ Opinion.*

Bellini, M. I., Graham, Y., Hayes, C., Zakeri, R., Parks, R., & Papalois, V. (2018). A woman's place is in theatre: Women's perceptions and experiences of working in surgery from the Association of Surgeons of Great Britain and Ireland Women in Surgery working group. *BMJ Open*. PMID:30617103

Bellini, M. I., Adair, A., Fotopoulou, C., Graham, Y., Hutson, A., McNally, S., Mohan, H., Vig, S., Parks, R., & Papalois, V. (2019). Changing the norm towards gender equity in surgery: The women in surgery working group of the Association of Surgeons of Great Britain and Ireland's perspective. *Journal of the Royal Society of Medicine*.

Chapter 1
Supporting Surgeons to Have Families:
Fertility, Pregnancy, Parental Leave, and Return to Work

Rhiannon L. Harries
Department of General Surgery, Morriston Hospital, Swansea, UK

Rebecca Spenser Nicholas
Department of Plastic and Reconstructive Surgery, Guy's and St. Thomas' NHS Trust, UK

Helen M. Mohan
Department of General Surgery, University Hospital Limerick, Ireland

ABSTRACT

Surgical training often overlaps childbearing years. It is important that those considering a career in surgery know it is possible to combine a career in surgery with having children—and are supported to do so. With the changing demographic of the surgical workforce in the UK, it is increasingly common that surgeons are trying to combine surgical training and pregnancy, or indeed consultant posts and pregnancy. It is crucial that there is a culture within a surgical department and training programme whereby surgeons feel supported in their fertility, pregnancy journey, return to work, and childrearing. It is imperative that trainees feel comfortable asking for and are given adequate time off for fertility issues and early and mid-trimester pregnancy loss. Support systems should be in place to provide emotional and practical support to both female and male surgeons who experience fertility problems, pregnancy loss, and stillbirth, as well as those who are pregnant, returning to work following parental leave and balancing childrearing with a surgical career.

DOI: 10.4018/978-1-5225-9599-1.ch001

BACKGROUND

An important part of maintaining an outstanding surgical workforce in the UK, and more widely, is retaining the best talent. Surgical training often overlaps childbearing years. As with many other careers, childcare requirements and the associated factors relate to a significant dropout rate. This chapter focuses on issues regarding fertility, pregnancy and maternity/paternity leave from a UK perspective, especially regarding surgical training. Whilst an increasing trend for shared division of parental responsibility between the genders is to be applauded, this issue does still predominantly affect females; In the UK, although women account for 70% of medical school admissions, this percentage drops at each stage of surgical training: 30% of core surgical trainees, 22% of higher surgical trainees and only 10% of consultant surgeons are female (Mohan et al., in press; Harries et al., 2016). It is important that those considering a career in surgery know it is possible to combine a career in surgery with having children and are supported to do so (Troppmann et al., 2009). With the changing demographics of the surgical workforce, it is increasingly common that surgeons are trying to combine surgical training and pregnancy, or indeed consultant posts and pregnancy. No matter whether a surgeon is pregnant during training or following completion of training when in consultant or attending posts, there are unique challenges which must be recognised in order to develop strategies to better support women and to harmonise family and career aspirations. There are increasing numbers of women entering surgical training and the gender gap at the top echelons has yet to balance out (GMC, 2016; Seemann et al., 2016). A British Medical Association (BMA) report found that the average female surgeons earn 20% less than her male counterpart, and even after using regression analysis to control for different characteristics of respondents and adjusting for hours worked, an unexplained gap still remains (£92,250 vs £73,482) (Dean, 2017). This may be due in part to challenges surrounding this intersection between childbearing and surgical training, with a lack of support of surgical trainees contributing to attrition and burnout. Supporting surgeons during pregnancy and return to work is essential.

Every woman's experience of pregnancy is different, and indeed no two pregnancies are the same. Some surgeons may have no difficulties with one pregnancy but have complications and significant issues with another pregnancy. When designing strategy and policy to empower pregnant surgeons, it is important that this spectrum of experience is recognized. It is tempting to just say "you can have it all", but non-surgeons and surgeons alike experience complications and symptoms of pregnancy, the devastation and the struggle of pregnancy loss, and infertility problems. Therefore, rather than saying "you can have it all", what the surgical workplace needs to be saying is "we will support you in whatever your fertility/pregnancy journey is and ensure that your job is not an impediment to your aspirations to have a family. If you are pregnant, we will support you and help you balance your surgical training/career and your health." In addition to supporting female surgeons, it is also essential to consider the impacts of fertility issues, pregnancy loss and childrearing responsibilities on male trainees. If we are serious about making progress towards gender equality in the surgical workforce, options such as shared parental leave and flexible working among male counterparts should be actively encouraged (Eaton, 2018).

Fertility and Pregnancy Loss

Fertility

Fertility is often a taboo subject and is not talked about sufficiently. Arghavan Salles recently drew attention to this in a powerful article in Time magazine (Salles, 2019). Delaying having a family is not unique to surgeons but there are many surgeons who do report delaying having a family due to their career. This may be due to not having had the opportunity to meet a partner or choosing to delay childbearing until after a certain stage in their career. Indeed, some surgeons may wait on an optimum time to have children before realising that there is never a "good time" and that it is a juggle at any stage. The surgical lifestyle with long hours, academic pressure and frequent house moves can make it more difficult to form and maintain a relationship with a partner. In a survey by the Association of Surgeons in Training (ASiT), eighty-six per cent of the 939 respondents believed that surgical training had negatively affected their ability to maintain a relationship (O'Callaghan et al., 2017).

Infertility can affect a woman at any age. Finding out that there is a low chance of conceiving or carrying a child to term can be devastating, as outlined by Salles (2019). Many people may need to undergo medically assisted reproduction in order to have a family. Fertility investigations and treatments can be difficult to balance with a surgical career. It is important to create a supportive culture where surgeons can feel comfortable discussing fertility issues and requesting breaks for treatments even if they are not comfortable discussing the specifics.

There are many ways of becoming a parent - aside from fertility treatment and assisted reproduction, people may meet a partner with children and become a step parent, others may adopt. It is important that all of these major life transitions are supported and that surgeons feel they can adjust the pace of their professional life to cope with the change and the unique challenges, heartbreak or joys that their circumstances may bring. Equally, not all pregnancies are planned- surgeons may need support to cope with a crisis pregnancy.

Pregnancy Loss

One in four of all pregnancies end in pregnancy loss, with over 10% of known pregnancies resulting in miscarriage (ACOG, 2015). Pregnancy loss can be at any stage of pregnancy, ranging from early losses to mid trimester losses, late trimester losses and stillbirth. In our society, early pregnancy loss traditionally has been shrouded in silence. This has made it more challenging for women to seek support and help at a time when they need it. It is a deeply personal decision whether to share details of a pregnancy loss with colleagues, but it is critical that the surgical working environment creates a culture where doing so is met by support and humanity. It is important that trainees feel comfortable asking for and are given adequate time off to allow physical and emotional recovery. Exact provisions for time off varies between countries, and depending on the stage of pregnancy at which the loss occurred. Surgical department leads and surgical trainers should advocate for their staff and trainees to ensure that surgeons have the time off that they need.

Although pregnancy and miscarriage physically affect females, it is important to also recognise the impact these, alongside fertility issues, have on male partners and the importance of compassionate leave and paternity leave in such circumstances (Mohan et al., in press; Eaton & Jackson, 2018).

Surgical Training and Pregnancy

Physical Implications of Pregnancy and Surgical Jobs

The physical effects of "normal pregnancy" are quite considerable on the human body. Indeed, a recent study of limits of human endurance have shown a rise in basal metabolic rate in pregnancy that is comparable to that of endurance athletes (Thurber et al., 2019). Normal pregnancy involves significant changes in the physiology of every organ system and metabolic and endocrine changes, resulting in an increased heart rate, increased work of breathing, dilution and hormonal changes. For many women, these changes are associated with significant pregnancy symptoms. Sickness of pregnancy (or morning sickness as it is often known as, despite occurring at any time of the day or night) can be severe, and its most severe form, hyperemesis gravidarum, affects 1 percent of pregnancies. It can be associated with significant psychological morbidity, for example increased rates of depression and anxiety are noted from hyperemesis gravidarum (Mitchell-Jones et al., 2017).

It is increasingly recognised that surgeons are not superhuman - although many trainees report working until final stages of pregnancy and not coming off onerous emergency cover rotas until late in pregnancy. The safety of this approach is increasingly under the spotlight. Indeed pregnant trainees can feel under enormous external pressure but also internal pressure from themselves to continue to work excessively during pregnancy. Rogers *et al* found that the risk of adverse pregnancy events is significantly higher for a female pregnant surgeon, than for a non-surgical partner of a male surgeon (Rogers et al., 2019). Indeed, they suggest that the risk of adverse events by being a surgeon may be equivalent to that of smoking. There is a need for high quality evidence to guide what constitutes safe working in pregnancy, but it is difficult to design a study that will adequately answer the question. Some jurisdictions such as Germany have quite strict laws on what pregnant women can do. These laws can in turn impede women's career progression. Other jurisdictions such as the UK and the USA lack clear guidance, and pregnant trainees frequently work long hours until late in pregnancy, potentially putting themselves at risk of complications. Women should feel comfortable reducing hours in pregnancy and following the advice of their obstetrician to come off emergency shift work or to finish work entirely, whenever this is deemed necessary. One hypothesis is that the development of the spiral arteries in the placenta between 24 and 32 weeks constitutes a critical phase and this may be affected by prolonged standing, such as during operating or endoscopy lists. Some female surgeons, however, may choose to continue working emergency shift work at night during the second and third trimester, and therefore rest facilities should be made available to support this decision. Women may, by choice or circumstance, defer having children until later due to their surgical career. This is not without risk as increasing maternal chronological age is associated with increased pregnancy complications (Richardson et al., 2019).

Industrial Hazards in the Surgical Workplace

There are specific hazards encountered by surgeons in the workplace. There are clear dangers with the use of cytotoxic drugs and 5-alpha reductase inhibitors, and these should be avoided (Hall & Williams, 2017). Although contested (Hamilton, 2018), there is also some evidence that topical use of povidone-iodine during the first trimester results in a sudden increase in urinary excretion of iodine and short-term variation in concentrations of thyroid hormones in maternal serum, which could have consequences for the embryo and foetus during crucial stages of development (Velasco et al., 2009). Therefore, it has been recommended that frequent use of iodine-based hand wash should be avoided during pregnancy (Hall, 2017).

The use of ionising radiation is another concern and there have been calls for clearer guidelines on pregnancy and occupational exposure (Shaw et al., 2012). The key time for pregnant women to avoid ionising radiation exposure is between 8-15 weeks of pregnancy - a crucial stage in foetal development (Shaw, 2011). There are general guidelines published by the UK Health and Safety Executive for any expectant or breastfeeding mother working with ionising radiation, recommending that exposure is limited to a dose of 1 millisievert for the duration of pregnancy (HSE, 2015). However, to our knowledge there are no agreed national guidelines that explain how this applies specifically to surgical training and practice, published either by the Royal Colleges, National Health Service (NHS), any of the Health Education authorities or readily-available source in the UK. Ionising radiation exposure affects certain specialties, in particular, trauma and orthopaedics, plastic surgery, vascular surgery and urology. Reassuringly, a survey of interventional radiologists found no increased risk of radiation associated adverse effects compared to the general population (Ghatan et al., 2016). The key is ensuring that radiation protections are rigorous during procedures in the environment where ionising radiation is used. This should protect both the pregnant and non-pregnant healthcare workers (Marx, 2018). One concern is that surgeons have been shown in previous surveys to have a low awareness of radiation safety (Walsh et al., 2019). It is imperative that anyone using ionising radiation in the operating theatre is appropriately educated in radiation safety and remains vigilant at all times to mitigate risk to pregnant and non-pregnant co-workers and themselves.

There is a risk of exposure to infection in the surgical environment. Immunisation against seasonal influenza is particularly important in pregnancy, and perhaps even more so in pregnant healthcare workers who are more likely to be exposed to those with influenza. Surgeons should already be immune to Hepatitis B, based on prior vaccination prior to commencing surgical work, but if there is any doubt, they should check their status. Immunisation against Pertussis is recommended for all pregnant women in every pregnancy. In the UK and Ireland this is between 16 and 32 weeks, but specific immunisation schedules may vary depending on the country.

There is also the omnipresent and real risk of assault in pregnancy in the hospital environment. It is important that the hospital is a safe space for all healthcare workers and that violence against staff is not tolerated.

Non-Physical Challenges Faced by Surgeons in Pregnancy

Unfortunately, negative attitudes, unsupportive comments and bullying of female surgeons having children and being pregnant are still common (Chen et al., 2013; Turner et al., 2012). A recent survey by ASiT[1] showed that 27.1% of surgical trainees felt unsupported during pregnancy. This is similar to the findings of a survey by the Irish Medical Organisation (IMO, 2017) that showed 18.4% of trainees did not feel supported by their employer during pregnancy. Rangel et al found that one of the factors associated with professional dissatisfaction of surgical trainees was a perception of stigma associated with pregnancy, due to requirement for time off and inability to work as long hours as non-pregnant counterparts (Rangel et al., 2018). This can only be compounded by rota gaps and internal pressure leading female trainees to feel they must keep working long and night shifts so that they do not "let the side down". Another article reported alarming findings relating to trainees seeking abortion as a means of dealing with pregnancy, indicating lack of support (Garza et al., 2017). Bullying in surgery has been shown to be frighteningly common (Pei & Cochran, 2019).

Pregnancy can bring significant physical challenges as discussed above. In this context, pregnancy represents a particularly vulnerable time for surgical trainees in the workplace for bullying and microaggressions towards them. The physical challenge of a difficult pregnancy can disarm a surgeon emotionally and render the job extremely challenging in terms of psychological reserve and emotional well-being. Going to work every day while battling pregnancy symptoms or complications can be hugely draining. This makes it even more important that a surgical department creates a supportive environment for pregnant trainees and has zero tolerance for sexist and discriminatory behaviour and bullying.

Training and Pregnancy

Balancing surgical training and pregnancy can be a challenge. The physical challenges mentioned above can impede pregnant trainees from fully participating in their normal activities and trainees need to be supported and not put at risk of harming themselves or their foetuses. Striking the balance between supporting trainees and their surgical training can be difficult. In order to fulfil their training goals for the year, a trainee should sit down with their educational supervisor and work out together what they need to do to achieve this. That may mean reducing other service commitments that have no or low training value and prioritising the aspects that are beneficial for their training goals. It is worth revisiting this frequently with meetings every few weeks as what the trainee can do may change throughout pregnancy as symptoms come and go and as complications occur. It is important that surgical departments make contingency plans if a pregnant trainee is unable to carry out certain commitments, so that the remaining trainees are not overburdened with the additional workload, which can in turn lead to negative sentiments towards the pregnant trainee.

For trainees in the UK and Ireland, time taken for maternity leave is added onto training and therefore the trainee's CCT (Certification of Completion of Training) date is extended. However, in some surgical specialties, it may be possible to apply for 3 months of one-off exceptional leave that does not need to be "paid back" during training. Trainees are advised to check the Joint Committee on Surgical Training website for information on their specialty (https://www.jcst.org).

Prematurity

Having premature babies is more common among surgeons than other occupations. Prematurity brings its own unique challenges. Ireland recently introduced legislation that extended maternity leave for those who have premature babies (thejournal.ie, 2017). However, this is not yet standard across jurisdictions. Clearly it is important to give surgeons they time they need for their premature baby.

Supporting Surgeons During Return to Work

Following a prolonged period of parental leave, it is common to be apprehensive about returning to work. Colleagues should be aware that it often takes some time for confidence levels to return to what they were pre-parental leave. Only 62% of surgical trainees in a recent study (n=118/193) felt that this had occurred at 6 months following their return to work from maternity leave[1]. The various challenges faced by returners have been well documented by the Association of Medical Royal Colleges' (AoMRC) 2016 Maternity / Paternity Survey and include concerns about their clinical competence and knowledge, as well as being concerned about colleague perceptions (AoMRC, 2016). Supported Return to Training (SuppoRTT) is one recently-launched initiative by Health Education England (HEE) that is seeking to offer support to enable those who have taken time out of training to return safely and confidently (HEE, 2017). Through a process of consultation with trainees and employers, the British Medical Association Junior Doctors AoMRC, the programme identified a number of concerns cited by returners (Figure 1) and suggested a range of mitigating actions that can support returners (Figure 2).

Confidence and self-perception of capability were reported as the utmost concern for returners from leave. Culture was reported as a major barrier to addressing issues faced when returning to training, as was the availability and cost of childcare. Provisions that could potentially mitigate the reported issues included a supernumerary period, phased return to work (e.g. gradual re-introduction of on call commit-

Figure 1. Returner issues reported, supported return to training (HEE, 2017).
Source: Health Education England. Supported Return to Training. 2017

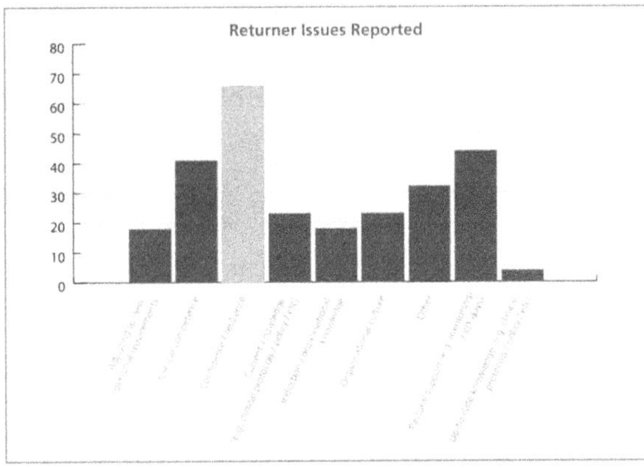

Figure 2. Mitigating actions to support returners, supported return to training
Source: Health Education England. Supported Return to Training. 2017

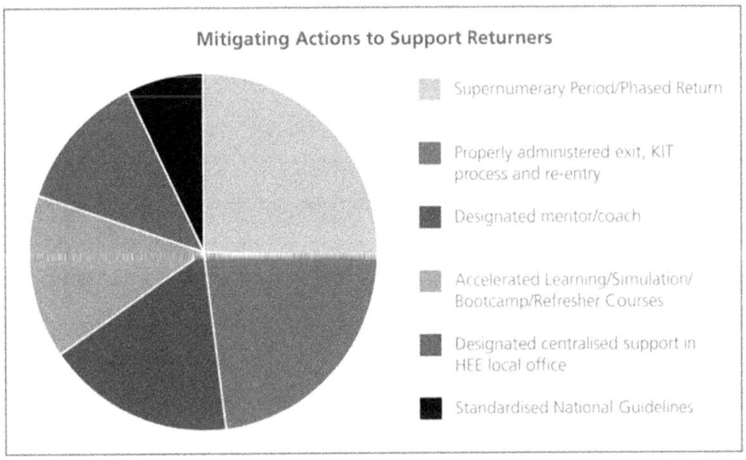

ments or flexible training), and pastoral support, including "Keeping In Touch" (KIT) days and access to a designated mentor or coach. Simulation and refresher training were also cited as useful for confidence building by enabling returners to brush up on clinical knowledge and skills. It is acknowledged that "one size does not fit all", and the amount of support that is required is dependent on the individual and specific circumstances (HEE, 2017).

Supporting Surgeons During Return from Parental Leave: 'Keeping in Touch' (KIT) Days

Within the UK, employees can do up to 10 days paid work during their parental leave, and these days are referred to as KIT days. These are optional and both the employee and employer should agree on them. It should be noted that parental leave pay should not be affected by taking these KIT days.

Supporting Surgeons During Return from Parental Leave: Flexible Working Options

There is a growing appetite for flexible working arrangements amongst junior doctors in training. In the 2017 General Medical Council (GMC) training survey 10.7% (n=5,642) of postgraduate trainees responded to say they were in LTFT (GMC, 2017). This is in comparison to just 8.0% in 2012 (BMA, 2015a). This trend has also been seen in other countries globally (Heuss & Haenggeli, 2003; Jerg-Bretzke & Limbrecht, 2012; Kaderli et al., 2010; Gordon et al., 2008; Carling et al., 1999; Saalwachter et al., 2006; Nomura et al., 2015; Mahady, 2011; Henry et al., 2012; McDonald et al., 2013; Gardener et al., 2002).

It is important that flexible working options are available to all surgeons - male and female, and for the full range of potential reasons. A significant proportion of trainees returning from parental leave may wish to consider flexible training options. Less than full-time training (LTFT) was first described in the Oxford region in the UK in 1966 for married females (Rue, 1967). Following the Calman reforms and the introduction of the specialist registrar grade, LTFT has been made available to all doctors in national training programmes. LTFT is postgraduate training whilst working a reduced number of hours, expressed as a percentage of full-time. It results in an increase in the number of years spent to complete postgraduate medical training.

LTFT can be granted to eligible trainees on the basis of 'well-founded reasons' for not being able to work full time (Table 1) (BMA, 2015b).

Table 1. Less than full-time training eligibility criteria (BMA, 2015b)

Category 1
· Disability or ill health (including IVF programmes)
· Responsibility for caring for children or a dependent
Category 2 – *"Unique opportunities for personal or professional development"*
· Sports training e.g. training for national/international sporting event
· Religious commitment e.g. training for a particular religious role
· Non-medical professional development e.g. fine arts course, law course etc

Approval for LTFT is required from the trainee's postgraduate Local Education and Training Board (LETB). Applications within category 1 will generally have priority, with all LETBs aiming to support these applications. Applications within category 2 will be dependent on the individual circumstances and the availability of funding. All applications for flexible training should be treated positively and if an application for LTFT is declined, the trainee has the right to appeal the outcome (BMA, 2015b).

LTFT is usually equal or greater than 50% equivalent of full-time training, though it can be less if agreed by all interested parties in extenuating circumstances. Day-time working and out of hours duties should be undertaken on a pro rata basis to that of those in the equivalent full-time post. Once approved, LTFT is organised and funded by both the LETB and the local hospital; with the educational component of basic pay from the LETB and the on-call banding arrangement of pay from the local hospital (BMA, 2015b).

Surgical trainees find it more difficult to obtain suitable LTFT posts compared to trainees from non-surgical specialities (Gray et al., 2001). The 2017 GMC training survey revealed that LTFT trainees were more common in certain specialties compared to others, with surgery having the lowest percentage (3%, n=257) (GMC, 2017). There is a duty from all interested parties (Royal Colleges, Surgical Training Committees and Training Programme Directors) to ensure that there is equal access to LTFT across all specialties, and that there is adequate information available on LTFT for trainees. Each LETB now outlines details of a local consultant within the trainee's specialty who is the nominated LTFT advisor. The Royal College of England also has a LTFT advisor who has personal experience of flexible working, who can be contacted for further information (please see www.rcseng.ac.uk for details).

Unfortunately, there is still some way to go with respect to reforming surgical culture in order to support flexible working. A recent study found that 53.8% of LTFT trainees within surgery have experienced undermining behaviour from work colleagues from what they perceived to be a direct result of their LTFT working[2]. Negative sentiments to those either interested in LTFT or currently working within LTFT in surgical specialties has no place in modern training and needs to be reported via the necessary channels. The recent campaigns to eliminate bullying behaviour within surgery, such as #HammerItOut and #LetsRemoveIt, all go some way to help highlight this issue and attempt to improve trainees morale and wellbeing (RCSEd, 2018; BOTA, 2017).

In 2017, 91.2% of all LTFT trainees were females, with 83% citing childrearing as the reason (GMC, 2017); However, LTFT is a gender-neutral concept, being accessible to both male and female trainees. Movements to support shared parental leave may see an increase in the number of males interested in accessing LTFT for childcare duties. There is considerable data about the general working population suggesting that when men are offered the opportunity of part-time work to enable them to be more involved in childrearing there is a high take up. According to the Office for National Statistics 27% of the UK workforce currently works part-time and this figure is steadily increasing (ONS, 2017; Fisher, 2018). This was also confirmed by ASiT's national LTFT survey of surgical trainees, where 33% male respondents said they would consider flexible training future[2].

The current training system supports three ways in which LTFT can be undertaken: LTFT in a full-time training post, supernumerary, or sharing of a training post with another Higher Surgical Trainee (slot-share arrangement). Slot-sharing is popular from the hospital trusts' point of view, as there is minimal, if any, impact on the service provision. However, in reality it can be logistically difficult to find appropriately matched trainees in the same region with compatible training needs. If a trainee is planning to commence LTFT following a period of maternity, or shared parental leave, it is recommended that a discussion with the training programme director takes place at the earliest possible time (ideally at the 25th week of the pregnancy for those undergoing maternity leave) to ensure appropriate planning and to arrange a suitable training placement allocation to meet future learning needs. Trainees should be aware that administration of a LTFT application by the LETB can take around three months duration (BMA, 2015b).

Educational, clinical supervisors, and rota coordinators should endeavour to ensure that trainees undertaking LTFT in a full-time training post are not expected to perform 100% of the full-time commitment workload within their LTFT hours. Any LTFT post needs to gain approval from the Royal College via the training programme director to ensure the educational content is equivalent in quality to full-time training. Once in a LTFT post, an annual assessment is made to ensure that LTFT is still required (BMA, 2015b).

Of course, flexible working is not limited to just those within training, but can occur whilst in a non-training post or after training is completed and working as a consultant. In addition, parental leave policies should be highlighted and made available to all staff, which entitles all working parents in the UK to take 18 weeks unpaid leave per child up to their 18th birthday. This can facilitate making childcare feasible during school holidays, periods of sickness or frequent hospital visits (Crown Copyright, 2019). Improved resourcing of surgical services is needed to improve flexible working options.

Supporting Surgeons During Return From Parental Leave: Facilitating Breastfeeding

Parents must be supported in whatever manner they choose to feed their child. For women who choose to continue to breastfeed on returning to work, this should be supported. This should include provision of facilities and time to pump e.g. a private space to pump and a fridge in which to store breast milk. There is wide variation in how supported trainees feel about breastfeeding at work. There is a higher rate of breastfeeding in those specialties which report better support (Gupta et al., 2019).

Supporting Surgeons During Return From Parental Leave: Placement and Childcare

Training programme directors should carefully consider the impact of training post location for childcare in preventing attrition in surgery. For example, allocating a trainee a placement which is a one-hour commute away from their childcare may lead to difficulties for that trainee to be able to collect their child at a reasonable time. Trainees need adequate notice of placements far away in order to make appropriate plans for childcare or swap placements to find more suitable arrangements closer to home. The availability of quality, accessible, and affordable childcare is a key issue for surgical trainees returning to work, given the unpredictable nature of surgical hours and the anti-social hours being expensive for childcare. Hospitals and the wider health service should endeavour to make their hospital more attractive to staff who are working parents, e.g. by ensuring childcare facilities exist on-site, with flexible drop-off and collection times that are suitable to accommodate the unpredictable nature of the finish time of theatre lists (Shaw et al., 2012).

RECOMMENDATIONS

- Create a culture within a surgical department and training programme whereby surgeons feel supported in their fertility, pregnancy journey and return to work.
- Ensure trainees feel comfortable asking for and are granted adequate time off for fertility issues and early and mid-trimester pregnancy loss.
- Ensure there is adequate education of surgical trainees, trainers and the training bodies regarding the risks of pregnancy and surgical training and the need to support pregnant trainees.
- Surgical Royal Colleges should work with trainees and the NHS to develop policy and a nationally-agreed "go-to" resource to better support trainees through their fertility, pregnancy and parenting journeys. Advocating to improve resourcing of surgical services is crucial in order to facilitate supporting flexible working patterns and parental leave.
- Ensure support systems are in place to provide emotional and practical support to surgeons who experience pregnancy loss and stillbirth.
- Ensure adequate pumping facilities and support of breastfeeding trainees.
- Encourage continued research in this area is needed to inform and develop clearer guidelines.
- Provide better support of paternity leave and shared parental leave.

REFERENCES

ACOG (The American College of Obstetricians and Gynaecologists). (2015). Early pregnancy loss. Available at https://www.acog.org/Patients/FAQs/Early-Pregnancy-Loss?IsMobileSet=false

AoMRC (The Academy of Medical Royal Colleges). (2016). Maternity/Paternity Survey Results. Available from http://aomrc.org.uk/wp-content/uploads/2016/06/Maternity_paternity_survey_200416-1.pdf

BMA (British Medical Association). (2015a). Less-than-full-time training guidance update. Available from https://www.bma.org.uk/news/2015/august/less-than-full-time-training-guidance-update

BMA (British Medical Association). (2015b). Less than full time guidance. Available at https://www.bma.org.uk/-/media/files/pdfs/developing%20your%20career/bma%20less%20than%20full%20time%20guidance.pdf

BOTA (British Orthopaedic Trainees Association). (2017). Cut it out/ Hammer it out. http://www.bota.org.uk/hammer-it-out/

Carling, P. C., Hayward, K., Coakley, E. H., & Wolf, A. M. (1999). Part-time residency training in internal medicine: Analysis of a ten-year experience. *Academic Medicine*, *74*(3), 282–284. doi:10.1097/00001888-199903000-00020 PMID:10099652

Chen, M. M., Yeo, H. L., Roman, S. A., Bell, R. H. Jr, & Sosa, J. A. (2013). Life events during surgical residency have different effects on women and men over time. *Surgery*, *154*(2), 162–170. doi:10.1016/j.surg.2013.03.014 PMID:23889946

Crown Copyright. (2019). Unpaid parental leave. UK Government. Available at https://www.gov.uk/parental-leave/print

Dean, E. (2017). The Gender Pay Gap in Surgery. *Royal College of Surgeons Bulletin*, *99*(1), 12–14. doi:10.1308/rcsbull.2017.12

Eaton, E. & Jackson, C. (2018). Want to improve gender equality at work? Help men take parental leave. *Mercer*. Available at https://www.mercer.com/our-thinking/want-to-improve-gender-equality-at-work-help-men-take-parental-leave.html

Fisher, D. (2018). Want men to share parental leave? Just give them equality. The Guardian. Available at https://www.theguardian.com/commentisfree/2018/feb/15/men-share-parental-leave-entitlement-women-equality-fathers

Gardner, S. V., James, M. F., & Evans, N. R. (2002). Gender issues among South African anaesthetists. *South African Medical Journal*, *92*(9), 732–736. PMID:12382361

Garza, R. M., Weston, J. S., & Furnas, H. J. (2017). Pregnancy and the Plastic Surgery Resident. *Plastic and Reconstructive Surgery*, *139*(1), 245–252. doi:10.1097/PRS.0000000000002861 PMID:28027263

Ghatan, C. E., Fassiotto, M., Jacobsen, J. P., Sze, D. Y., & Kothary, N. (2016). Occupational Radiation Exposure during Pregnancy: A Survey of Attitudes and Practices among Interventional Radiologists. *Journal of Vascular and Interventional Radiology*, *27*(7), 1013–20.e3. doi:10.1016/j.jvir.2016.03.040 PMID:27236211

GMC (General Medical Council). (2017). Training Environments 2017: Key findings from the national training survey. Available at https://www.gmc-uk.org/about/what-we-do-and-why/data-and-research/-/media/documents/nts-report-20173_pdf-72689147.pdf

GMC (The General Medical Council). (2016). The State of Medical Education and Practice in the UK 2016. Executive Summary. Available at http://www.gmcuk.org/GMC_SOMEP_2016___Executive_summary.pdf_68137466.pdf

Gordon, M. B., McGuinness, G. A., Stanton, B. F., Brooks, S., Chiang, V. W., Vinci, R., & Sectish, T. C. (2008). Part-time training in pediatric residency programs: Principles and practices. *Pediatrics*, *122*(4), e938–e944. doi:10.1542/peds.2008-0719 PMID:18809596

Gray, S., Alexander, K., & Eaton, J. (2004). Equal opportunity for all? Trends in flexible training 1995-2001. *Medical Teacher*, *26*(3), 256–259. doi:10.1080/0142159042000191993 PMID:15203504

Gupta, A., Meriwether, K., & Hewlett, G. (2019). Impact of training specialty on breastfeeding among resident physicians: A National Survey. *Breastfeeding Medicine*, *14*(1), 46–56. doi:10.1089/bfm.2018.0140 PMID:30346796

Hall, S. J., & Williams, S. T. (2017). The pregnant urologist. *BJU International*, *120*(5), 731–734. doi:10.1111/bju.13927 PMID:28581066

Hamilton LC. The lesser-spotted pregnant surgeon. *RCS Bull.*, *100*(4), 172-175.

Harries, R. L., Gokani, V. J., Smitham, P., & Fitzgerald, J. E. F. (2016). Less than full-time training in surgery: A cross-sectional study evaluating the accessibility and experiences of flexible training in the surgical trainee workforce. *BMJ Open*, *6*(4), e010136. doi:10.1136/bmjopen-2015-010136 PMID:27091819

HEE (Health Education England). (2017). Supported Return to Training. Available at https://www.hee.nhs.uk/sites/default/files/documents/Supported%20Return%20to%20Training.pdf

Henry, A., Clements, S., Kingston, A., & Abbott, J. (2012). In search of work/life balance: Trainee perspectives on part-time obstetrics and gynaecology specialist training. *BMC Research Notes*, *5*(1), 19. doi:10.1186/1756-0500-5-19 PMID:22233566

Heuss, L. T., & Haenggeli, C. (2003). Open access to part-time specialist training- the Swiss experience. *Swiss Medical Weekly*, *133*(17-18), 263–266. PMID:12833197

HSE (Health and Safety Executive). (2015). Working safely with ionising radiation: Guidance for expectant and breastfeeding mothers. Available at http://www.hse.gov.uk/pubns/indg334.pdf

IMO (Irish Medical Organisation). (2017). IMO Position Paper on Women in Medicine. Available at https://www.imo.ie/policy-international-affair/documents/IMO-Position-Paper-on-Women-in-Medicine-Final.pdf

Jerg-Bretzke, L., & Limbrecht, K. (2012). Where have they gone?- a discussion on the balancing act of female doctors between work and family. *GMS Zeitschrift für Medizinische*, *29*(2), 19. PMID:22558025

Kaderli, R., Guller, U., Muff, B., Stefenelli, U., & Businger, A. (2010). Women in surgery: A survey in Switzerland. *Archives of Surgery*, *145*(11), 1119–1121. doi:10.1001/archsurg.2010.245 PMID:21079102

Mahady, S. E. (2011). Adding flexibility to physician training. *The Medical Journal of Australia*, *194*(9), 460–462. PMID:21534903

Marx, M. V. (2018). Baby on Board: Managing Occupational Radiation Exposure During Pregnancy. *Techniques in Vascular and Interventional Radiology*, *21*(1), 32–36. doi:10.1053/j.tvir.2017.12.007 PMID:29471998

McDonald, R. E., Jeeves, A. E., Vasey, C. E., Wright, D. M., & O'Grady, G. (2013). Supply and demand mismatch for flexible (part-time) surgical training in Australasia. *The Medical Journal of Australia*, *198*(8), 423–425. doi:10.5694/mja12.11685 PMID:23641991

Mitchell-Jones, N., Gallos, I., Farren, J., Tobias, A., Bottomley, C., & Bourne, T. (2017). Psychological morbidity associated with hyperemesis gravidarum: A systematic review and meta-analysis. *British Journal of Obstetrics and Gynaecology*, *124*(1), 20–30. doi:10.1111/1471-0528.14180 PMID:27418035

Mohan, H., Ali, O., Gokani, V. J., McGoldrick, C., Smitham, P., Fitzgerald, J. E. F., & Harries, R. L. (in press). Surgical trainees experience of pregnancy, maternity and paternity leave: A cross-sectional study. *Postgraduate Medical Journal*.

Nomura, K., Yamazaki, Y., Gruppen, L. D., Horie, S., Takeuchi, M., & Illing, J. (2015). The difficulty of professional continuation among female doctors in Japan: A qualitative study of alumnae of 13 medical schools in Japan. *BMJ Open*, *5*(3), e005845. doi:10.1136/bmjopen-2014-005845 PMID:25818268

O'Callaghan, J., Mohan, H. M., & Harries, R. L.Council of the Association of Surgeons in Training. (2017). The non-monetary costs of surgical training. *Annals of the Royal College of Surgeons of England (Suppl)*, *100*(8), 339–344. doi:10.1308/rcsbull.2018.339

ONS (Office for National Statistics). (2017). UK Labour Market: Estimates of employment, unemployment, economic inactivity and other employment-related statistics for the UK. Available at https://www.ons.gov.uk/employmentandlabourmarket/peopleinwork/employmentandemployeetypes/bulletins/uklabourmarket/jan2017

Pei, K. Y., & Cochran, A. (2019). Workplace Bullying Among Surgeons - the perfect crime. *Annals of Surgery, 269*(1), 43–44. doi:10.1097/SLA.0000000000003018 PMID:30247324

Rangel, E. L., Lyu, H., Haider, A. H., Castillo-Angeles, M., Doherty, G. M., & Smink, D. S. (2018). Factors Associated with Residency and Career Dissatisfaction in Childbearing Surgical Residents. *JAMA Surgery, 153*(11), 1004–1011. doi:10.1001/jamasurg.2018.2571 PMID:30073246

RCSEd (The Royal College of Surgeons in Edinburgh). (2018). Anti-bullying and undermining campaign. Available at https://www.rcsed.ac.uk/professional-support-development-resources/anti-bullying-and-undermining-campaign

Richardson, A., Mascarenhas, M., & Balen, A. (2019). Is a woman's chronological age or 'ovarian age' more important in determining perinatal outcome after assisted reproductive treatment? *Human Fertility (Cambridge, England)*, 1–7. doi:10.1080/14647273.2019.1597987 PMID:31038011

Rogers, A. C., Wren, S. M., & McNamara, D. A. (2019). Gender and Specialty Influences on Personal and Professional Life Among Trainees. *Annals of Surgery*, *269*(2), 383–387. doi:10.1097/SLA.0000000000002580 PMID:29099401

Rue, R. (1967). Employment of married women doctors in hospitals in the Oxford Region. *Lancet, 1*(7502), 1267–1268. doi:10.1016/S0140-6736(67)92730-4 PMID:4165051

Saalwachter, A. R., Freischlag, J. A., Sawyer, R. G., & Sanfey, H. A. (2006). Part-time training in general surgery: Results of a web-based survey. *Archives of Surgery*, *141*(10), 977–982. doi:10.1001/archsurg.141.10.977 PMID:17043275

Salles, A. (2019). "I Spent my Fertile Years training to be a Surgeon. Now, it might be too late for me to have a Baby". Available at https://time.com/5484506/fertility-egg-freezing/

Seemann, N. M., Webster, F., Holden, H. A., Carol-anne, E. M., Baxter, N., Desjardins, C., & Cil, T. (2016). Women in academic surgery: Why is the playing field still not level? *American Journal of Surgery, 211*(2), 343–349. doi:10.1016/j.amjsurg.2015.08.036 PMID:26723836

Shaw, P. M., Vouyouka, A., & Reed, A. (2012). Time for radiation safety program guidelines for pregnant trainees and vascular surgeons. *Journal of Vascular Surgery*, *55*(3), 862–8.e2. doi:10.1016/j.jvs.2011.11.045 PMID:22277686

Thejournal.ie. (2017). Mothers of premature babies to be given extended paid maternity leave. Available at https://www.thejournal.ie/premature-babies-extended-leave-3627843-Oct2017/

Thurber, C., Dugas, L. R., Ocobock, C., Carlson, B., Speakman, J.R., & Pontzer, H. (2019). Extreme events reveal an alimentary limit on sustained maximal human energy expenditure. *Science Advances, 5*(6).

Troppmann, K. M., Palis, B. E., Goodnight, J. E. Jr, Ho, H. S., & Troppmann, C. (2009). Women surgeons in the new millennium. *Archives of Surgery*, *144*(7), 635–642. doi:10.1001/archsurg.2009.120 PMID:19620543

Turner, P. L., Lumpkins, K., Gabre, J., Lin, M. J., Liu, X., & Terrin, M. (2012). Pregnancy among women surgeons: Trends over time. *Archives of Surgery*, *147*(5), 474–479. doi:10.1001/archsurg.2011.1693 PMID:22351877

Velasco, I., Naranjo, S., Lopez-Pedrera, C., Garriga, M. J., Garcıa-Fuentes, E., & Soriguer, F. (2009). Use of povidone-iodine during the first trimester of pregnancy: A correct practice? *BJOG*, *116*(3), 452–455. doi:10.1111/j.1471-0528.2008.02059.x PMID:19187379

Walsh, D. F., Thome, A. P., Mody, K. S., Eltorai, A. E. M., Daniels, A. H., & Mulcahey, M. K. (2019). Radiation safety education as a component of orthopedic training. *Orthopedic Reviews*, *11*(1), 7883. doi:10.4081/or.2019.7883 PMID:30996841

Chapter 2
Parental Leave During Surgical Training:
Gender Equity, Parental Leave, Parental Policies, Childbearing, Conciliation, Surgery

Patricia Maria Saez Carlin
Hospital Clínico San Carlos, Universidad Complutense de Madrid, Spain

ABSTRACT

Work-family conciliation is currently in vogue. However, reality demonstrates that there is still a long way to go before being forced to make a choice between work, family, or personal life. Can a balance be achieved among the three? In relation to the medical profession, is there currently an adequate conciliation policy? Can these strategies be extrapolated to the training period? The proposal in this chapter consists in carrying out an up-to-date analysis on the parental leave situation during medical training as one of the main aspects of conciliation, by analysing parental leave policies and barriers faced by surgical trainees.

CURRENT STATE OF GENDER PARITY IN THE HEALTH SYSTEM

Gender balance in the medical workforce is changing (World Health Organization [WHO], 2006) and currently, the presence of female doctors in daily medical care is a fact. However, it has taken many centuries to recognize women as medical professionals and to change people´s mindset in terms of gender equity.

The figure of a woman as a healer goes back to ancestral times. Yet, women´s role in the story of medicine has remained in the background for years and has not been recognized until a few decades ago. Because of women`s particularly feminine qualities such as altruism or delicacy, in combination with skills gained and fulfilled during motherhood and childcaring, they have been implicated throughout history in taking care of the sick and the needy, an occupation which has been described as "caring-

DOI: 10.4018/978-1-5225-9599-1.ch002

work". However, due to traditional superiority of men over women, their work was usually disdained and relegated to the treatment of patients who lacked economic resources and could not afford the cost of a male doctor. Therefore, *women-healers* were mainly requested by patients as a last resort to treat their diseases and were, for a long period of time, dismissed and even considered to be witches.

The 19th century brought the era of "modern medicine" and the idea of professionalisation began to gain importance in every job sector (Witz, 1992). Yet, only men were included in the medical workforce as women were still not allowed to entry medical schools. Therefore, this major progress in the evolution of professional education implied the creation of new barriers for women, who were again excluded from training and from access to university. This situation led to women sometimes seeking their own opportunities and training and working incognito.

It was not until the end of the century that the first female medical school was created. From then on, there has been an increase in the number of women practicing medicine (Blackmore, 2013). This was mainly motivated by the arrival of global social changes during the 20th century in terms of improvements in gender equity. Additionally, female access to medical education was also favoured by the World Wars. The need for qualified personnel to join the armed forces resulted in opening the quota of women to access medical training. However, despite these advances, women continued to be economically dependent on their husbands and were limited by household chores. Their mandatory and sole responsibility over family and domestic chores has been, after their access to university education, one of the principal obstacles of women´s incorporation into the workplace. It must be highlighted that this obstacle remains unresolved as will be commented later in the chapter.

During the last decades, and linked to the idea of professionalization mentioned above, society has demanded a qualification system for professionals, in which doctors in the health sector have been equally included. This modus operandi promotes professional certification based on the results of impartial exams and on the achievement of career merits which has secondarily, decreased gender, sex or social class inequalities. Consequently, the improvements in gender barriers achieved by the mentioned system has increased the number of female medical university enrolments. The good marks accomplished by female students in school, better than male in the majority of centres, have consolidated a progressive entry of women in medical schools, once the gender restriction has been overcome.

With all this, the latest data reveal that female medical graduates in the United States reached 47.3% in 2017 (Association of American Medical College [AAMC], 2018) with similar statistics in European countries (45% in the United Kingdom, (Medical´s Women Federation [MWF], n.d.)) and comprised more than 40% of general surgery residents. Nevertheless, in many countries, the distribution of women by occupational category tends to lean in favour of nurses and midwives and other 'care' jobs as community health workers. Accordingly, women are often underrepresented in other categories, for example, doctors, dentists, pharmacists and managers (WHO, 2008).

However, although absolute barriers to women accessing the medical profession based on gender have disappeared in most countries, new barriers are coming to light (Elston, 2009). With regard to this, one of the principal barriers currently under debate is related to pregnancy and childcare. Motherhood is a reality that essentially affects the female sex and as a consequence, indirectly and mandatorily represents a challenge for women when deciding a professional career. Various studies show that even among the most highly educated women (those with a master's degree or higher), 80% have had their first child by age 34 (Livingston, 2015), which coincides with the medical training period. Female medical students and trainees still face comments that discourage them from choosing surgery, with sexist comments such as "do you not want to have a family" not infrequent. Secondarily, lower rates of advancement of women into leadership positions in the medical workforce compared to men have been achieved, as would be predicted by the number of female enrolments in medical schools for the past three decades. This does not mean that women want to stop having children and renounce their figure as mothers. But they also want to be able to participate and succeed in any type of professional career as men do if they are talented for it, without external barriers that stop their professional aspirations. For this, there is still work to do in order to satisfactorily achieve an adequate gender equity regime in the sector.

In summary, in spite of the great advances in the last two centuries in terms of gender equity in the medical profession, there are still some barriers to solve in order to achieve equal opportunities for women in the medical workforce, work-family conciliation being one of the major issues which will be discussed below.

The Need of Conciliation Strategies: Why?

As mentioned previously one of the current barriers for women in the medical workforce is parenthood. Today´s young men and women professionals are strongly demanding a balance between work and family for their personal lives. Can this really be achieved? Should it be a social change promoted by organizations and authorities?

New generations are putting into value other factors in life not exclusively related to work. As reported by surveys carried out in 2017-2018, young workers value flexibility over salary (Taylor 2017) (Clemente, 2018) which allows them to reconcile and organise their time more autonomously and without strict ties. In this sense, the typical definition of a good leader capable of putting work before everything else, is declining. Instead, a new figure is becoming much more powerful: a person who is able to successfully balance family or personal life (sports, travelling, cultural activities or other interests…) with a professional career. That is what is considered the truly effective manager, with authentic leadership.

Many studies have reported the variables that shape professional success, and which include: individual differences, the organization (the company and society) and the family (Chinchilla, 2018). An adequate combination of the three factors permits a favourable environment to achieve stable and lasting career success. It is essential to focus on these for the development of adequate family-work-life balance policies based on the person and needs.

Conciliation is born from the person itself. The human being is not transformed into different people depending on whether they are at work, at leisure or in a family environment. It is always the same person playing different roles. Conciliation means achieving a harmonious situation between the different areas, integrating them into one life. In this way, the main resource of conciliation is the person him-herself. The construction of a single upright project which defines the life trajectory of each individual and that integrates the different areas, is the base of an adequate family and work conciliation policy. In this sense, it is essential that national authorities worldwide contribute to the enrichment of work, family and personal life, since they are fundamental, irrevocable and complementary dimensions in the lives of today´s men and women.

For this, the organization (company and society) must be able to respond with flexibility to the worker´s personal needs being capable to combine all the features of the worker[6]. This appeal has already seeped in the industry in the past years, and large companies have recently launched better strategies toward more family-friendly employment policies (e.g. Google, Facebook (Cohen, 2015), Amazon (Tepper Nov 2015) and Netflix (Tepper Aug 2015)). Therefore, this change in mentality must be spread through all sectors, including the medical workforce.

Another aspect to take into account is that, even though when thinking of conciliation, the idea is usually related to improvements in female policies, many of the changes that women need in order to remain in the workforce are equally sought by younger male professionals. In this sense, as noted previously, generational and societal changes also affect men or non-childbearing parents in terms of desire for time and involvement with family. Conversely, parenthood and consequently parental leave situations involve maternity leaves mainly, but also other situations that have to be considered outside the traditional male-female relationships as same-sex partnerships, non-married unions or adoption.

In terms of the medical workforce, there has been recent interest over the last decades in carrying out improvements with regard to gender equity and family-work policies, mainly motivated by women´s medical associations (Medical Women´s Federation, Women in Surgery of the Royal College of Surgeons, Group on Women in Medicine and Science (GWIMS) of the Association of American Medical Colleges (AAMC)...). Even though it is not a problem unique to medicine it is particularly problematic in this sector, because of patients' need for 24-hour care.

This interest comes from the ideal of achieving a real gender equity itself. However, there is another urgent and fundamental problem that must be borne in mind, which is related to the incessant change in gender in the medical workforce.

In this sense, it is essential to emphasise the increasing number of female doctors in the healthcare system, which will in the near future largely exceed the amount of men doctors. Because of this, an innovative workforce planning and financial modelling which includes female doctor´s demands and needs must be evaluated and carried out in order to preserve a quality standard of care. Particularly, it may represent important defiance in fields that attract large numbers of women (e.g. Obstetrics and Gynaecology) as well as a taking into account a potential decrease in applications to currently male-dominated specialties such as surgery.

Directly linked to this, there is, at present, a lack of women in senior positions. As an example, according to AAMC data, women represent 17% of tenured professors, 16% of full professors, 10% of department chairs, and 11% of medical school deans at United States academic medical centres (AAMC, 2015). Statistics confirm there are lower rates of advancement of women into leadership positions in the medical workforce as would be predicted by the number of female enrolments in medicine schools in previous decades. This suggests that there are other reasons apart from their later incorporation into the field.

In this sense, several authors have reported that the underrepresentation of women in senior positions in medicine has been many times related to family reasons (Carnes, 2008). Female doctors may opt for part-time or other forms of flexible working in order to achieve family-work conciliation as suggested by Taylor and colleagues (Taylor, 2009). A lack of male support for household chores and childcare can consequently affect female medics career aspirations or make work-life integration more challenging (Gjerberg, 2003) (Reed, 2001). This may contribute to male doctors developing their professional careers more rapidly than their female colleagues.

At present, some countries have implemented strategies in this subject. As an example, the 'Quality Worklife Quality Healthcare Collaborative' (QWQHC, 2007) in Canada is an association, formed by 12 healthcare organizations, which aims to improve health professionals' work-life balance to ultimately improve patient outcomes and service delivery. Additionally, Women´s Medical Associations in various countries worldwide work to improve the disparity between male and female doctors, promoting conciliation programmes and encouraging and enabling women to fulfil their career ambitions by encouraging the use of flexible working arrangements and support in childbearing (Deech, 2009). Encouraging less than full time training options and flexible working arrangements for men may also improve the gender divide- this is discussed further in the chapter on pregnancy and less than full time training.

Another example is the Harvard Brigham and Women's Hospital in Boston, Massachusetts. Their experience clearly demonstrates that local action can ameliorate in many ways these barriers for female doctors. By creating an Office for Women's Careers, which is actively engaged in the promotion of women to senior positions, they have seen that the number of female professors has doubled (Nadelson, 2006).

Policymakers must think of new ways of reorganising the existing stock of doctors rather than increasing and rotating employers with every parental leave. Innovative human resources' strategies should be considered in order to achieve current and future doctors´ demands in terms of conciliation. Some of the measures have already been reported by women working groups in medicine (Women doctors: making a difference) as for example: improving access to mentoring and career advice, identifying female role models, creating female leadership courses, competency based training programmes, improving access to part-time working and flexible training, thinking of innovative job design which adequate to doctor´s needs, increases in job shares or enhancing access to childcare helps. Part-time schedules have been broadly discussed in literature (Laurance, 2004) (McKinstry, 2008). As an example, a study comparing flexible trainees with full-time trainees found that the outcomes of training were very similar: 92% of flexible trainees obtained a certificate of completion of training (CCT) compared with 90% of full-time trainees, with flexible trainees more likely to take part-time consultant posts after they finished their training(Gray, 2005).

In summary, there is a real necessity of adaption to young worker´s demands, as they make up the majority of the working population. Culture shifts towards support and increase of flexible and "family-friendly" strategies, coupled with formal parental leave policies from leaders, are needed in order to allow women to achieve senior positions in medicine, which in turn guarantees the continuity of a high-quality health system.

Parental Leave During Medical Training: Current Situation and Obstacles

In order to improve gender equity and family-work conciliation it is imperative to understand the role that pregnancy and parenthood play amongst doctors, especially women. Parental leave is still a taboo topic due to a lack of consolidated policies and internal and external pressures faced by the trainee in this situation. These aspects will be therefore explained and analysed.

Doctors still face real challenges during their training programs as they coincide with their childbearing years. As commented previously (Livingston, 2015), the majority of women have their first child during their early 30s and expecting them to delay pregnancy until after their long training period isn't reasonable, given the increased risk of infertility and pregnancy complications among older women. In addition, it has been repeatedly reported that female residents have increased rates of complications during pregnancy compared with the general population regarding pregnancy-induced hypertension, pre-eclampsia, intrauterine growth restriction and miscarriage (Walker, 2006) (Klebanoff, 2000) (Merchant, 2011) → can be deleted or changed to another chapter if considered. The ability to conciliate a successful medical career with family duties becomes an even more complex challenge in hospital-based specialties as they often imply long and unpredictable hours, being on call, and scarcity of part-time work options. Furthermore, the situation is exacerbated in surgical specialties, were barriers for women are even more accentuated.

In European Union Countries, EU Maternity Leave Directive (92/85/EEC) declares that women have the right to a minimum of 14 weeks (3 months) maternity leave, of which at least two weeks are compulsory, and can be allocated before and/or after giving birth. This applies equally for doctors during their training period. However, the directive serves only as guidance for EU countries and therefore there is still significant variation in the way that maternity leave policy is organised by each state. In terms of length of leave, there are differences not only with regard to the number of weeks available, but also whether the leave is mandatory, non-mandatory, or a combination of both. The RAND Europe report provides an overview of current maternity leave policies across European countries, which vary from 6 to 52 weeks in respect of post-natal maternity leaves, being the shortest identifiable total leave length given by Spain (6 mandatory leave weeks → Spanish legislation says that of the total 16 weeks permitted, only the first 6 weeks after birth are mandatory for the mother. The father can request the remaining 10 weeks) while the longest is given by Bulgaria (52 non-mandatory weeks) (Strang, n.d).

On the other hand, in the US, parental leave policies during doctor´s training are organised in an autonomous way by each institution and varies depending on the specialty. American Medical Colleges do not have a unique and defined schedule. As revealed for example in a recent systematic review (Humphries, 2017), the American College of Graduate Medical Education (ACGME) does not have a formal parental leave policy that GME programmes must follow. As a consequence, leave time for family purposes was taken from unpaid or sick leave, annual leave, or disability.

Another obstacle is in relation to breastfeeding. The World Health Organization recommends exclusive breastfeeding up to 6 months, with continued breast feeding up to 2 years, since exclusive breastfeeding provides babies with the perfect nutrition for healthy growth and brain development, and protection from various health threats (Agostoni, 2009) (Chung, 2007). However, with today's policies, this objective is very difficult to achieve. Research confirms that mothers who plan to return to work sooner, especially earlier than 12 weeks, are less likely to have exclusive breastfeeding plans (Mirkovic, 2014). Paternity leaves are also related to the subject, as children whose fathers did not take time off to help with childcaring during the first year were significantly less likely to be breastfed at 2, 4, and 6 months of age (Flacking, 2010).

However, a good example of conciliation policies has been developed by Nordic European countries who have implemented national strategies which properly favour WHO´s recommendations. As an example, Sweden has long maternity and paternity leaves, with 480 days (16 months) shared between father and mother receiving 80% of the salary up to 390 days. The approximately equal numbers of male and female physicians in Scandinavia have coincided with the emergence of progressive work–life policies, the belief that motherhood and employment can be combined, and changing expectations of work-life balance (Aditi Ramakrishnan, MA 2014).

In summary, there is a lack of parity for having children during medical training programmes which is perpetuated by the different positions of the centres that vary from hostile, to indifferent, to supportive in a few exceptions. Current parental leave policies are insufficient in most of the countries worldwide in order to achieve an adequate care of both parents and newborn babies, not even allowing the minimum recommended time for breastfeeding. Therefore, there is a need for organised programmes with consolidated parental policies which can offer a suitable solution to trainees, colleagues and programme directors.

What are the Unique Aspects of Surgical Practice That Make Parental Leave Different to Other Medical Specialties?

Parenthood and a successful career in surgery are eminently possible to combine. However, as mentioned previously, there are still major barriers for women when choosing surgical specialties, some of them related to childbearing. Even though female-mother roles in surgery are becoming more popular and equally capable to men, a surgeon´s personality implies a strong work ethic and commitment to patients which may make the decision to have children difficult initially, especially during training (Bass, 2004) (Willett, 2010). In contrast, there are a number of benefits of having a surgeon who is also a parent, acknowledging that some of the traits that help one succeed as a parent are also incredibly valuable in the surgical field.

Another factor unique to surgeons is the constant pressure of maintaining their surgical skills (Smith, 2013). There is not an established time that a surgeon can be away from practice, but the longer it is, theoretically the more difficult it will be to restart. However, it is a reality that surgical trainees routinely take breaks from clinical surgery for other reasons such as research or external rotations and go back to the operating theatre after being away sometimes for several years. In this sense there is a need for re-entry support after parental leave that satisfy the trainee and trainers. It is vital for planning and for the best use of women's talents that their re-entry into the profession is at the forefront of arrangements for maternity leave and thereafter. It is essential that women have a clear and unambiguous mechanism to step off and then get back on the specialist training ladder, so that the value of the training they have already completed is not lost and that their skills can be topped up on return to full-time practice. As an example, in countries like UK, trainees have the option of progressive training before incorporation from maternity leave which permits an adequate transition to work duties. Other options are that trainees on maternity leave have the option of attending technical skills courses and conferences having the same access to funding as their working colleagues and that these activities are baby friendly.

On the other hand, surgical departments are extremely competitive and unconscious bias and outdated attitudes still remain. In this sense, parenthood has classically been considered an obstacle during training because it can entail negative perception by programme directors, colleagues and indeed sometimes the trainee herself which is still present in today´s medical departments (Sayres, 1986) (Braun, 1992) (Franco, 1983). In a recent survey on the opinion of general surgery programme directors carried out in 2016 (Sandler, 2016), 61% of the directors considered that becoming a parent negatively affected female trainees' work, including increased strain on fellow residents (33%), fewer scholarly activities (9%), fewer clinical activities (8%), less dedication to patient care (6%) and decreased timeliness (5%). In addition, directors responsible for general surgery programmes considered that becoming a parent had a negative effect on female resident´s work more than male´s (61% vs. 34%) and thought that having children decreased female resident´s well-being more often than that of male residents (32% vs. 9%). Furthermore, 15% of general surgery programme directors said they would not recommend that female residents have children during their training programme. The authors also report that female residents were less likely to be covered by their surgical colleagues during formal maternity leave period when comparing to paternity leave policies taken by male colleagues (50%vs 70%). This is due to the lack of information on the issue amongst the trainees themselves. In this sense, another study (Dixit, 2015) shows how both male and female residents without children are usually unaware of parental leave policies and therefore not supportive of their fellow parenting colleagues. Consequently, awareness of these policies among trainees is crucial, as they directly affect the good running of the department.

Taking into account the above the above, pregnancy and childbirth strongly affect trainee´s choices on medical programmes, career plans and willingness to take additional degrees more often for women than for men (Blair, 2015). The negative perception prompted by programme directors who should act as the trainee´s mentor has a strong impact on the resident´s career, resulting in delay in childbearing for many female residents across specialties (Holliday, 2015). An American survey recently published on 347 female surgeons who had one or more pregnancies during residency, found that 39% strongly considered leaving their programme and 29,5% said they would not recommend a surgical career to female medical students because of the difficulties of balancing pregnancy and motherhood with training (Rangel, 2018). This was enhanced by a high percentage of women (85.6%) who worked with an unmodified schedule until birth and another big group (63.6%) who were concerned that their work schedule could affect their health or the health of their unborn child. On the other hand, this same study reported the lack of mentorship by 66.8% of the respondents, who would have wished for more effective coaching on how to reconcile a surgical career with motherhood and pregnancy. These issues highlight the importance of support for female trainees with regard to pregnancy and maternity leave and the need to challenge overt sexism and unconscious bias.

In a recent survey for women of the Association of Surgeons of Great Britain and Ireland carried out in 2017 (Bellini MI, 2019), 31% of them reported feeling that surgical professions did not make motherhood easy. On the other hand, 16% said that surgical departments felt like an "old boys´club" and noted the disadvantage of childcaring. Out of all the survey respondents, 42% agreed that access to more flexible career and training programmes would improve the presence of women in surgical sectors, while a third of them pointed out that these types of measures are currently frowned upon. Thus, there is a need of a fundamental change in hospital culture, which permits doctors of both genders to be more involved in family life without it being detrimental to their career. A more equal division of domestic and childcare obligations and better opportunities in hospital-based specialties to adjust work to family responsibilities when having small children, would reduce the gender differences and allow more women to complete specialization.

However, the above data is based on a subjective perception by programme directors and trainees but when analysing in detail, there are other studies published to date which report the opposite. As an example, a recent study on surgical trainees did not find any relation between sex or incidence of childrearing during training and academic productivity (Brown, 2014). Residents with children born during training did not demonstrate fewer total case numbers, exam scores or research work rates compared with residents who did not have children during training. Women who had children during training were more likely to pursue fellowship (87.5%) than those who did not (66.7%). Another study on Gynaecology & Obstetric residents demonstrates that Pregnancy and delivery did not decrease surgical experience major procedures in the programme (Lashbrook, 2003).

Thus, supported by these results, which clearly are opposite to subjective negative perceptions mentioned previously, there is a need to change negative attitudes toward trainee parents and females in particular, and encourage a culture change toward an environment of support to promote their success.

Currently, most specialty boards require a mandatory "time-spent" training in order to graduate and achieve a professional degree. Allowing trainees to extend their training in order to take maternity leave should be facilitated. However, the amount of "time spent" involved in clinical activity during training maybe should be replaced by quality of "time spent" favoured by a competency-based program. This is not new, as the idea of professionalization was firstly mentioned in "modern medicine" in the 19th century, as previously commented. Indeed, in the UK training is moving towards a competency-based approach.

The length and rigour of surgical residency are necessary to train skilled surgeons, especially in setting limitations on duty hours. A move towards competency-based education, rather than strict quotas of weeks worked may provide additional flexibility for residents, improving parenting trainees' quality of life and will attract more talented students without sacrificing educational excellence.

In summary, surgical residency programmes need to consider creating parental leave guidelines that are compatible with their schedule and adapt to their residents' needs. Surgical residency is unique in that it may be more physically demanding, may require longer hours, may have specific occupational hazards (as for example needlestick injury and exposure to anaesthetic vapours), and may not have the same flexibility in scheduling enjoyed by other residency programmes. A maternity/parenting policy for surgical residents must account for these unique concerns of surgical training and should address the following issues deemed important by resident responders: clinical expectations in the third trimester including on-call duties, flexible rotation scheduling, use of vacation time toward maternity/parenting, and clear delineation of how time off for maternity/parental leave may impact length of training. This may reduce resident´s pressure and allow for planning parental leave. Moreover, the existence of such guidelines is relevant to the recruitment of future trainees, particularly with regard to surgical specialties.

CONCLUSION

- Gender balance in the medical workforce is changing and the number of female doctors is increasing.
- One of the major barriers for women in the medical workforce is parenthood, especially when choosing and staying in surgical specialties.
- New generations of men and women professionals strongly demand policies which reconcile work and family life.
- Family care is still disproportionately carried by women resulting in a slower progression in their medical careers and an underrepresentation of women in senior positions.
- Innovative workforce planning which includes female doctor´s needs must be evaluated in order to preserve a quality standard of care.
- Doctors face real challenges during their training programmes as they coincide with their child-bearing years.
- Parental leave during medical training is still a taboo topic due to a lack of consolidated policies and internal and external pressures faced by the trainee in this situation.
- There are factors unique to surgical specialties which make parental leave different to other specialties: maintaining surgical skills and negative perceptions by colleagues with unconscious bias still a major issue.
- Pregnancy and childcare are negatively perceived by programme directors, colleagues and the trainee herself.
- The lack of support for parenthood has a strong impact on the resident´s career, resulting in delaying in childbearing by many female residents.
- Surgical trainees demand more effective coaching on how to reconcile a surgical career with motherhood and pregnancy.

- Recent studies have not identified a relationship between sex or incidence of childrearing during training and academic productivity in surgical residents.
- A move towards competency-based education may provide additional flexibility for residents, improving parenting trainees' quality of life and will attract more talented students without sacrificing educational excellence.

REFERENCES

AAMC. (2005). *Women in U.S. academic medicine statistics and medical school benchmarking, 2004–2005*. Washington, DC: Association of American Medical Colleges.

Aditi Ramakrishnan, M. A., Dana Sambuco, M. P. P. A., Reshma Jagsi, M. D., & Phil, D. (2014). Women's Participation in the Medical Profession: Insights from Experiences in Japan, Scandinavia, Russia, and Eastern Europe. *Journal of Women's Health*, *23*(11), 927–934. doi:10.1089/jwh.2014.4736 PMID:25320867

Agostoni, C., Braegger, C., Decsi, T., Kolacek, S., Koletzko, B., Michaelsen, K. F., ... van Goudoever, J. (2009). Breast-feeding: A commentary by the ESPGHAN Committee on Nutrition. *Journal of Pediatric Gastroenterology and Nutrition*, *49*(1), 112–125. doi:10.1097/MPG.0b013e31819f1e05 PMID:19502997

Association of American Medical College. (2018). Retrieved from www.aamc.org

Bass, B. L., & Napolitano, L. M. (2004). Gender and diversity considerations in surgical training. *The Surgical Clinics of North America*, *84*(6), 1537–1555. doi:10.1016/j.suc.2004.06.008 PMID:15501274

Bellini, M. I., Graham, Y., Hayes, C., Zakeri, R., Parks, R., & Papalois, V. (2019). A Woman´s place in theatre: women´s perceptions and experiences of working in surgery from the Association of Surgeons of Great Britain and Ireland. Women in Surgery working group. *BJM Open. 7;9*(1). doi:10.1136/bmjopen-2018-024349

Blackmore, S. (2013). *Elizabeth Blackwell: the first woman to qualify as a doctor in America*. University of Bristol. The Wellcome Trust 2013. Retrieved from http://blog.wellcome.ac.uk/2013/07/22/elizabeth-blackwell/

Blair, J. E., Mayer, A. P., Caubet, S. L., Norby, S. M., O'Connor, M. I., & Hayes, S. N. (2015). Pregnancy and Parental Leave During Graduate Medical Education. *Academic Medicine*, *1*(November). doi:10.1097/ACM.0000000000001006 PMID:26606722

Braun, D. L., & Susman, V. L. (1992). Pregnancy during psychiatry residency: A study of attitudes. *Academic Psychiatry*, *16*(4), 178–185. doi:10.1007/BF03341390 PMID:24435425

Brown, E. G., Galante, J. M., Keller, B. A., Braxton, J., & Farmer, D. L. (2014). Pregnancy-Related Attrition in General Surgery. *JAMA Surgery*, *149*(9), 893. doi:10.1001/jamasurg.2014.1227 PMID:25029501

Carnes, M., Morrissey, C., & Geller, S. E. (2008). Women's health and women's leadership in academic medicine: Hitting the same glass ceiling? *Journal of Women's Health*, *17*(9), 1453–1462. doi:10.1089/jwh.2007.0688 PMID:18954235

Chinchilla, N. (2018). *Integrar la vida. "Integrate life*. Barcelona, Spain: Ariel.

Chung, M., Raman, G., Chew, P., Magula, N., Trikalinos, T., & Lau, J. (2007). Breastfeeding and maternal and infant health outcomes in developed countries. *Evidence Report/Technol Assessment., 153*, 1–186. PMID:17764214

Clemente, P. (2018). *El poder de flexibilizar dinámicas*. El mundo. Retrieved from http://www.elmundo.es/economia/innovadores/2018/12/20/5c17e4e721efa0e31d8b461e.html

Cohen, D. (2015). Facebook Offers All Employees 4 Months' Parental Leave. AdWeek. Retrieved from http://www.adweek.com/digital/four-months-parental-leave/

Deech, R. (2009). *Women doctors: making a difference. Report of the Chair of the National Working Group on Women in Medicine*. London, UK: Department of Health.

Dixit, A., Feldman-Winter, L., & Szucs, K. (2015). Parental leave policies and pediatric trainees in the United States. *Journal of Human Lactation, 31*(3), 434–439.

Elston, M. A. (2009). *Women and medicine: the future*. London, UK: Royal College of Physicians. Retrieved from www.rcplondon.ac.uk/pubs/brochure.aspx?e=277

Flacking, R., Dykes, F., & Ewald, U. (2010). The influence of fathers' socio- economic status and paternity leave on breastfeeding duration: A population-based cohort study. *Scandinavian Journal of Public Health, 38*(4), 337–343. doi:10.1177/1403494810362002 PMID:20147577

Franco, K., Evans, C. L., Best, A. P., Zrull, J. P., & Pizza, G. A. (1983). Conflicts associated with physicians' pregnancies. *The American Journal of Psychiatry, 140*(7), 902–904. doi:10.1176/ajp.140.7.902 PMID:6859310

Gjerberg, E. (2003). Women doctors in Norway: The challenging balance between career and family life. *Social Science & Medicine, 57*(7), 1327–1341. doi:10.1016/S0277-9536(02)00513-0 PMID:12899913

Gray, S. F., Goodyear, H. M., & Jones, M. J. T. (2005). Outcomes of flexible training compared to full time training during the Specialist Registrar Grade in the UK. *Med Educ Online*. Retrieved from www.med-ed-online.org/pdf/10000007.pdf

Holliday, E. B., Ahmed, A. A., Jagsi, R., Stentz, N. C., Woodward, W. A., Fuller, C. D., & Thomas, C. R. Jr. (2015). Pregnancy and Parenthood in Radiation Oncology, Views and Experiences Survey (PROVES): Results of a Blinded Prospective Trainee Parenting and Career Development Assessment. *Radiation Oncology Biology, 92*(3), 516–524. doi:10.1016/j.ijrobp.2015.02.024 PMID:25892584

Humphries, L., Lyon, S., Garza, R., Butz, D., Lemelman, B., & Park, J. (2017). Parental leave policies in graduate medical education: A systematic review. *The American college of surgeons*.

Klebanoff, M. A., Shiono, P., & Rhoads, G. (1990). Outcomes of pregnancy in a national sample of resident physicians. *The New England Journal of Medicine, 323*(15), 1040–1045. doi:10.1056/NEJM199010113231506 PMID:2215563

Lashbrook, D. L., Frazier, L. M., Horbelt, D. V., Stembridge, T. W., & Rall, M. J. (2003). Pregnancy during obstetrics and gynecology residency: Effect on surgical experience. *American Journal of Obstetrics and Gynecology*, *189*(3), 662–665. doi:10.1067/S0002-9378(03)00877-9 PMID:14526288

Laurance, J. (2004) The medical timebomb: too many women doctors. Retrieved from http://www.independent.co.uk/life-style/health-and-families/health-news/the-medicaltimebomb too many-women-doctors-6260011.html

Livingston, G. (2015, July 6). For most highly educated women, motherhood doesn't start until the 30s. Washington, DC. Retrieved from http://www.pewresearch.org/fact-tank/2015/01/15/for-most- highly-educated-women-motherhood-doesnt-start-until-the-30s/

McKinstry, B. (2008). Are there too many female medical graduates? Yes. [Medical's Women Federation. n.d.]. *BMJ (Clinical Research Ed.)*, *336*(7647), 748. doi:10.1136/bmj.39505.491065.94 PMID:18390524

Merchant, S., Hameed, M., & Melck, A. (2011). Pregnancy among residents enrolled in general surgery (PREGS): A survey of residents in a single Canadian training program. *Canadian Journal of Surgery*, *54*(6), 375–380. doi:10.1503/cjs.015710 PMID:21939607

Mirkovic, K. R., Perrine, C. G., Scanlon, K. S., & Grummer-Strawn, L. M. (2014). In the United States, a mother's plans for infant feeding are associated with her plans for employment. *Journal of Human Lactation*, *30*(3), 292–297. doi:10.1177/0890334414535665 PMID:24868017

Nadelson, C. (2006). *A Model for Women's Career Development: An Office for Women's Careers*. Queensland, Australia: Presentation at Griffith University.

Quality Worklife Quality Healthcare Collaborative. (2007). *Within Our Grasp: A Healthy Workplace Action Strategy for Success and Sustainability in Canada's Healthcare System*. Ontario, Canada.

Rangel, E., Smink, D., Castillo-Angeles, M., Kwakye, G., Changala, M., Haider, A. H., & Doherty, G. M. (2018). Pregnancy and Motherhood During Surgical Training. *JAMA Surgery*, *153*(7), 644–652. doi:10.1001/jamasurg.2018.0153 PMID:29562068

Reed, V., & Buddeberg-Fischer, B. (2001). Career obstacles for women in medicine: An overview. *Medical Education*, *35*(2), 139–147. doi:10.1046/j.1365-2923.2001.00837.x PMID:11169087

Sandler, B. J., Tackett, J. J., Longo, W. E., & Yoo, P. S. (2016). Pregnancy and Parenthood among Surgery Residents: Results of the First Nationwide Survey of General Surgery Residency Program Directors. *Journal of the American College of Surgeons*, 1–7. doi:10.1016/j.jamcollsurg.12.004 PMID:26776357

Sayres, M., Wyshak, G., Denterlein, G., Apfel, R., Shore, E., & Federman, D. (1986). Pregnancy during residency. *The New England Journal of Medicine*, *314*(7), 418–423. doi:10.1056/NEJM198602133140705 PMID:3945268

Smith, C., Galante, J. M., Pierce, J. L., & Scherer, L. A. (2013). The Surgical Residency Baby Boom: Changing Patterns of Childbearing During Residency Over a 30-Year Span. *Journal of Graduate Medical Education*, *5*(4), 625–629. doi:10.4300/JGME-D-12-00334.1 PMID:24455012

Strang, L. & Broeks, M. RAND Europe report. (n.d.). Maternity Leave Policies. European Commission. Europa EU.

Taylor, K. S., Lambert, T. W., & Goldacre, M. J. (2009). Career progression and destinations, comparing men and women in the NHS: Postal questionnaire surveys. *BMJ (Clinical Research Ed.)*, *338*(jun02 1), b1735. doi:10.1136/bmj.b1735 PMID:19493938

Taylor, T. (2017, Dec. 7). Workplace Flexibility For Millennials: Appealing To A Valuable New Generation. *Forbes*.

Tepper, T. (2015). Amazon's Parental Leave: The New Free Soda? *Money*. http://time.com/money/4098026/amazon-paid-parental-leave-benefits/

Tepper, T. (2015). *The Pros and Cons of Netflix's New Parental Leave Plan*. Retrieved from http://time.com/money/3985632/netflix-unlimited-parental-leave/

Walker, J. J. (2000). Pre-eclampsia. *Lancet*, *356*(9237), 1260–1265. doi:10.1016/S0140-6736(00)02800-2 PMID:11072961

Willett, L. L., Wellons, M. F., Hartig, J. R., Roenigk, L., Panda, M., Dearinger, A. T., ... Houston, T. K. (2010). Do women residents delay childbearing due to perceived career threats? *Academic Medicine*, *85*(4), 640–646. doi:10.1097/ACM.0b013e3181d2cb5b PMID:20354380

Witz, A. (1992). *Professions and Patriarchy*. London, UK: Routledge. doi:10.4324/9780203167786_chapter_2

World Health Organization Databases. (2006). Global Atlas of the Health Workforce: Gender Distribution on Selected Health Professions. Geneva.

World Health Organization Databases. (2008). Gender and Workforce statistics.

Chapter 3
Representation of Gender Equality From the Perspective of the Medical Trainee and its Ripple Effect:
Highlighting Gender Inequality in Medical Student Experiences

Lap Yan Leung
St George's University Hospitals NHS Foundation Trust, UK

ABSTRACT

It comes as no surprise that to tackle gender inequality in the future of the medical profession, the experiences of those who will become it must first be reviewed. Gender inequality is rife throughout all aspects of medical student life; from the classroom to clinical placements, from other healthcare professionals and public alike, for both male and female students. This chapter will discuss these, review literature, and share experiences. Consequently, this has an impact on their career choices, attrition, and mental health. By improving experiences and encouraging diversity, the hope is to reduce the negative effects discussed within the chapter, and break the cycle of inequality.

INTRODUCTION

The desire for gender equality in the medical profession has never been more transparent and public as currently. It comes as no surprise that to tackle the future of the medical professions, we must first review the experiences of those who will become it.

From the perspective of a medical trainee, gender inequality affects the day-to-day experience and training, varying treatment from both healthcare professionals and the public and differing advice from seniors, colleagues and the wider community. Consequently, it has an impact on career choices, attrition and mental health.

DOI: 10.4018/978-1-5225-9599-1.ch003

The chapter will review the changes in medical student intake; describe medical student experiences both in the classroom and on placement, followed by the consequences of these experiences. Although gender issues are acknowledged on an international stage, there is limited information as to the rationale behind why they occur, particularly in relation to medical trainees and students. Furthermore, in aid of making change, this chapter will try to not only identify areas of gender inequality but attempt to suggest strategical methods in which we can implement change.

With the primary goal of identifying and challenging gender inequality within medical school, the hope is to tackle the problem at the core as a preventative measure breaking the cycle, instead of a reactive stance.

As with most aspects of gender inequality, typically the limelight demonstrates that inequality is greater amongst women. However, there are areas in which gender inequality is more evident in men and the aim is to highlight these as equally important as those affecting women.

A Long Journey: Acceptance of Women in Medicine

Welcoming women into medicine has been a slow and at times a frowned upon process. From being considered witches and being burned at the stake, to now being Presidents of medical societies; women have come a long way. (Arrizabalaga, Abellana, Viñas, Merino & Ascaso, 2014; "Women in medicine", n.d.)

Women's way into formal medicine was through nursing, with others like Margaret Buckley masquerading as a male doctor for 46 years. The first ever woman to gain official entry into medicine was Elizabeth Blackwell (USA) in 1849 ("Women in medicine", n.d.). Since then the proportion of women entering medicine continues to rise. In 1996 more women were being accepted into medical school than men within Australia, the United Kingdom (UK) and the United States of America (USA) (Reynold, 2018). Female physicians now form 26% of the UK workforce compared to 6% in 1950 ("Timeline of women in medicine", 2018) but there is clear disparity between percentage entering medical school (>50%) and those working (26%).

Research consistently tells us that gender stereotypes and childhood aspirations emerge early in childhood and continue throughout adolescence (Legewie & DiPrete, 2014). Although encouraging that both genders are permitted to study medicine, entry into medical school is not the only obstacle they face. It is of equal important that deliverers of medical education and training address the gender inequalities within medical school itself.

It is clear from reviewing history that gender stereotypes have drastically changed over time. From the right to vote in 1918 and the women in the workforce post World War II, society began to understand women too can contribute to more than just the home. Physical ability continued to be questioned and famously in 1967, Katherine Switzer became the first woman to officially complete the full Boston marathon, not without an element of 'race drama'. Freedom to be independent was demonstrated in 2018 by Saudi women being allowed to drive, previously prevented by Saudi Arabian law. This stated that women should always have a male guardian and therefore would never need to drive. This change in law became necessary as the female workforce increased who needed to be able to drive independently.

Medicine is a widely acknowledged vocation which involves intellect, physical stamina and independence to make decisions. Women, with these skills, have a proven track record in leadership roles within the political arena across the world. These changes above as well as many more have demonstrated women's capabilities and have generated momentum for change towards women as leaders in healthcare.

There is no clear legislation specifying gender discrimination in education, however many fundamental principles are held in a variety of combined international legislation (Bagheritari & David, 2013). Despite all these, young activists exist because true equality does not. Famously Malala Yousafzai was shot in the head in Pakistan in 2012 by Taliban fighters, more than 100 girls were kidnapped from school in Nigeria in 2014 and only rescued in 2017. Even if legislation allows it, other factors (including war) will mean real access to education is not truly equal.

Despite all the improvements across the globe, it is clear that there is still a way to go. In 2018 it became evident that a prestigious medical school in Tokyo was deliberately altering scores of female candidates so preventing success. This tampering was felt to be appropriate since women would have shortened careers due to having children; suggesting an undertone they were not worth training. The President explained: "I suspect that there was a lack of sensitivity to the rules of modern society, in which women should not be treated differently because of their gender". He further explained that "women were not treated differently once they were accepted but acknowledged that some people believed women should not be allowed to become surgeons" (McCurry, 2018).

Gender stereotypes and progression throughout history are multifactorial. We can see that huge milestones have been reached yet much is still needed to achieve true equality. With more women entering the medical profession, how do we break the cycle of gender discrimination?

This chapter aims to review medical education in the context of gender equality, not just to improve those of women, but to review it holistically and consider ways to look forward and not repeat history.

Medical Student Experiences: Within the Classroom

Universally, medical school training is a minimum of four years. In America, minimum entry requirements include at least one pre-medical undergraduate degree. In the UK there are multiple entry points; either after secondary school (until aged 18) entering a minimum 5 year undergraduate or after another undergraduate degree usually science based, entering the shortened four-year graduate entry programme. These differences will of course bring a heterogeneous student population, in which diversity brings new dynamics and challenges.

Nationally each country will have governing bodies for medicine. These will set the curricula defining the expected outcomes of a student and govern the standards for medical schools. However, there is a huge variety within each medical school as to their course structure and training; providing very different experiences for not just each university or college but each individual trainee.

Traditionally more historic universities, such as Oxford and Cambridge within the UK, consist of pre-clinical lectures or classroom-heavy learning of basic clinical sciences, physiology and basic anatomy. These are usually supplemented by more bookwork and reading time. If the student progresses they will enter 'clinical years' where they enter clinical placements on hospital wards, surgical environments and within the community. Training has shifted towards a more integrated approach to learning with different higher education providers mixing clinical work into the earlier 'pre-clinical years'. The amount and method in which this is done varies on an individual university basis.

Reviewing how genders engage with the varying course structures and their differing experiences in different learning environments, i.e. classroom or placement, will highlight areas that educators can hopefully tackle, innovate change and reduce any gender gap.

As most medical schools start with more classroom-based teaching, we shall first review students' experiences here.

Pedagogical Approaches Based on Neuroscience

Pedagogy is the academic study of the method and practice of teaching and learning. Different pedagogical approaches have been reviewed over time, each with individual benefits for specific scenarios, learning topic and dependent on who is being taught. Increasing interest in neuroscience and pedagogical approaches has led to extensive research into neurological function whilst learning. The ability to use non-invasive neuroimaging in the form of functional Magnetic Resonance Imaging (fMRI), Electroencephalograms (EEG) and Positron Emission tomography (PET) scanning has allowed dynamic live research of how the different genders learn. It is clear that both the neuroanatomy itself and physiological functioning of the brain varies between genders (Magon, 2013). If we are able to understand these ingrained neurological differences, we can delineate how best to adjust teaching style, pedagogy and encourage the best of the students we teach.

Structurally, the brain becomes relatively permanent after 26 weeks gestation, males have larger cerebral volumes and women have more white matter (consisting of the network connections) as opposed to grey matter (contains the cell bodies). Functionally, there are stark differences between the genders. Males tend to demonstrate better natural ability with fine and gross motor whereas female students tend to demonstrate better language skills. This could suggest men engage easier with practical activities whilst women are better at comprehension. Despite a natural lenience for male students to partake practically, research demonstrates that active learning is beneficial for both genders and by increasing elements of true active learning; the gender gap is closed (Laws, Rosborough & Poodry, 1999; Lorenzo, Crouch & Mazur, 2006).

Popular beliefs that men are more 'left brained', associated with being logical and objective, compared to women 'right brained', associated with intuitive and emotional states, can be confusing and backdated; leading to a very black and white stereotype of each gender. Scientifically, both genders use both hemispheres via the corpus callosum; the neurological network that transmits signals between the hemispheres. Interestingly however, the connections do vary between genders. FMRI imaging shows during tasks, women will use a more symmetrical hemispheric pattern, suggesting why women are, arguably, able to multi-task easier. Additionally, there is evidence that despite wanting to avoid stereotyping women, they do score higher on empathy tests, social sensitivity and emotion recognition (Schulte-Rüther, Markowitsch, Shah, Fink & Piefke, 2008).

Girls develop their pre-frontal cortex (used in higher order thinking, rationale and complex thinking) earlier allowing for better concentration at a younger age. Males have large Amygdalas (needed for processing emotions) so in practical terms may be 'stuck in emotions' for longer. In practice if a male student is struggling with a concept and experiences feelings of negativity, it may be more difficult to break this. Similarly, this disparity may lead to male students being more impulsive where women will act slower with a more thorough response and talk themselves out of their emotions. Practically it may seem male students are naturally driven towards more stressful, higher turnover and less emotive specialties.

Furthermore, from the age of 4 girls will tend to show a significantly longer gaze towards adults than boys. Boys will act more on their own accord, with less weight on those watching (Magon, 2013). Within the medical student context, we can see how female students may look towards mentors and role models more than male students, and male students may therefore appear more independent.

So, what does this mean for the classroom and learning styles? If they are so different, should we have single-gender teaching? Although there are benefits to this and practice of this is seen commonly in secondary education, it is generally frowned upon within higher education, particularly in teaching medicine. For physicians, the ability to develop strengths demonstrated of both genders is essential. Thus, integration is embraced to develop skills whilst encouraging neuroplasticity; the brain's ability to create new networks. As medical educators, awareness of these differences will still aid in individual approaches and understanding of behaviours.

With regards to hormones women tend to have higher serotonin levels. Higher serotonin levels are linked to anxiety and insecurities. In practice this means women may be more insecure about their abilities, and thus despite the same credentials as male colleagues, be less willing to volunteer and create opportunities. Unfortunately in medicine, appearing confident increases your patient's confidence in you and also gives you more opportunities within the teams. A male and female surgeon may be the same in competency, but the female may ask for their senior to be in the theatre for reassurance and male equivalent will not. Thus the man will appear more competent through increased confidence alone.

Even so there are day-to-day adjustments that can be made in response to better understanding:

- Increasing active learning within the classroom will help both genders stay attuned and when done effectively can completely reduce the gender gap in learning.
- Women may be less inclined to answer questions in a wider cohort compared to the male students who may be more impulsive with their answers. Using the strengths of both genders in discussion can help all understand a topic better. However, it may explain why women seem shier and are less likely to offer as volunteers or make opportunities.
- Men, who may thrive off more stressful situations, may enjoy learning by testing. Whereas women may find that method of teaching intimidating.
- Women will look to their superiors more than their male peers. Having mentors, positive role models and leaders who women can turn to is crucial in their development, confidence and reassurance.
- Natural functional and structural differences of male and female students may explain why, generally speaking, they might drift towards certain specialty choices. This is discussed in more detail later.

Hidden Curriculum

Higher education institutes are obligated to clearly inform students and teachers alike of the course curriculum as outlined in their higher education documents. These consist of scheduled teaching sessions, rotations, assessments and professional expectations. An aspect of medical school however that is less obvious is the hidden curriculum. The hidden curriculum is that which is not stated outrightly, but through observing cultures, beliefs and behaviours, they are passed onto to the next generation (Hill, Bowman, Stalmeijer & Hart, 2014).

Research at the Association of Medical Education describe different ways in which this 'hidden curriculum' might be presented. Within their research, they discuss how medical students see the entry path into their desired specialty. The cycle involves initially building networks within the chosen specialty through relationships, then acquiring the essential accolades associated. Once these have occurred, the students must learn to fit in and 'walk the talk' in order to be identified as 'one of the club', thereby being invited to participate. Once invited the cycle restarts. It is clear that within surgery, as with this study, the ability to participate, often associated with 'scrubbing in' is a clear distinguishing way to 'partake' and without passing this threshold it is unlikely they will further proceed (Hill et al., 2014). The inability to

Figure 1. Shows an illustration of the cycle
(Hill et al., 2014).

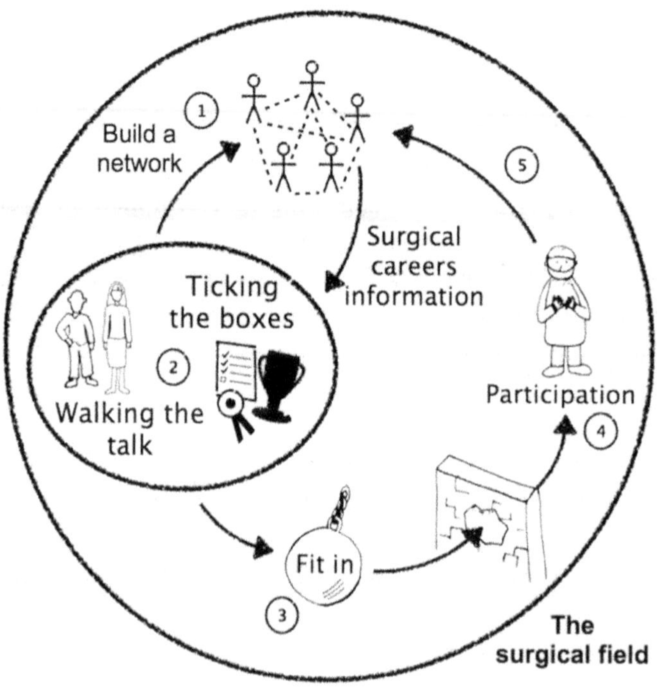

'play the game' and 'fit into the specialty mould' will lead to fewer future opportunities. Unfortunately, this aspect of hidden curriculum is not obviously laid out and thus many students do not recognise this, or very late into their medical student life.

The hidden curriculum can also become evident through formal teaching via the language that is used. This can often be ingrained in culture as demonstrated by Taiwanese medical students. Taiwanese students, pre-Facebook, used an online discussion board and the comments over a 10-year period were analysed for gender-related postings (Cheng & Yang, 2015).

In 2004 Taiwan recognised the presence of male dominated culture and implemented the Gender Equality Act to overcome this. Despite this Act, research showed that students still noted 'benevolent sexism' and 'hostile sexism'. An example of benevolent sexism (to act in a 'caring' manner) was for an educator to consider, 'I won't ask XX female student if they want to do this research project as they must be very busy with their families'. Although this may sound accommodating and forward thinking, it is made on the assumption of how that student feels without even asking and offering the same opportunities. Another example demonstrated was where male Professors did not prompt for more answers when teaching female students if the answer was incorrect, which they would normally do with a male student 'as they did not want to publicly embarrass her'. Again, the paternalistic protection leads to exclusion from gaining knowledge. These assumptions are then witnessed and absorbed by surrounding colleagues and medical students; both self-esteem and learning opportunities are missed.

'Hostile sexism' is perhaps the more widely acknowledged form of sexism stemming from emphasis of the power of patriarchy and actively emphasising negative female values. Hostile sexism may be unwelcomed sexual comments/innuendos, objectification and degrading attitudes. The research in

Taiwan described common jokes about 'taming women'. One description describes one teacher asking for '2 strong men' to help move equipment, a not uncommon phrase to hear. It stereotypes women as the weaker gender, or other examples where the women do more 'caring work'. This not only reinforces gender stereotypes of women but in hidden undertones, suggests men are not allowed to be 'caring' outwardly and if not physically strong are not considered 'men'.

One further issue derived from the research is the difficulty of women to speak up. Even on an online and possibly anonymous platform, it was evidently difficult for women to speak up about the discrimination felt after a nude image of a woman was used as a joke. Her response depicts hesitancy and knowledge that colleagues may dismiss her concerns as merely 'making too much of a fuss over nothing'. This shows the hidden curriculum occurs in both formal and informal settings, both language and acts, but the ability to point them out and challenge them are within itself a challenge. A safe welcome environment in which these are discussed and addressed is essential to moving forwards. Communication is key to understanding how language is used and assumptions are made. The quote from a Professor demonstrates this well: "The aorta is an active one so is located at the left to spine, vena cava is a quiet one so at the right. Why is the liver on the right of the spine? Because it produces the extra blood women need for their monthly periods". Here men are depicted as active, women are passive and should remain quiet as receivers and have periods. Although this may appear harmless anecdotal method of remembering anatomy, the language clearly perpetuates and reinforces gender stereotypes.

Gender Bias in Medicine

Society is increasingly aware that gender does not equate to the sex of an individual. The sex of an individual is dependent on the last chromosome of typically 23 pairs of chromosomes. These chromosomes contain the DeoxyriboNucleic Acid (DNA) and thus the genetics of the human body. The female genotype has XX as the last chromosomes, men have XY as the last chromosome, and genetic variety will occur leading to genetic pathologies. In some cases, babies will be born with ambiguous genitalia and thus raised as either gender; male or female as chosen by the carer.

Although the sex of the individual tends to be more clear cut; XX = female and XY = male, except for circumstances described, gender is a more fluid term in which society recognises is rapidly changing and dynamic. Despite the changes, there is real gender bias in medicine. Gender bias can occur when the assumption is made that men and women are equal, when they are not. Or when assumptions are made that there are differences and there aren't (Risberg, Johansson & Hamberg, 2009).

Sex and Gender Based Medicine (SGBM) is defined as the practice of medicine based on the understanding that biology (dictated by sex chromosomes) and social roles (gender) are important in and have implications for prevention, screening, diagnosis, and treatment in men and women (Jenkins et al., 2016). A survey sent to over 35,000 students across multiple medical schools in USA demonstrate that less than half of respondents had SGBM teaching and 96% agreed understanding improves patient care (Jenkins et al., 2016).

There are fundamental differences in biology and physiology of men and women, not just 'women's health' or 'reproductive health'. Teaching and understanding this will help the profession as a whole and will improve the health of all patients. Clear differences exist in the cardiovascular, respiratory, pharmacology medicine to list but a few examples (Regitz-Zagrosek, 2012).

Cardiovascular diseases are the main cause of death for men and women in western industrial nations. (Totals might not be 100 owing to rounding up or down of data. (Office of National Statistics Berlin" 2005)

Figure 2. Shows percentage breakdown of causes of death for men and women in Germany

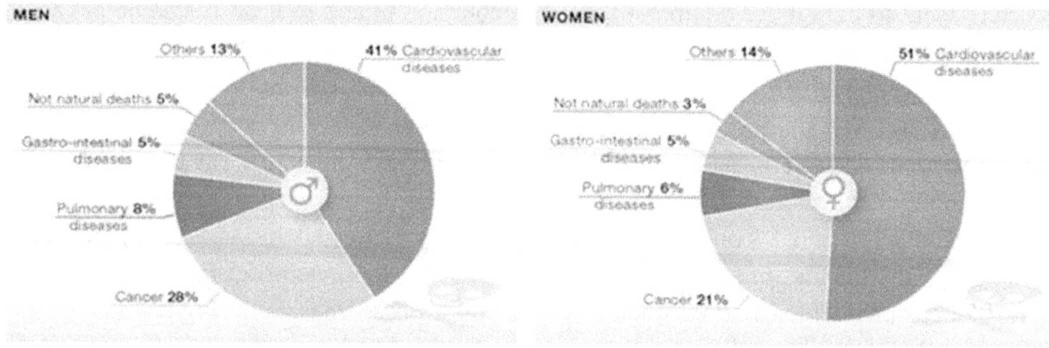

Furthermore, varying health outcomes exist for different genders with the same condition. Women are less likely to be offered the same treatment as men, and men are more likely to receive more advantaged diagnostic and therapeutic interventions (Hamberg, 2008). Specific examples include women obtaining dialysis later than men, undergo fewer kidney transplants (Jindal, Ryan, Sajjad, Murthy & Baines, 2005; Kausz et al., 2000) and women will receive less guidance-based diagnosis and less-invasive treatment than men (Regitz-Zagrosek, 2006). Comparatively, osteoporosis and depression are generally considered female diseases and can be under-diagnosed in men (Kautzky-Willer A, 2012).

If medical students and professionals are less aware of gender and sex problems within our own institutions, they are also at risk of implementing gender bias in their practice of medicine. Evidence demonstrates curriculum inclusion would increase awareness and rippling would improve patient outcomes (Hamberg, K, 2008).

Medical Student Experience: On Placement

As explained, medical students will have multiple years of clinical placements. During these years the students rotate through different specialties; interact and learn to assess patients and continue to absorb more of the hidden curriculum. Placement life is very different to pre-clinical work and it can be a shock to the system. These changes to 'real–world' medicine highlight new gender inequalities and here we aim to tackle them.

Harassment During Clinical Placements

Gender discrimination unfortunately occurs during clinical rotations. It is considered to be the conveying of hostile or degrading attitudes. In some workplaces this may include bribery or threats in exchange for sexual cooperation, though fortunately there is no evidence that this occurs for medical students. Gender harassment can take the form of unwanted sexual attention in both verbal and non-verbal forms (O'Hare, E., O'Donohue, W, 1998)

There is clear evidence that gender discrimination is very real for medical students. Large percentages of men (83.2%) and women (92.8%) experienced, observed, or heard about at least one incident of gender discrimination and sexual harassment during medical school. Compared with men, significantly (p </= 0.01) more women report exposure to gender discrimination and sexual harassment (Stratton,

McLaughlin, Witte, Fosson & Nora, 2005). Clinically this may represent a female medical student or doctor placing a male urinary catheter and receiving inappropriate sexual comments, or patients commenting they enjoy being touched by the student whilst performing an examination.

Research shows that women who identify as more feminine on the Bem Sex-role inventory (Bem, 1974) are more likely to be victims of harassment. These consist of what society called 'feminine traits' and includes examples such as understanding, flatterable and gentle. Male traits are considered as 'independent, leadership ability, makes decisions easily, defends own beliefs' (O'Hare, E., O'Donohue, W, 1998). Although societal constructs of gender are changing, there is still much rooted generalisation of what it means to be feminine or masculine. Interesting, this research was conducted on self-completed questionnaires, implying women will identify with these stereotypical traits. Perhaps this demonstrates unconscious bias of gender resulting in women discriminating against their own sex.

Despite women experiencing more discrimination and sexual harassment, correlations between exposure to gender discrimination and self-assessed impact on career decisions tended to be larger for men. This suggests that although fewer men are generally affected, they may weigh such experiences more heavily on their choice of specialty and residency program (Stratton, McLaughlin, Witte, Fosson & Nora, 2005)

Treatment From Patients and Families

As medical professionals our job is to provide the best 'patient centred care' possible. However, it is not uncommon for patients and/or their families to not treat the healthcare workforce as non-discriminately. Usually misunderstanding comes from ignorance and not malice. These tend to stem from their own exposure which, unless they have family members in healthcare or have healthcare exposure, comes from media.

For medical students, this commonly presents as female medical students being assumed to be nurses or other healthcare professionals despite not wearing the equivalent uniform or having already introduced themselves as the doctor. In fact 75% of female doctors have been called a nurse or non-clinical title in their careers (Sara, 2017).

To make matters more complicated, research demonstrates females will be less likely to self-advocate. Female colleagues should feel able to speak up in a non-confrontational manner and male colleagues should advocate on their behalf. It is not uncommon for a female doctor to approach a patient with a male medical student and for the patient to immediately assume the male medical student is the senior clinician (Rabinowitz, 2018). Unfortunately, conformity and non-disruptive behaviour is key to professional advancement, whistleblowing is still frowned upon in practice, so perhaps in reality it appears simpler to simply 'not make an unnecessary fuss'. There needs to be institutional widespread changes in ethos and values for this to change.

Although anecdotal evidence is not solid, discussions between female medical students and doctors show that these are common problems faced by them. Further research should be undertaken to formalise these anecdotal comments and experiences. For example, female doctors may be called 'a good female doctor' or a 'good female surgeon', but the desire is to simply hear 'good doctor' or 'good surgeon' irrespective of gender.

As introduced, media continues to play a huge role in what the medical profession looks like. It would be reassuring to know that the community has moved from the traditional opinion that Sir Lancelot Spratt, a TV character of a demanding white male surgeon, has changed. Unfortunately, this image has been difficult to dispel as demonstrated by a scenario the British Broadcasting Corporation asked the British population (*Do you have a gender-bias?*, 2017)

A father and son are in a car crash. The father dies at the scene and the boy is taken to hospital and needs an operation. The surgeon says "I cannot operate on this boy. He is my son." Who is the surgeon?

The British population suggested the son was adopted so it might be his biological son, or the father's ghost or even the mother had an affair with the surgeon. Few came to the conclusion the surgeon was the mother. Though simplified and crudely put, this possibly demonstrates people believe a father's ghost is a more likely option than a surgeon being female.

Although it may seem insignificant that someone is called an incorrect title, the effects of this are larger than understood as these misunderstandings are laced with other unconscious connotations. For example, one may also have their competency, knowledge or ability to lead a team questioned. One social media article in the public sector described an event where a male and female colleague swapped names when corresponding in emails. The result and discussion of which demonstrated that by simply having a female name, their competency is more likely to questioned and respect was not assumed. This can in itself take time so female students can often take longer to complete tasks simply because more effort and time is needed in first gaining respect and trust. Although it highlighted what women already know to be true, it also highlighted that it often takes a man to explain for people to listen in the first place (Natalie, 2017). All these factors play a large role in gender inequality and thus the medical school experience.

Treatment From Healthcare Professionals

It would be reassuring to say that gender inequality stops at the workplace door, limiting it to be an act from the public through ignorance. Unfortunately, evidence shows this is not true and gender inequality is also a result from other healthcare professionals. Up to 88% of those in medical school or residency training and 91% within practice in the USA reported gender discrimination, inappropriate comments or lack of respect from within the medical team (Bruce, Battista, Plankey, Johnson & Marshall, 2015).

In some cases, evidence demonstrates that in an environment which is one-sided-gender heavy, individuals may receive more harassment as the minority is singled out. For example, a female medical student on a surgical rotation. On the other hand, contrary evidence demonstrates gender discrimination is more common in environments of more equal percentages due to the increased chances of gender interactions. This could be the case for Internal Medicine.

Anecdotally, and for unknown reasons, male doctors tend to be treated with more respect and overall better by female nurses. These comments come from both male and female colleagues and medical students. Furthermore, comments from both genders describe how female medical students can often be degraded more by female consultants than male consultants. It would be suggested that evidence-based academia is conducted to confirm or reject these feelings from common but anecdotal comments. Unfortunately, it is known that increased abuse does affect performance, it increases stress and eventually cycles. Evidence shows how this can further lead to negative views from their supervisors (Walton, 2015).

The role of clinical placements is for the student to gain as much experience, both consolidating their knowledge into the clinical workplace and experience in potentially specialty-specific practical procedures. A university in America used portfolios to review whether there was gender equality on placements. It demonstrated that male medical students had fewer opportunities to perform gynaecological exams (Isaac, Chertoff, Lee & Carnes, 2011). Although this might be expected as female patients may be less likely to consent, the striking finding was that often the doctors responsible for that medical student did not even ask the patient. It is the responsibility of the medical educators on placement to be aware of their assumptions, not assume a patient may or may not consent, and not withhold learning opportunities. This paper highlights how the use of portfolios can monitor not only competencies but potential gender inequalities.

Furthermore, the American university reviewed the letters written by Deans for medical students, analysing the language used in the letters and noticed a stark difference. Language used for men and women show an underlying and persuasive discrimination. Men were "excellers (sic) and eager beavers" whilst women were "enthusiastic worker bees", men tended to "take initiative" whilst women "were enthusiastic". Fortunately, these differences did not affect the ranking or choice of residency but the undertone that women are more passive exists. Unconscious bias continues to be evident in all aspects of medical student life, often from the very people paid to train and develop them. It raises the wider question of whether all senior clinicians are suitable to be clinical supervisors or whether supervision should be an accredited role, given time, dedication and appropriate selection (Isaac, Chertoff, Lee & Carnes, 2011).

Medical Students Within the Minority: Culture, Belief, Race

Healthcare is an environment which should have no barriers, from gender to race, from culture to religion, it should always be accessible. Similarly, many countries have increasing diversity in their healthcare workforce alongside the increasing diversity in the population that they treat.

The General Medical Council (GMC), the governing body of UK medical professionals, 2018 report shows a 50% rise in international medical graduate applications following the removal of Visa Tier 2, 'skilled worker' requirements . There has also been an increase of 22% black and minority ethnics, and a 132% increase in those affiliating as Muslim ("The state of medical education and practice in the UK", 2018). With this changing population, there are new challenges in ensuring all are able to excel to their best abilities. We will briefly mention new challenges that may not have been previously prevalent that need more attention and a unified action plan.

The commonest problem faced by Muslim female medical students, whose beliefs say they should cover their forearms, is the 'bare below the elbow' policy in place as an infection control measure. Although the Department of Health has produced clear equality and diversity guidelines on the issue, individual trusts still have varying guidance on what this means in practice. Many women will be expected to either abide by rolling up their sleeves in the event of patient contact, going against their beliefs, or be expected to pay for and wear disposable arm covers. Similarly, Sikh students may remove their Kara, a religious bracelet, in the event of patient contact or wear it elsewhere on their body. Guidance is sparse between trusts and often independent societies are created in the absence of clear guidelines, for example the British Islamic Medical Association ("Hijabs & Bare Below the Elbows Toolkits", 2017).

Similarly, those who abide by wearing a Hijab, an Islamic head covering the head and neck, have no national guidance regarding what they should do in operating theatres, leaving it to individual trust policies which are often limited in information and practical solutions. Despite there being research that shows headgear has no effect on theatre bacterial count (Humphreys, Russell, Marshall, Ricketts & Reeves, 1991), uncertainties can lead to other theatre staff reporting patient safety concerns, meaning the medical student feels unwelcomed and is uncertain as to how to proceed. For example, in 2016 one NHS Anaesthetic consultant was suspended for confronting a Muslim surgeon who refused to remove her Hijab. He was later reinstated after understanding he was trying to follow health and safety protocols ("'The hijab has no place in NHS hospitals', argues Muslim writer", 2016). It is clear how these uncertainties can lead to students missing valuable learning opportunities or leading to exclusion of that as a specialty, as further expressed by several surgical trainees at a Women in Surgery conference. In some trusts it is acceptable to change into a fresh Hijab before operating and wear the Orthopaedic scrub hats that also cover the neck. This is what Sikh men who wear Dastaars will typically do.

Across the globe, depending on a country's own religious and cultural beliefs, there are varying guidelines. The president of Cairo University in Egypt recently banned the wearing of Niqab, face covering wear, for all healthcare staff including medical students as he believed patients have the right to know who is treating them and also to aid in effective communication ("'The hijab has no place in NHS hospitals', argues Muslim writer", 2016).

What we can see here is the need to be sensitive to diversity and individual beliefs, but also a clear demonstration that local guidelines are insufficient. There is a need for unified standards across the nation consistent with the country's beliefs. This will reduce misunderstanding between team members, uncertainties of medical students on their placements, their exposure to certain specialties and their interaction with patients who may also have bias.

The Consequences of Gender Inequality Within Medical School

From the chapter so far, it is hoped that it is clear gender inequality does exist in all aspects of medical school and affect both genders.

Highlighting the experiences and having suggested some combat methods for those specific problems is important. However, we would like to further proceed by demonstrating some wider problems that gender inequality within medical school can contribute to. Consequences include the impact on the medical students' future specialty choice, healthcare attrition and burnout, to name a few.

Specialty Choices

Gender inequality obviously affects the individual being discriminated against and this will become clear regarding specialty choice for them. However, it is extremely important to also recognise the impact this will have on that specialty as a whole and thus reduced diversity of the medical profession altogether.

According to the American Medical Association (AMA), women will make up larger percentages of the workforce in family medicine (58%), Paediatrics (75%) and O&G (85%). The data shows male residents prefer to specialize in surgery (59%), Emergency (62%) and Radiology (73%) (Lyndra, 2015). These figures seem consistent throughout the globe with some sub-specialities showing even further disparities ("Statistics — Royal College of Surgeons", 2018). There are many reasons for these, and gender inequality is one influencing factor.

Having discussed medical school exposure, we know that although different genders should be timetabled similar exposure to each specialty, their experiences are very different. Research demonstrates that one key contributor to future specialty choice is what their early exposure to a specialty is like. Earlier exposure to both a specialty and opportunity for research is a key motivator and when coupled with mentorship a student is 13 x more likely to prefer that specialty than others (Berger, Giacalone, Barlow, Kapadia & Keith, 2017). Furthermore, simply earlier exposure to basic surgical skills, will increase the likelihood of someone considering that career. This could be as little as a one-day course (Leung, LY., 2018)

Figure 3. Shows percentage of consultants who are female within the following specialties ("Statistics — Royal College of Surgeons", 2018)

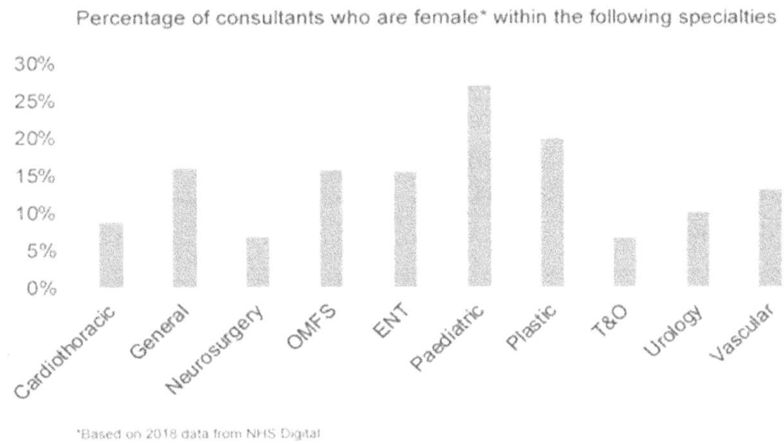

Mentorship and role models are both important but are different. Mentorship is taking an individual under your wing to develop and guide, often when one is appointed a specific tutor. However, role models can be anyone and everyone irrespective of their seniority or frequency of contact (Healy, Cantillon, Malone & Kerin, 2012). The British Medical Journal describes how students may find it difficult to become 'something you cannot see'. In this way it can be difficult for men to imagine being Obstetrics and Gynaecology consultants or female students believing they can become Trauma and Orthopaedic surgeons as they do not see seniors they can aspire to become. Anecdotal and literature evidence show female students hold a lack of confidence and seriously consider what a 'good career' for a woman will be (Reynold, E., 2018: Martin & Barnard, 2013). Female medical students report a strong desire for mentors to be female as to understand and discuss gender specific issues in search for advice (Risberg, Johansson, Westman & Hamberg, 2003). Although there may be preferences, evidence shows that an effective role model does not have to be the same gender as who they are modelling to (Piccinato, Rodrigues, Rocha & Troncon, 2017). Again, we ask for all medical educators, whether will be a one-off situation role model, or well-known mentor to advocate and be role models for all genders.

Equally, representation of genders on committees and leadership roles is important for the younger generation to see. There have been initiatives to propagate enthusiasm for gender equality for example the Athena SWAN charter to encourage and recognise women in science. Unfortunately, formal national societies fall short of true representation with women only accounting for 8% of presidents and 19% of executive surgical committees in surgical societies within the UK, despite accounting for 27% of the surgical workforce (Skinner H, 2018). It is important to emphasise the aim is not to simply have a 50: 50 ratio of men: women across societies, but that people should be awarded positions based on merit alone. However, it is difficult to believe that women fall so short on this as no evidence exists to demonstrate women are less competent at their roles.

A Canadian study surveyed medical students in attempt to understand their rationale for specialty choices and split them into major, intermediate and minor factors. Major factors included their undergraduate experience (including their curriculum layout and time dedicated to each specialty, as well as emphasis of that specialty within their exams) (Pianosi K, Bethune C, Hurley K, 2016). They also described their personal exposure to the specialty on rotation, public perceptions and recruitment. Influences including teacher influences and partner factors were considered major. As both men and women report wanting to take time out in training for children, considering this in their training and future plans has an influencing factor ("More residents building families during training", 2016). Research within the Netherlands shows that the most important factor for their specialty choice was in fact lifestyle factors, with the biggest determinant being gender (Heiligers, 2012). With certain specialties being well known for longer working hours, for example acute hospital training or surgery, it is no wonder that 67% of female foundation doctors in 2015 did not think surgery was a suitable career for women ("sexism-in-surgery-females-being-put-off-becoming-surgeons-by-men", 2016).

Unfortunately, these negative experiences are echoed by qualitative findings of trainees who have been unable to take flexible training and do experience discrimination at a number of levels (Meghen K, Sweeney C, Linehan C, O'Flynn S, Boylan G, 2013). When students see this, they are less inclined to follow suit. These experiences can come in positive remarks, e.g. female General Practitioners advising that it is a good work-life balance. Or can take place in negative feedback for example a female surgeon explaining they are not confident in operating after taking 6 months maternity leave (S. Williams, 2018). Despite both genders desiring parental leave, commonly men will take on average 1 week of paternity leave whilst women will take 6-8 weeks ("More residents building families during training", 2016). This has obvious different consequences for the trainees and medical students recognise this early on in their studies.

With the gender construct paradigm shifting, research based on typical 'female or male personalities' becomes less founded. However, there has been much evidence that does demonstrate certain personalities match certain specialties, and some personalities still follow the more traditional male or female stereotypes. For example, according to a study using Myers Briggs personality typing, women are more introverted and feeling-based which lends well to family medicine. In contrast men are extraverted and will lend to Emergency departments (Stilwell, N 2000).

Overall, there are many reasons for specialty choice but in all those elements above, students may face gender inequality and thus do not have true equal access and support to enter a given one. Medical school may be the sole exposure to a specialty, particularly in progression structures similar to that of the USA where specialty choice happens straight after medical school. Medical students will continue to change their choices throughout medical school (Compton M, Frank E, Elon L, Carrera J, 2008) and will continue to change even during postgraduate training (Goldacre, Laxton, & Lambert, 2010). However, some specialties have higher percentage follow through and attrition. For example, the commonest specialty for students to choose and then remain in after 10 years is surgery. Whereas 50% of hospital medics will change to GP within 10 years of foundation training. It is therefore important that medical educators and role models exist for medical students and trainees at all stages alike. There is clear need to evaluate why this change exists and to allow flexibility within the system (Goldacre, Laxton, & Lambert, 2010).

Attrition Rates

As briefly mentioned before, and in more detail within other chapters, attrition is a huge problem within the medical profession. This describes how large percentages will leave the workforce or not progress the 'ladder' the same. The consequences are huge, not just in representation for medical students but for the wider workforce and lack of progression for unclear reasons. The Association of American Medical Colleges shoes that despite half of medical students being female, only 20% of Professors and 16% of Deans are Professors ("Overcoming gender obstacles in medicine", 2016).

Figure 4. Shows the attrition throughout surgical training
(Moberly, 2018).

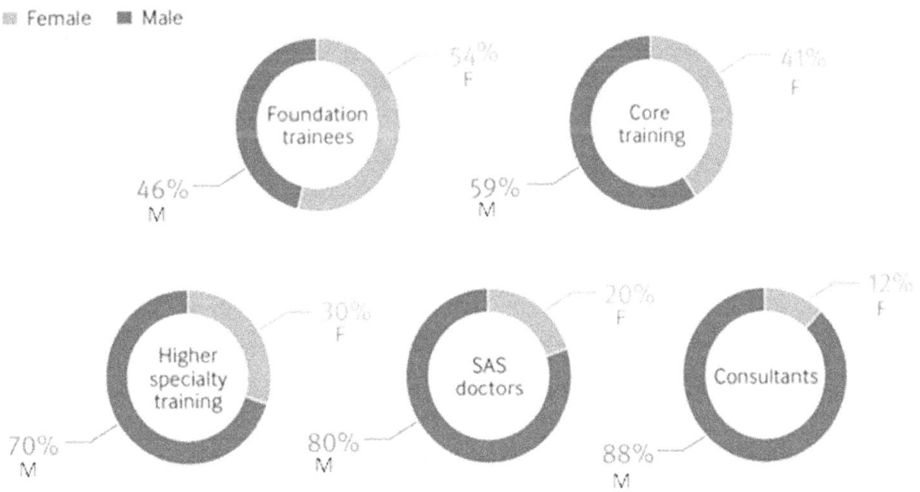
Female
Male
Foundation trainees
54%
F
46%
M
Core training
41%
F
59%
M
Higher specialty training
30%
F
70%
M
SAS doctors
20%
F
80%
M
Consultants
12%
F
88%
M

The gender gap has improved over time; in 1993 only 3% of surgical consultants were female whereas now 12% are but there are stark differences in subspecialty choices; only 6% of Trauma and Orthopaedic doctors are female compared to 27% of paediatric surgeons ("Statistics — Royal College of Surgeons", 2018).

Burnout

Medical school is a very stressful time, full of new and very advanced experiences. At medical school building resilience is key. Unfortunately, external factors can greatly impact individuals in different ways and lead to dire consequences. The Office of National Statistics in the UK report that 430 healthcare professionals took their own life between 2011 and 2015, with only one UK confidential service for doctors. To rub salt in the wound; only those working in London can self-refer leaving everyone else at loss ("Suicides in the UK Statistical bulletins - Office for National Statistics", 2017). It is well known that sadly suicides are not limited to graduates but also medical students.

Burnout of the workforce is a national disaster and the GMC have recognised this. 70% of doctors report working more hours every week than rostered, 25% are asked to act up to a senior position each week, 50% are asked to act down to fill gaps. In response, 25% have taken reduced hours to cope with the pressures which lead to increase rota gaps and thus more pressure. Alongside an increased workload, 60% feel reduced work satisfaction, 25% witness reduced patient care at least once a week and 50% recorded a decrease in satisfaction of their work-life-balance. Despite raising concerns, 25% of trainees believe their concerns won't be appropriately dealt with, 30% feel unsupported by both managers and senior clinicians each week and a 30% reduction in mentoring has been provided. All this leads to not just a reduced workforce as people retire early, leave the country or work reduced hours, but increased mental health problems ("The state of medical education and practice in the UK", 2018; Arrizabalaga, P., 2014). Alongside both national and trust-wide governmental and political problems, recent events regarding the medical manslaughter case involving Dr Bawa-Garba has sent shockwaves through the profession across the globe. It has driven increased anxiety and concerns of those in the workforce as patients are increasingly encouraged to make complaints ("The state of medical education and practice in the UK", 201; *Factsheet Dr Bawa-Garba*, 2018). In America, only half of USA physicians report they would study medicine again, down from 70% the previous year (Susan, 2012)

All these factors together lead to higher burnout with 48% of women and 38% of male peers reporting burnout. These figures are extremely concerning; not just through the mere statistics but in knowing that there are usually underreported statistics. In the national American survey in 2018 reported that their work is the highest contributor (Sara, 2018).

The NHS Practitioner Health Programme report that female practitioners have four times higher risk of suicide than the average population ("Practitioner Health Programme", 2017). Women are more likely to ask for help than men, who will try to reduce stress by engaging in physical activity (Sara, B. 2018). In the average population, men have a higher suicide risk as they are less likely to ask for help in part due to toxic masculinity, described as the suppression of emotions to cope with harsh conditions. Here gender inequality is clear and men are disadvantaged. Medical school and educators need to dismantle the beliefs that asking for help, particularly of men who will be more resistant to it, is weak. As proof of this need, the Hippocratic Oath first written in 1949 was changed in 2017 to include an element of the importance of self-care, and is now recited by all medical students who graduate from medical school ("NZ doctor's Hippocratic Oath change passed", 2017).

CONCLUSION

Gender inequality is clear throughout the medical profession and this chapter has sought to describe the perspectives of medical students, highlighting areas of particular concern with the aim of strategically tackling them. We have seen how the impact of gender equality is huge for both the individual themselves and also the wider healthcare workforce and widespread across the globe.

Within all aspects of medical school life, there are ways in which we can address and shift the gender equality paradigm. For medical students in the classroom, medical educators need to become aware of and reveal the hidden curriculum to students, ensure exposure to all specialties for all students and work towards ensuring their exposure is equivalent for both genders. To dispel the myth that women's health is simply reproductive health, SGBM needs to be taught and thus patient care will be improved in the future. Medical educators should be an accredited role where they receive teaching about the differences of learning styles by male and female students, how this impacts pedagogy and their engagement with course structure. Perhaps, in certain higher education institutes, the course structure itself should be reviewed to incorporate more active learning which reduces gender-gap. Of top-most importance, is ensuring leaders who have the power to change all this also want to and know how to. Swedish research demonstrates that male leaders agree that gender inequality in medical school is an important topic but they are either reluctant due to other priorities or at lost as to how (Risberg et al., 2011).

Once on placement, gender inequality can become evidence through day-to-day experiences from the way patients or families treat them, other health-care professionals treat them or again through witnessed hidden curriculum. Using portfolios and reviewing assessments, we can see where the gender gaps are, and by accrediting medical student educators we can try to reduce unconscious bias and assumptions that lead to reduced student exposure and opportunities. With an increasingly diverse medical student population we must learn to address their beliefs in a sensitive and practical way. The way forward is for national consistent guidance instead of local non-distributed information that can lead to misunderstanding and compromise of patient care.

To further reduce the gender gap, we should continue to collect data and share experiences, as we are with this book, transforming anecdotal experiences into a more academic evidence-based approach. By encouraging everyone, irrespective of gender, to firstly recognise that they are role models and then embracing the role can help further encourage medical students. Mentoring schemes should be accessible to all and not just to those who seem to 'fit in', and tackling the causes for poor attrition and poor representation can show younger trainees they too can become what they see, or encouraged to become that person who is the change.

Throughout the last few years, social media has become an essential tool to distributing experiences to both healthcare professionals but also the public. Twitter hastags including #Ilooklikeasurgeon challenge the concept that only men can become a surgeon, (Logghe, Jones, McCoubrey & Fitzgerald, 2017), Facebook groups can now widely disseminate events to wider audiences and videoing live conferences mean that those with family commitments do not have to choose between attending or leaving their child at home.

It is true that the medical profession has come a long way in in terms of gender equality, however the journey continues. Gender inequality is present for both women and men in different but profound ways. These have a ripple effect on both the individual but also the wider healthcare population. It is the responsibility of all those within the healthcare profession, particularly education providers, to firstly accept these events and then set the precedent for change. If we as educators do not do so, the next

Figure 5. #the NewYorker frontpage for #Ilooklikeasurgeon
(Mouly et al., 2017)

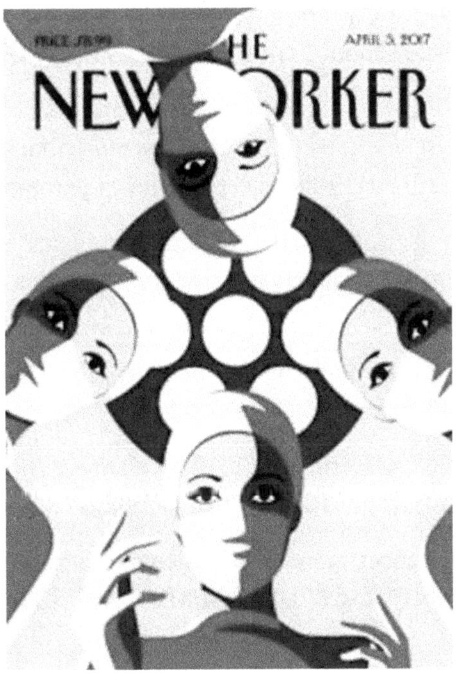

generation of doctors will continue to follow in our footsteps and the cycle will continue. Let us work together to reduce the gender gap, increase diversity and improve the health of our own workforce but also the patients we aim to treat.

REFRENCES

Arrizabalaga, P., Abellana, R., Viñas, O., Merino, A., & Ascaso, C. (2014). Gender inequalities in the medical profession: Are there still barriers to women physicians in the 21st century? *Gaceta Sanitaria, 28*(5), 351–438. doi:10.1016/j.gaceta.2014.03.014 PMID:24889702

Bagheritari, M. & David, M. (2013). Legislation and Policy – GEA – Gender and Education Association. Retrieved from http://www.genderandeducation.com/resources-2/legislative-frameworks/

Berger, A., Giacalone, J., Barlow, P., Kapadia, M., & Keith, J. (2017). Choosing surgery as a career: Early results of a longitudinal study of medical students. *Surgery, 161*(6), 1683–1689. doi:10.1016/j.surg.2016.12.016 PMID:28161006

British Broadcasting Corporation. (2017). *Do you have a gender-bias?* [Video]. Retrieved from https://www.youtube.com/watch?v=J69HkKz9g4A

Bruce, A., Battista, A., Plankey, M., Johnson, L., & Marshall, M. (2015). Perceptions of gender-based discrimination during surgical training and practice. *Medical Education Online, 20*(1), 25923. doi:10.3402/meo.v20.25923 PMID:25652117

Cheng, L., & Yang, H. (2015). Learning about gender on campus: An analysis of the hidden curriculum for medical students. *Medical Education, 49*(3), 321–331. doi:10.1111/medu.12628 PMID:25693991

Compton, M., Frank, E., Elon, L., & Carrera, J. (2008). Changes in U. S. Medical Students' Specialty Interests Over the Course of Medical School. *J Gen Intern Med Jul; 23*(7), 1095–1100. doi:10.100711606-008-0579-z

General Medical Council. (2018). *Factsheet Dr Bawa-Garba* [Ebook]. Retrieved from https://www.gmc-uk.org/-/media/documents/20180419-factsheet---dr-bawa-garba-case-final_pdf-74385491.pdf

Goldacre, M., Laxton, L., & Lambert, T. (2010). Medical graduates' early career choices of specialty and their eventual specialty destinations: UK prospective cohort studies. *BMJ, 341*(jul06 1). doi:10.1136/bmj.c3199

Hamberg, K. (2008). Gender Bias in Medicine. *Women's Health (London, England), 4*(3), 237–243. doi:10.2217/17455057.4.3.237 PMID:19072473

Healy, N., Cantillon, P., Malone, C., & Kerin, M. (2012). Role models and mentors in surgery. *American Journal of Surgery, 204*(2), 256–261. doi:10.1016/j.amjsurg.2011.09.031 PMID:22621833

Heiligers, P. (2012). Gender differences in medical students' motives and career choice. *BMC Medical Education, 12*(1), 82. doi:10.1186/1472-6920-12-82 PMID:22913471

Hijabs & Bare Below the Elbows Toolkits. (2017). [Society Guidance] Retrieved from http://www.britishima.org/hbbe-toolkits/

Hill, E., Bowman, K., Stalmeijer, R., & Hart, J. (2014). You've got to know the rules to play the game: How medical students negotiate the hidden curriculum of surgical careers. *Medical Education*, *48*(9), 884–894. doi:10.1111/medu.12488 PMID:25113115

Humphreys, H., Russell, A., Marshall, R., Ricketts, V., & Reeves, D. (1991). The effect of surgical theatre head-gear on air bacterial counts. *The Journal of Hospital Infection*, *19*(3), 175–180. doi:10.1016/0195-6701(91)90221-S PMID:1685505

Isaac, C., Chertoff, J., Lee, B., & Carnes, M. (2011). Do Students' and Authors' Genders Affect Evaluations? A Linguistic Analysis of Medical Student Performance Evaluations. *Academic Medicine*, *86*(1), 59–66. doi:10.1097/ACM.0b013e318200561d PMID:21099389

Jenkins, M., Herrmann, A., Tashjian, A., Ramineni, T., Ramakrishnan, R., Raef, D., ... Shatzer, J. (2016). Sex and gender in medical education: A national student survey. *Biology of Sex Differences*, *7*(S1), 45. doi:10.118613293-016-0094-6 PMID:27785347

Jindal, R., Ryan, J., Sajjad, I., Murthy, M., & Baines, L. (2005). Kidney Transplantation and Gender Disparity. *American Journal of Nephrology*, *25*(5), 474–483. doi:10.1159/000087920 PMID:16127268

Kausz, A. T., Obrador, G. T., Arora, P., Ruthazer, R., Levey, A. S., & Pereira, B. J. (2000). Late initiation of dialysis among women and ethnic minorities in the United States. *Journal of the American Society of Nephrology*, *11*, 2351–2357. PMID:11095658

Kautzky-Willer, A. (2012). Sex and gender differences in endocrinology. In S. Oertelt-Prigione & V. Regitz-Zagrosek (Eds.), *Sex and Gender Aspects in Clinical Medicine* (pp. 125–149). London, UK: Springer. doi:10.1007/978-0-85729-832-4_9

Laws, P., Rosborough, P., & Poodry, F. (1999). Women's responses to an activity-based introductory physics program. *American Journal of Physics*, *67*(S1), S32–S37. doi:10.1119/1.19077

Legewie, J., & DiPrete, T. (2014). The High School Environment and the Gender Gap in Science and Engineering. *Sociology of Education*, *87*(4), 259–280. doi:10.1177/0038040714547770 PMID:27857451

Leung, L. Y. (2018). Encouraging female undergraduate student to consider a surgical career [Abstract]. *Association of Surgeons of Great Britain and Ireland, 53*(Winter), 88-89. Retrieved from http://asgbi.org/Journals/Winter%202018%20JASGBI.pdf

Logghe, H., Jones, C., McCoubrey, A., & Fitzgerald, E. (2017). #ILookLikeASurgeon: Embracing diversity to improve patient outcomes. *BMJ (Clinical Research Ed.)*, *j4653*. doi:10.1136/bmj.j4653 PMID:29018031

Lorenzo, M., Crouch, C., & Mazur, E. (2006). Reducing the gender gap in the physics classroom. *American Journal of Physics*, *74*(2), 118–122. doi:10.1119/1.2162549

Lyndra, V. (2015). How medical specialties vary by gender. Retrieved from https://www.ama-assn.org/residents-students/specialty-profiles/how-medical-specialties-vary-gender

Magon, A. (2013). Gender, the brain and education: do boys and girls learn differently? [University Library] Retrieved from https://dspace.library.uvic.ca/handle/1828/1411

Martin, P., & Barnard, A. (2013). The experience of women in male-dominated occupations: A constructivist grounded theory inquiry. *SA Journal of Industrial Psychology*, *39*(2). doi:10.4102ajip.v39i2.1099

McCurry, J. (2018). Tokyo medical school admits changing results to exclude women. Retrieved from https://www.theguardian.com/world/2018/aug/08/tokyo-medical-school-admits-changing-results-to-exclude-women

Meghen, K., Sweeney, C., Linehan, C., O'Flynn, S., & Boylan, G. (2013) Women in hospital medicine: facts, figures and personal experiences. [Abstract] *Ir Med J. Feb;106*(2):39-42.

Moberly, T. (2018). A fifth of surgeons in England are female. *BMJ (Clinical Research Ed.), k4530.* doi:10.1136/bmj.k4530 PMID:30377150

More residents building families during training. (2016). [Medical Society Research] Retrieved from https://www.ama-assn.org/residents-students/resident-student-health/more-residents-building-families-during-training

Mouly, F., Bormes, G., Wiley, C., Roupenian, K., Berry, P., Cassidy, J., ... (2017). The New Yorker Cover That's Being Replicated by Women Surgeons Across the World. Retrieved from https://www.newyorker.com/culture/culture-desk/the-new-yorker-cover-thats-being-replicated-by-women-surgeons-across-the-world

Natalie, G. (2017). What Happened When A Man And Woman Swapped Names At Work. Retrieved from https://www.refinery29.com/en-gb/2017/03/144692/man-woman-swap-names-workplace-sexism

NZ doctor's Hippocratic Oath change passed. (2017). Retrieved from https://www.radionz.co.nz/news/world/341592/nz-doctor-s-hippocratic-oath-change-passed

O'Hare, E. & O'Donohue, W. (1998). Sexual Harassment: Identifying risk factors. *Archives of Sexual Behaviour; New York, 27*(6), 561 – 80.

Office of National Statistics Berlin. (2005). [National Statistics] Retrieved from http://www.rki.de/EN/Content/Health_Monitoring/Health_Reporting/GBEDownloadsT/mittleres_lebensalter.pdf?__blob=publicationFile

Overcoming gender obstacles in medicine. (2016). [Medical Society Advice] Retrieved from https://www.ama-assn.org/practice-management/physician-diversity/overcoming-gender-obstacles-medicine

Pianosi, K., Bethune, C., & Hurley, K. (2016). Medical student career choice: A qualitative study of fourth-year medical students at Memorial University, Newfoundland. *CMAJ Open*, *4*(2), E147–E152. doi:10.9778/cmajo.20150103 PMID:27398357

Piccinato, C., Rodrigues, M., Rocha, L., & Troncon, L. (2017). Characteristics of role models who influenced medical residents to choose surgery as a specialty: Exploratory study. *Sao Paulo Medical Journal*, *135*(6), 529–534. doi:10.1590/1516-3180.2017.0053030517 PMID:29116309

Practitioner Health Programme. (2017). Retrieved from https://php.nhs.uk/

Rabinowitz, L. (2018). Recognizing Blind Spots— A Remedy for Gender Bias in Medicine? *The New England Journal of Medicine*, *378*(24), 2253–2255. doi:10.1056/NEJMp1802228 PMID:29897846

Regitz-Zagrosek, V. (2006). Therapeutic implications of the gender-specific aspects of cardiovascular disease. *Nature Reviews. Drug Discovery*, *5*(5), 425–439. doi:10.1038/nrd2032 PMID:16672926

Regitz-Zagrosek, V. (2012). Sex and gender differences in health. *EMBO Reports*, *13*(7), 596–603. doi:10.1038/embor.2012.87 PMID:22699937

Regitz-Zagrosek, V., Oertelt-Prigione, S., Seeland, U., & Hetzer, R. (2010). Sex and Gender Differences in Myocardial Hypertrophy and Heart Failure. *Circulation Journal*, *74*(7), 1265–1273. doi:10.1253/circj.CJ-10-0196 PMID:20558892

Reynold, E. (2018). Why I want to be a colorectal surgeon: the importance of role models in influencing women to pursue surgery [Abstract]. *Association of Surgeons of Great Britain and Ireland, 53*(Winter): 90-91. Retrieved from http://asgbi.org/Journals/Winter%202018%20JASGBI.pdf

Risberg, G., Johansson, E., & Hamberg, K. (2009). A theoretical model for analysing gender bias in medicine. *International Journal for Equity in Health*, *8*(1), 28. doi:10.1186/1475-9276-8-28 PMID:19646289

Risberg, G., Johansson, E., Westman, G., & Hamberg, K. (2003). Gender in medicine – an issue for women only? A survey of physician teachers' gender attitudes. *International Journal for Equity in Health*, *2*(1), 10. doi:10.1186/1475-9276-2-10 PMID:14613502

Sara, B. (2017). In patient satisfaction scores, what role does bias play? [Wedblog] Retrieved from https://www.ama-assn.org/practice-management/physician-diversity/patient-satisfaction-scores-what-role-does-bias-play

Sara, B. (2018). How does gender impact physician burnout? 3 key takeaways. Retrieved from https://www.ama-assn.org/practice-management/physician-health/how-does-gender-impact-physician-burnout-3-key-takeaways

Schulte-Rüther, M., Markowitsch, H., Shah, N., Fink, G., & Piefke, M. (2008). Gender differences in brain networks supporting empathy. *NeuroImage*, *42*(1), 393–403. doi:10.1016/j.neuroimage.2008.04.180 PMID:18514546

Sexism-in-surgery-females-being-put-off-becoming-surgeons-by-men. (2016). [Online Newspaper] Retrieved from https://wwww.telegraph.co.uk/news/health/11903476/sexism-in-surgery-females-being-put-off-becoming-surgeons-by-men.html%OA

Skinner, H. (2018). Gender discrimination in leadership roles in surgical specialties in the UK. *Association of Surgeons of Great Britain and Ireland, 53*(Winter): 95. Retrieved from http://asgbi.org/Journals/Winter%202018%20JASGBI.pdf

Statistics — Royal College of Surgeons. (2018). [National society Report] Retrieved from https://www.rcseng.ac.uk/careers-in-surgery/women-in-surgery/statistics/

Stilwell, N., Wallick, M., Thal, S., & Burleson, J. (2000). Myers-Briggs Type and Medical Specialty Choice: A New Look at an Old Question. *Teaching and Learning in Medicine*, *12*(1), 14–20. doi:10.1207/S15328015TLM1201_3 PMID:11228862

Stratton, T., McLaughlin, M., Witte, F., Fosson, S., & Nora, L. (2005). Does Students?? Exposure to Gender Discrimination and Sexual Harassment in Medical School Affect Specialty Choice and Residency Program Selection? *Academic Medicine*, *80*(4), 400–408. doi:10.1097/00001888-200504000-00020 PMID:15793027

Suicides in the UK Statistical bulletins - Office for National Statistics. (2017). Retrieved from https://www.ons.gov.uk/peoplepopulationandcommunity/birthsdeathsandmarriages/deaths/bulletins/suicidesintheunitedkingdom/previousReleases

Susan, A. (2012). Why Do So Many Doctors Regret Their Job Choice? Retrieved from https://www.forbes.com/sites/susanadams/2012/04/27/why-do-so-many-doctors-regret-their-job-choice/#e3c420737fae

'The hijab has no place in NHS hospitals', argues Muslim writer. (2016). [Online Newspaper] Retrieved from https://www.dailymail.co.uk/health/article-3561324/The-hijab-no-place-hospitals-Muslim-writer-says-medicine-free-religion-health-hazard-clothing-banned.html

The state of medical education and practice in the UK. (2018). Retrieved from https://www.gmc-uk.org/about/what-we-do-and-why/data-and-research/the-state-of-medical-education-and-practice-in-the-uk

Timeline of women in medicine. (2018). [Museum Information] Retrieved from https://www.ama-assn.org/practice-management/physician-diversity/timeline-women-medicine

Walton, M. (2015). Sexual equality, discrimination and harassment in medicine: It's time to act. *The Medical Journal of Australia*, *203*(4), 167–169. doi:10.5694/mja15.00379 PMID:26268278

Williams, S. (2018). Guiding the higher surgical trainee return to work: a deanery perspective [Abstract]. *Association of Surgeons of Great Britain and Ireland, 53*(Winter), 91-92. Retrieved from http://asgbi.org/Journals/Winter%202018%20JASGBI.pdf

Women in medicine. (n.d.). Retrieved from http://broughttolife.sciencemuseum.org.uk/broughttolife/themes/practisingmedicine/women

Chapter 4
Training Martians and Venusians on Jupiter:
Gender Equity in Medical Training

Stella Vig
Croydon University Hospital, UK

Paul Dent
Croydon University Hospital, UK

ABSTRACT

The challenge of diversification in the medical workforce cannot be ignored. Society and societal norms have also progressed at pace and terms and attitudes that were acceptable are now outdated. Trainers must be professionalised to ensure that training of trainees remains an exemplar role. It is accepted that boys and girls learn differently but have the same potential. Equity of opportunity ensures that the modern society retains and values all genders. By exploring whether these differences continue into the post-graduate education system, the medical profession can accommodate and mitigate to ensure equity. This chapter will explore the need for professional trainers, the educational needs of the modern-day medical trainee, and the challenges that need to be accommodated to ensure that the medical workforce retains a passion long into their careers.

TRAINING MARTIANS AND VENUSIANS ON JUPITER

Master Craftsmen and Professional Trainers

Medical Education is key to ensuring that skills and communication developed by the profession are passed on from generation to generation. The apprentice model was embedded as a tool to enable this, with an apprentice defined as a person who is learning a trade from a skilled employer, having agreed to work for a fixed period at low wages. The term apprentice is derived from the French, appendre, to learn and applications were made to become an apprentice to learn from the expert. The expectation of the learner was that they would continue with the teacher until the craft was learnt.

DOI: 10.4018/978-1-5225-9599-1.ch004

The time spent in training enabled an individual to experience a wide range of clinical conditions. In surgical specialities, this would allow the apprentice to participate through assistantships and then through supervised operating finally to independent surgical operating. This required a relationship to be developed between the master and the apprentice which was largely subservient. The relationships were often male to male as the medical profession initially excluded the female gender. A social and educational medical hierarchy and language developed to facilitate this. This norm was unchallenged and was acceptable before the millennium where the medical profession embraced diversity.

The diversification has occurred at pace and is in terms of 'feminisation' as well as reaching out across social classes. The change in acceptance in educational and social norms dictate that educational theory, learning styles and delivery methods are changed to accommodate the new medical generation.

This chapter will explore the need for professional trainers, the educational needs of the modern-day medical trainee and the challenges that need to be accommodated to ensure that the medical workforce retains a passion long into their careers.

Diversification in the Medical Workforce

Data from the Universities and Colleges Admissions Service show that across the UK 59.0% of those accepted to medical school in 2017 were women with an increase since the late 1990s (Moberly, 2018). In the USA, a third of practising medical professionals are female (Kaiser, 2018) with 50% of medical students being female (Association of American Medical Colleges, 2017). Despite the investment of time in ensuring that there is widening participation is the medical profession, there is attrition in the non-male medical workforce, so that men continue to be over-represented both in clinical senior roles as well as in academia. The number of women entering the surgical professions has increased over the last 10 years in the USA as well as the UK. The pace of change at senior level and across surgical specialities has been relatively slow and movements such as the #ILookLikeASurgeon and #HowIBecameAWomanInSurgery Twitter hashtags, "New Yorker Cover Challenge," and the American Women in Surgery have highlighted the need for change.

The diversification is compounded by a societal change. The generations until the Millennium were brought up considering three stages of life (Gratton & Scott, 2017). These were education, career and then retirement. For many in the medical profession, this developed an institutionalisation of the workforce who were devoted to the care of their patients and their career.

The current generations consider their lives in a very different way. The trainees are keen to develop portfolio careers and are not afraid to undertake gap years. Many students will take a break between their final year in school prior to the university degree. In the UK, the medical students who continue into the first two years of their medical careers (The Foundation Programme) decide to take a career break rather than continue into speciality training (Table 1) (Foundation Programme, 2017).

Table 1. Percentage of trainees entering speciality training in the UK from the foundation programme

	2011	2012	2013	2014	2015	2016	2017
Trainees entering Speciality Training	71.3%	67%	64.4%	58.8%	52%	50.4%	42.6%

The trainees are choosing surgical specialties with an increasing number of women entering the specialities at junior level, but the surgical professions struggle to retain trainees especially in their final years. The factors that challenge are the perception that surgical hours remain arduous and are inflexible, especially with on calls (Wolfe, 2017). The trainees wish to enjoy a work life balance and consider having a rewarding family life the norm. The society outside of the work environment also evidences changing societal perceptions as to appropriate career choices for women. Government guidelines are now embedded in law regarding maternity and paternity leave. The Joint Committee on Surgical Training (JCST) and Health Education England (HEE) have set standards for ensuring that trainees are successful when returning from a period of absence regardless of gender (JCST, 2017).

Rassie (2017) suggests that in the apprentice model, the student becomes familiar with the culture, processes and expectations of the medical workforce. The curricula based medical training that is currently embedded in the medical profession continues to rely on surgical trainers training juniors and so the underlying tenet still applies. The challenge faced is that as the societal norms have changed, the medical culture, processes and expectations may cause dissonance with the outside world.

Professionalising Medical Trainers

The Hippocratic Oath and expected duties of a doctor expect that a clinician will take part in clinical teaching: "to impart precept, oral instruction, and all other instruction … to indentured pupils who have taken the physician's oath" (Hippocrates, 1923). The credibility develops on the calibre of the clinical skill rather than the fact that the individual has been taught to teach (Watling et al., 2013; Watling et al., 2014). Watling compared the music teacher who may not be musically gifted but the ability to teach music is paramount but that having both a musical and teaching talent underpinned an excellent teacher.

In the UK, the GMC have mandated that there is an accreditation process for those that teach but this still relies on brief, infrequent sessions which often may be done online. A formal process needs to be embedded not only to enable teaching but also to understand that the learning styles of the generation below maybe very different to current trainers who will need to adapt.

Watling (2014) also described the disadvantage of the lack of long-term interactions. He states that the musical students felt that the continuity of their relationship with their teachers was central to meaningful and effective feedback: "the longitudinal relationship with the music teacher facilitated the perception of feedback as not only accurate and well-informed, but also firmly well-intentioned. Within such trusting relationships, feedback could be more direct, more critical and at times harsher, while remaining influential". He then compared this to the medical student experience where medical students and supervisor relationships were necessarily much shorter-term and described receiving feedback that was more superficial and felt easier to discard. This feedback was "less likely to be perceived as credible and thus less likely to be accepted and acted upon."

The surgical environment is still male dominated at senior level, as this reflects the surgical fraternity of the previous generation. As women become more senior, they do appear to be more likely to be engaged with trainees and training but as the numbers are still small. Klingensmith and Anderson (2006) performed a cross-sectional survey of membership of the Association for Surgical Education and evidenced the percentage of women who have participated in the American College of Surgeons' "Surgeons as Educators" course was 20.4% over 11 years, 32% for the Association for Surgical Education's "Surgical Education Research Fellowship" over 10 years. They postulated that the data confirmed that women are more likely to seek advanced educational training.

A study reviewing the motivation of teachers entering teaching found that men were interested in teaching a subject whilst women were interested in shaping the future of the children and making a social contribution (Figure 1) (Wyatt-Smith et al., 2017). There are no data in the medical specialties, but extrapolation feels appropriate in the medical profession. In the medical profession, data is required to understand whether gender of the trainer supports excellence in both appraisal and mentorship of medical trainees. Trainees are not widely exposed to non-male surgical role models or surgery at Medical School or during Foundation training and therefore the myths and fables of surgical trainers and careers continue. The surgical placements are also often short and therefore medical students do not develop mentoring relationships with surgical trainers whether male or female.

Gray (1992) states that women and men are fundamentally different psychologically both in terms of motivation but also in the way that they respond to stress and conflict. It is also suggested that women are taught to nurture whilst men are taught to assert and manage, so that the societal norms influence the way that women and men behave which influences motivation. Whichever theory is correct, there is no doubt that men and women do behave in different ways. This must apply to both trainers and trainees.

Qualified teachers are taught not only to recognise their own biases but also to recognise that they may have to use different techniques whilst teaching boys and girls. Whether these differences are due to the environment in which boys and girls are nurtured or whether these differences are due to nature maybe debated but what is important is that teachers ensure that all students develop to their fullest potential. It is reported that boys are more physical, need more space to learn and are not as good at concentrating when reading and writing whereas girls produce more drama, multitask better and will write with more detail. How do teachers and trainers ensure that all are catered for? Teachers are trained to teach but also to understand the learning and behaviour styles and needs of the students they teach. By understanding the group dynamics, they can understand how to achieve the best from every student.

Figure 1. Motivations of male and female teachers from learning sciences institute Australia

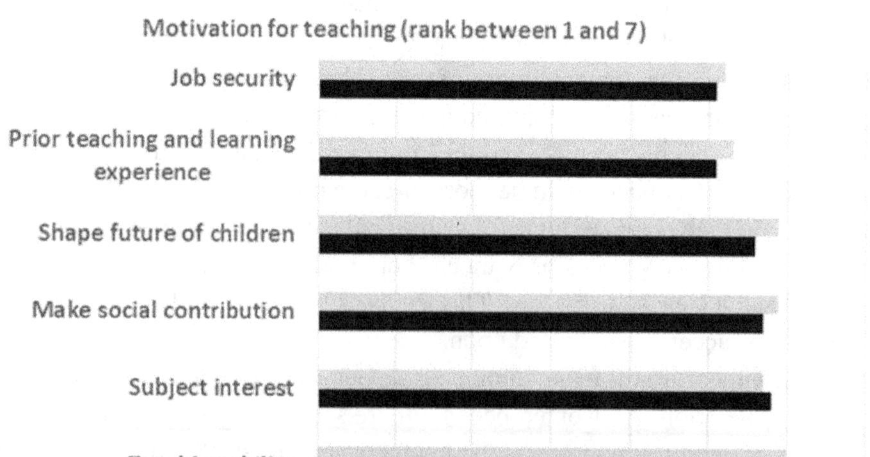

It is suggested that emotions develop with age as higher cognitive functions mature. A female body produces more serotonin and oxytocin at an earlier age which leads calmness and an ability to connect emotionally which leads to close friendships. The cerebral cortex (speech) and hippocampus (memory and language) is more mature, earlier in females. In boys, the spatial awareness element of the cerebral cortex tends to mature earlier than girls. These factors lead to an advantage to girls if they are asked to write creatively and when describing feelings and emotions. This also advantages boys who will learn at pace from practical and visual activities.

At school, boys are noted to participate in risk as this seems to put them at the front of the male hierarchy in the classroom and playground. This puts them at additional risk as they also overestimate their ability (Sax, 2017) are more likely to respond aggressively to situations.

Gross (2014) suggests that the differences are most pronounced in young children, and as children grow older, their home environment, their interests and their peers have the greatest influence over their behaviour. It is thought that by the 12th grade, the differences between boys and girls are very subtle. Understanding these subtle differences can help educators guide their students in a positive way, meeting them and their needs, and will differentiate between a good teacher and an excellent one.

Gross relates 'When little boys don't want to make eye contact and they fidget in their seats, and little girls are caught talking and sending notes, a savvy teacher can organize her classroom in which she takes into consideration that little boys need to move around, and little girls need to express themselves verbally, and interprets this as part of their biology rather than misbehaviour. A savvy parent can be sure that there are playtime opportunities during the day for both boys and girls to unwind and express themselves in a creative way. Further, allowing children to start school especially little boys a little later, perhaps even by a year, gives them an edge. A more mature child can handle school material in a much better way. '

Gross also suggests that 'In my years as a researcher and educator, I've found it to be true that boys and girls perceive their school problems in different ways. Girls tend to take their problems and failures personally and are much more self-critical. Boys, on the other hand, see their problems in more focused ways and will assign their failure to an area of study rather than over-generalize and see themselves as lacking. Ironically girls tend to do better in school than boys and are more likely to stay in school and graduate.'

By understanding the factors above, girls maybe encouraged to develop spatial awareness that may lend to a STEM (Science, Technology, Engineering, Mathematics) career which are still dominated by the boys. Boys maybe encouraged by utilising war and mythology to improve creative writing as well as utilising their desire to take risk and be competitive such as the junior entrepreneur programmes.

Trainees

It is accepted that there are differences in school children based on gender but that these become subtler as they mature. There appears to be a difference in students in Medical School as well as post graduate training. Personal reflection after 10 years as a Foundation Programme Director and as a General Surgery trainer and Programme Director suggest that men are still more likely to take risk and reflect on complications as a team cause whilst women tend to take personal blame and need more assurance that they are doing well.

Sandberg (2015) states that women appear to be underconfident and feel the impact of the 'imposter syndrome'. It is postulated that this may be due to underlying personality differences, but which need to be understood as medical training progresses especially in male dominated environments.

According to Carl G. Jung's theory of psychological types (Jung, 1971), people can be characterized by 3 preferences. These preferences are: general attitude: Extraverted (E), Introverted (I), perception: Sensing (S) vs. Intuition (N), judging: Thinking (T) vs. Feeling (F). A fourth type was introduced by Isabel Briggs Myers, a researcher and practitioner of Jung's theory, Judging (J) vs. Perceiving (P) (Briggs Myers, 1980).

These 8 preferences can give rise to 16 personality types and Myers Briggs has been used as an assessment of personality type.

In one study of 157 medical trainees (Martinou et al., 2014) found that the preferential profile across all groups was Extroversion (E), Sensing (S), Feeling (F), and Perception (P). The study demonstrated that trainees became more introvert and more reliant on data rather than gut feeling (S to N) as they became more senior. More foundation doctors favoured an extrovert and sensing personality when compared with core trainees (72% vs 60.4% and 77.4% vs 57.5%, respectively). More core surgical trainees appeared to prefer extroversion when compared with their medical counterparts (66.7% vs 54.2%). More core medical trainees favoured an intuitive behaviour when compared with their surgical colleagues (50% vs 35%). Significantly, more female trainees (83.3%) displayed an extrovert personality than male trainees (66.7%) did. The question raised is whether there are differential personality types between the genders.

Analysis of MBTI scores in the general population suggest that men and women do have different personality types. These are displayed in the table below (Table 2):

Women appear to be more likely to demonstrate an extroverted personality type. E type personalities enjoy the company of others whilst I types are more comfortable on their own. Men are more likely to be thinkers whilst women are more likely to be feelers, considering how interactions impact on others. It appears that women are more likely to be judgers and be organised whilst men are more likely to be perceivers, happy to plan as activities arise.

A study carried out prior to Martinou of 41 surgical residents in the United States (Swanson, 2010), demonstrated that the preferences of S, T and J were more likely as well as trainees being more introvert (54%). These trainees were born between 1965 and 1980 and were labelled as generation X. Swanson compared the dataset to historic cohorts and suggested that the changing society and training environments were attracting a different personality type with a previous prevalence of ESTJ personality types (Schaubnut & Thompson, 2008). Swanson reflects that the I personality type indicates an individual who preferred to communicate through writing, learned through internal reflection, and distilled thought independently. In contrast, Swanson suggested that the E personality type favoured spoken over written

Table 2. MBTI personality type in men and women

MBTI type	Men	Women	Both
E		✓	
I	✓		
S			✓
N			✓
F		✓	
T	✓		
J		✓	
P	✓		

communication, learned through action and discussion, and was stimulated through interactions with other people. It is recognised that the difference in personality type may lead to communication break down and poor team dynamics which may impact both on learning as well as patient care.

It appears that the changing environment of the medical profession attracts different personality types. The original generation (mostly men) may have been extroverts and then environmental factors then began to attract more introvert individuals. As more women are entering medicine, so the E becomes more pronounced.

It is apparent that generations are not identical, and trainers need to be aware that their teaching methods cannot be as they learnt but need to be developed and adapted to the personality type of the trainees allocated to them. This will need to change between genders and individuals and the trainees need to be self-aware of their own personalities.

Does the personality type influence risk tolerance in the medical profession?

Contessa and colleagues (2013) investigated whether there was an association between surgical personality and risk tolerance. The Myers Briggs type indicator was correlated against and an assessment of risk tolerance measured by the Revised Physicians' Reactions to Uncertainty (PRU) and Physician Risk Attitude (risk aversion, PRA) scales.

This study concluded the following: 'In certain areas of risk assessment, it appears that surgeons with personality factors E (Extravert), T (Thinking), and P (Perception) demonstrated higher tolerance for risk. Conversely, as MBTI® dichotomies are complementary, surgeons with personality factors I (Introvert), F (Feeling), and J (Judgment) suggest risk aversion on these same measures. These findings are supported by at least 2 studies outside medicine demonstrating that personality factors E, N, T, and P are associated with risk taking.'

Learning styles have been demonstrated to be different in children. It is important to understand whether they continue to be different in adult life and as the clinicians become more senior. A study carried out over a decade ago investigated the change in learning style over a 12-year period (Mammen et al., 2007).

The Kolb Learning Style Inventory (KLSI) was administered yearly to general surgery residents at the University of Cincinnati from 1994 to 2006 (91 residents). KLSI considers 4 learning styles (Kolb et al., 1999). The converging learning style learns by actively solving problems, the accommodating learning style uses emotion and interpersonal relationships. The assimilating learning style learns by abstract logic and the diverging learning style learns best by observation. Professions tend to attract certain learning styles. Family residents or General Practitioners tend to be accommodators, whereas internal medicine residents or physicians tend to be more convergent (Sadler et al., 1978; Plovnick, 1975).

The data suggested that the prevalent learning style was converging (185, 57%), followed by assimilating (58, 18%), accommodating (44, 14%), and diverging (38, 12%). Early year trainees differed in learning style between the genders. Major differences were noted in the assimilating and accommodating learning styles, with 38% of female general surgery residents in the accommodating group as compared with 11% of their male counterparts ($p <$ or $= 0.001$, chi-square test). On the other hand, 26% of male general surgery residents demonstrated the assimilating learning style, whereas none of their female counterparts fitted into that category. The learning style did not seem to change as the trainees progressed, but a convergent axis did appear.

The differences in personality traits, risk management and learning style needs to be considered as trainers teach and curricula are developed. As the percentage of females in general surgery increases, so does the percentage of accommodating and convergent learners. The accommodating learners tends to learn best by performing tasks at their own pace after being given an assignment. Trainers should provide support by serving as a resource for consultation, but group learning is felt to be useful. Convergent learners learn better by performing tasks as individuals with assistance from an instructor as necessary with group projects and discussions off putting. It is therefore vital that the trainer understands the need of the trainee as there is a changing trainee population, the profession must expect a change in the expectations of trainees dependent on the gender.

The personality traits will also impact on the social and educational relationships on the medical and surgical teams. This may cause conflict between specialties and this was investigated by Sorenson and colleagues (1995). The study reviewed 135 first and middle level managers with gender, psychological type and conflict style questionnaires. Gender was related to psychological type as discussed previously: male respondents were predominantly "thinkers" and female respondents were predominantly "feelers." "Feelers" were more likely to choose an obliging style than were "thinkers." Male respondents had a higher obliging score than did female respondents. The data suggested that conflict style preference was complex and superseded both gender and personality type.

There is also evidence that suggests that the personality traits can be linked to the motivation to learn and this can be nurtured by trainers (Major et al., 2006). The traits can also be linked to stress and burnout (McManus et al., 2004) but the enjoyment of work and learning was associated with an extravert personality. In general practice, where the trainer, trainee interaction is very close and on a one to one basis, the understanding of personality and the need to nurture is very important. One study demonstrated that the trainee and trainer personality traits are now divergent (Joffe et al., 2016). In this study, trainees report that they are less emotionally resilient than their seniors. In addition, women appeared to have less emotional resilience than men.

Joffe suggests 'Offering all trainees the opportunity of completing psychometrics and receiving feedback may be a consideration for the training programme as it would increase insight into personal attributes that can support or impede the development of GP expertise, and identify more vulnerable individuals to guide targeted interventions from trainers to programme directors.'

To Achieve Excellence for All

If it is accepted that the learning styles are not uniform within the community of medical students and junior doctors, then the skills to manage the training of these doctors must be learnt. The gender composition of the seniors in the medical profession and especially academia is currently male dominant. The gender composition up of the students entering the profession is at least 50:50. This mismatch generates a level of unconscious bias and dissonance and maybe the cause of the lack of progression of females to more senior roles. There are clearly other factors such as career breaks and part time working (Taylor et al, 2009) which may mean that career progression becomes slower for females. The nature of part time working, especially in surgery, may reduce the ability to partake in opportunities both in the workplace as well as skill and non-surgical skill courses.

This unconscious bias may also develop in trainees who perceive that there are certain rules which will allow them to progress. This, in turn, may lead to poor motivation or resentment as their career progresses. A study of cardiothoracic trainees in 2015 stated that women accounted for 20% of residents and there were no differences between the genders related to specialty interest, academic versus private practice career, or pursuit of additional training (Stephens et al, 2016). Women were more likely to pursue additional training in minimally invasive thoracic surgery (10% versus 2.5%, $p = 0.001$) and less likely to perform research in their careers (65% versus 88%, $p = 0.043$). Although women were equally satisfied with their career choice, graduating women felt less prepared technically (77% versus 90%, p = 0.01) and for practicing independently (71% versus 87%, p = 0.01). Women were less likely to be married (26% versus 62%, p < 0.001) and have children (19% versus 49%, p < 0.001).

The expectation of the new generation is that they have fulfilled lives which include having a family and a work life balance and trainers will need to understand and accommodate these needs.

Unconscious bias exists within the medical profession and therefore trainers. Training in equality and diversity is mandatory within educational roles but there are many subtle unconscious biases held within the senior medical profession.

McNally discussed the need awareness of unconscious bias when dealing with juniors (McNally, 2016). The document, Avoiding Unconscious Bias, discusses bias arising in the workplace and how to reduce it. The document advises that bias is an entity that needs to be acknowledged and then understood. This is essential in order to mitigate and ensure that, especially trainers, find something in common and force themselves to appear as if there are no biases until they diminish and then do not exist (Thiederman, 2008).

Thiedeman suggests that this process can be broken down into seven steps:

1. Become mindful of one's biases
2. Put one's biases through triage
3. Identify the secondary gains of one's biases
4. Dissect one's biases
5. Identify common kinship groups
6. Shove one's biases aside
7. Fake it until one makes it (what we say can become what we believe)

This should become a normal process for any trainer or supervisor to consider once a trainee has been assigned. This would assure a process that if the trainee does not fit the image of who should be doing this role, then the trainer would have to understand why this feeling exists. By understanding this, the trainer would be able to reduce any discrimination or prejudice that may develop during the trainee/trainer interaction. This would also reduce the perception that the trainee may feel that they are being bullied or discriminated against.

The Royal Australasian College of Surgeons documented a 50% experience of bullying and discrimination including sexual harassment in their fellows and trainees. When the college challenged this, it found that the senior surgeons did not realise that their behaviour amounted to harassment. This led to the college to introduce its 'Lets operate with respect' campaign in 2016.

Trainers need to understand their own personality type and how they react to stress as well as that of trainees who are under stress. The data suggest that most senior male surgeons are introverts whilst most female surgical trainees are extroverts. Under stress, an introverted personality type may wish to take more control and internalise reflection. This personality type may feel that their way is the only way. Under the same conditions, the extroverted personality type, may wish to escape the situation by finding other things to do and avoid the now. This may develop a perception that they are insensitive and aloof although they may feel that they are personally responsible for what may have gone awry. Use of a 'prebrief', especially in the operating environment would allow both trainer and trainee to rehearse moments of stress induced by complex parts of the operation allowing a common language and understanding to be developed that would minimise real time stress.

Unconscious bias can lead to language being used that empowers the senior trainer and may have been acceptable a generation ago. As society has changed, the same language may be perceived as an attempt to belittle, undermine or humiliate trainees. Taking over a case in theatre rather than talking a trainee through a complication may lead to undermining in theatre and criticism of the trainee's competence. Normal surgical banter allows the building of a strong teams unless it is perceived as destructive innuendo and sarcasm, is personal, or inappropriate.

A strong trainer will ensure that the language used is carefully chosen to encourage the trainee considering the individual's learning style. In addition, the educational contract should be explicit as to how concerns can be raised and how discomfort can be raised discreetly but explicitly in real time.

Trainers may also need to be chosen according to the needs of the trainers and training environment rather than the current stance that everyone is a trainer.

This professionalisation of trainers is key to improving medical training. The trainers must evidence their teaching and clinical skills and ensure continued professional development. The support of the host organisation is also key. Trainers provide service at a variety of healthcare providers. Training takes time and therefore service needs will need to be reduced to allow a patient training environment to be developed. There should be protected time for reflection and feedback and development of training materials and environments. This is especially important when developing simulation and AR modules. This valuable training time will need to be reimbursed rather than be carried out on goodwill and gratis.

The Commission on the Future of Surgery has evidenced that the surgical environment and workload will evolve rapidly as technologies advance and aid or replace current surgical activities (Kerr, 2018). The Commission also suggest that training involves repeated modules throughout training that do not add to the knowledge base. It is suggested that training may be moved into an online platform to reduce the repetition, but this may dispassion the social, extrovert learner.

The Commission suggests that Human Factor training needs to be utilised for communication training as well as team skills. The report also states that new technologies such as data analytics, AR and VR will enhance training, with high-fidelity patient-specific simulation, and remote mentoring and proctoring. It is important that learning styles and gender differences are considered in advance of the revolution. One study has demonstrated that personalised web-based or human factor training appears to improve learning in females but makes no difference in men (Chen et al, 2016).

#ChangetheNorm: The Way Forward

The medical profession will need to learn from other training environments and embrace the new medical generation. Professional trainers should be handpicked and be invested in so that training becomes a valuable skill set. The personality traits and learning styles of the trainees should be understood as there are clear differences both between past and new generations but also between male and female individuals.

Pastoral support and mentoring will improve the environment and enable trainees to develop emotional resilience to allow long fulfilled medical careers. The medical training environment and work force planning will need to understand and address the expectations of the new generation, both male and female, to be successful in portfolio careers.

The need to change the norm at pace is vital to support trainees who are very different from their trainers. With the increase in female entrants to medical school, it should be expected that the workforce will become pregnant and need time to be mothers and that this will need to be accommodated within the educational timeline. Trainer support at these times is important and an understanding of the need for a change for both genders is key to the skills of an excellent trainer and workplace. Trainees need to be involved in the changes to curricula development and visions for the future, they are the trainers of the next generation.

It is accepted that boys and girls learn differently but have the same potential. Equity of opportunity ensures that the modern society retains and values all genders. By understanding that these differences continue into the post graduate education system, the medical profession can accommodate and mitigate to ensure equity to all genders.

REFERENCES

Association of American Medical Colleges. (2017). *More Women Than Men Enrolled in U.S. Medical Schools in 2017*. Retrieved from https://news.aamc.org/content/downloadable/117/

Briggs Myers, I., & Myers, P. B. (1995). *Gifts Differing: Understanding Personality Type*. Palo Alto, CA: Davies-Black Publishing.

Chen, S., Huang, P., Shih, Y., & Chang, L. (2016). Investigation of multiple human factors in personalized learning. *Interactive Learning Environments*, *24*(1), 119–141. doi:10.1080/10494820.2013.825809

Contessa, J., Suarez, L., Kyruakides, T., & Nadzam, G. (2013). The Influence of Surgeon Personality Factors on Risk Tolerance: A Pilot Study. *Journal of Surgical Education*, *70*(6), 806–812. doi:10.1016/j.jsurg.2013.07.014 PMID:24209660

Foundation Programme. (2017). *UK Foundation Programme Career Destinations Report 2017*. Retrieved from http://www.foundationprogramme.nhs.uk/sites/default/files/2018-07/2017%20F2%20Career%20Destinations%20Report_0.pdf

Gratton, L., & Scott, A. (2016). *The 100-year life Living and Working in an Age of Longevity*. London, UK: Bloomsbury Information Ltd.

Gray, J. (1992). *Men are from Mars, Women are from Venus*. London, UK: HarperCollins.

Gross, G. (2014). *Men are from Mars, women are from Venus... or are they? Are the differences between boys and girls really that great? Or is our biological determinism more of a self-fulfilled prophecy?* Human Behaviour, Parenting, and Education.

Joffe, M., MacLeod, S., Kedziora, M., & Main, P. (2016). GP trainers and trainees – trait and gender differences in personality: Implications for GP training. *Education for Primary Care*, *27*(3), 205–213. doi:10.1080/14739879.2016.1147135 PMID:27059247

Joint Committee on Surgical Training. (2017). *Guidance on the management of surgical trainees returning to clinical training after extended leave*. Retrieved from https://www.jcst.org/-/media/files/jcst/key-documents/return-to-work-guidance-final.pdf

<jrn>Kerr, R. (2018). Commission on the Future of Surgery. Royal College of Surgeons of England.

Jung, C. G. (1971). Psychological types. In *Collected works of C* (Vol. 6). G. Jung.

Kaiser, H. J. (2018). *Professionally active physicians by Gender*. Retrieved from https://www.kff.org/other/state-indicator/physicians-by-gender

Klingensmith, M., & Anderson, K. (2006). Educational scholarship as a route to academic promotion: A depiction of surgical education scholars. *American Journal of Surgery, 191*(4), 533–537. doi:10.1016/j.amjsurg.2006.01.007</jrn>

Kolb, D. A., Boyatzis, R. E., & Mainemelis, C. (1999) *Experiential learning theory: previous research and new directions*. Working Paper 99-98. Cleveland, OH: Case Western Reserve University Hippocrates of Cos, (1923) The Oath [Internet]. Loeb Classical Library. 1923; 147, 298–299. doi:10.4159/DLCL.hippocrates_cos-oath

Major, D. A., Turner, J. E., & Fletcher, T. D. (2006). Linking proactive personality and the big five to motivation to learn and development activity. *The Journal of Applied Psychology, 91*(4), 927–935. doi:10.1037/0021-9010.91.4.927 PMID:16834515

Mammen, J. M., Fischer, D. R., Anderson, A., James, L. E., Nussbaum, M. S., Bower, R. H., & Pritts, T. A. (2007). Learning styles vary among general surgery residents: Analysis of 12 years of data. *Journal of Surgical Education, 64*(6), 386–389. doi:10.1016/j.jsurg.2007.08.005 PMID:18063274

Martinou, E., Allan, H., & Vig, S. (2014). Personality Differences Among Junior Postgraduate Trainees in the United Kingdom. *The Journal of Surgery, 72*(1), 122–127. doi:10.1016/j.jsurg.2014.06.014 PMID:25091381

McManus, I. C., Keeling, A., & Paice, E. (2004) Stress, burnout and doctors' attitudes to work are determined by personality and learning style: A twelve year longitudinal study of UK medical graduates. *BMC Med., 18*(2), 29. Retrieved from http://www.biomedcentral.com/1741-7015/2/29

McNally, S. (2016) Sexual harassment and bullying in UK surgery: no room for complacency. *BMJ 354*. doi:10.1136/bmj.i4682

Moberly, T. (2018). Number of women entering medical school rises after decade of decline. *BMJ (Clinical Research Ed.), 360*, k254. doi:10.1136/bmj.k254

Plovnick, M. S. (1975). Primary care career choices and medical student learning styles. *Journal of Medical Education, 50*, 849–855. PMID:1171243

Rassie, K. (2017). The apprenticeship model of clinical medical education: Time for structural change. *The New Zealand Medical Journal, 130*(1461), 66–72. PMID:28859068

Sadler, G. R., Plovnick, M., & Snope, F. C. (1978). Learning styles and teaching implications. *Journal of Medical Education, 53*, 847–849. PMID:712775

Sandberg, S. (2015). Lean. In *Women, Work, and the Will to Lead*. New York, NY: Knopf.

Sax, L. (2017). *Why Gender Matters: What Parents and Teachers Need to Know about the Emerging Science of Sex Differences* (2nd ed.). New York, NY: Broadway Books.

Schaubnut, N. A., & Thompson, R. A. (2008). *MBTI type tables for occupations*. Mountain View, CA: CPP.

Sorenson, P. S., Hawkins, K., & Sorenson, R. L. (1995). *Gender*. Psychological Type and Conflict Style Preference. doi:10.1136/postgradmedj-2015-133919

Stephens, E. H., Robich, M. P., Walters, D. M., DeNino, W. F., Aftab, M., Tchantchaleishvili, V., ... Shah, A. A. (2016). Gender and Cardiothoracic Surgery Training: Specialty Interests, Satisfaction, and Career Pathways. *The Annals of Thoracic Surgery*, *102*(1), 200–206. doi:10.1016/j.athoracsur.2016.03.043 PMID:27157051

Swanson, J. A., Mara, B., D'Cunha, J., & Maddaus, M. A. (2010). Personality Profiling of the Modern Surgical Trainee: Insights into Generation X. *Journal of Surgical Education*, *67*(6), 417–420. doi:10.1016/j.jsurg.2010.07.017 PMID:21156301

Taylor, K. S., Lambert, T. W., & Goldacre, M. J. (2009). Career progression and destinations, comparing men and women in the NHS: Postal questionnaire surveys. *BMJ (Clinical Research Ed.)*, *338*(jun02 1), b1735. doi:10.1136/bmj.b1735 PMID:19493938

Thiederman, S. (2008). *Making Diversity Work*. New York, NY: Kaplan.

Watling, C., Driessen, E., van der Vleuten, C. P., & Lingard, L. (2014, July). Learning culture and feedback: An international study of medical athletes and musicians. *Medical Education*, *48*(7), 713–723. doi:10.1111/medu.12407 PMID:24909533

Watling, C., Driessen, E., van der Vleuten, C. P., Vanstone, M., & Lingard, L. (2013, August). Music lessons: Revealing medicine's learning culture through a comparison with that of music. *Medical Education*, *47*(8), 842–850. doi:10.1111/medu.12235 PMID:23837431

Wolfe, L. (2018). *Statistics on the number of women surgeons in the United States. Why is it tough to increase the number of women in surgery?* Retrieved from https://www.thebalancecareers.com/number-of-women-surgeons-in-the-us-3972900

Wyatt-Smith, C., Du Plessis, A., Hand, K., Wang, J., Alexander, C., & Colbert, P. (2017). *Why choose teaching? A matter of choice: Evidence from the field. A report prepared for the Queensland College of Teachers*. Brisbane, Australia: Learning Sciences Institute Australia. Retrieved from https://www.qct.edu.au/pdf/WhyChooseTeachingReport.pdf

Chapter 5
Understanding the Value of Gender Equity in Healthcare and How to Pursue It

Emma Adriana Gans
Leiden University Medical Center, The Netherlands

ABSTRACT

Female and male physicians practice medicine differently. Female physicians engage in different communication styles, allocate more time to preventative care, and show different leadership qualities. Because gender diversity is still lacking in the top academic and clinical positions, medical organizations are not fully benefiting from these strengths. This chapter will identify three barriers that prevent women from advancing to these positions: the double burden syndrome, sexism and sexual harassment, and gender bias. This chapter will take a critical look at organizational culture and propose changes that can contribute to the pursuit of gender equity.

INTRODUCTION

The importance of gender equity within medicine or any other field is a notion that resonates with most of us. It aligns with our value of providing equal opportunities for all and therefore seems apparent. Perhaps, because the philosophy of equality between the sexes fits so well within our modern society, we assume it is within reach and simply a matter of time. While this a noble thought, it reduces gender equity to a simple concept, which in fact, it is not at all. Continuing to regard gender equity in this manner will prevent us from moving forward.

In order to truly pursue gender equity in medicine, we need to first grasp how and why gender equity is of value to the medical profession. The value is greater than simply striving for equality between the sexes in general. The significance lies in the fact that female doctors bring specific qualities to the medical field that lead to great benefit. These qualities deserve to be recognized and then given the space to be fully expressed. Unfortunately, this is not yet the case today. Therefore, we need to have an honest

DOI: 10.4018/978-1-5225-9599-1.ch005

look at the medical world and identify barriers that prevent women from advancing. The significant presence of females in medical school unfortunately does not mean that the glass ceiling has been shattered. Identifying the barriers that are still in place will culminate in an opportunity to strategize how to revolutionize the medical profession.

THE GENDER GAP IN MEDICINE

For many years, in the pursuit of gender equality in the work domain, women had to prove that they were just as capable as their male peers in the jobs that everyone considered male professions for decades. Women first had to show that they were equipped with similar intellectual power and skill as men. Today, women are drawn to and welcomed into medical schools in large numbers suggesting that this goal has been achieved. However, when we take a closer look at the numbers, we see that a lack of gender diversity in many positions in the medical world persists.

For the past decade, in countries such as the United States and the Netherlands, females make up approximately half of all medical students.(AAMC, 2016. Capaciteitsorgaan, 2016.) Yet, somehow female doctors remain underrepresented in the top clinical and academic positions. In the United States, 38% of faculty members, 15% of department chairs and 16% of deans are female. In some departments the gender gap is even greater: less than 1% of surgical department chairs are female.(AAMC, 2016) In the Netherlands, 46% of medical specialists are female. Again, certain departments lag far behind: 11% of cardio-thoracic surgeons, 11% of orthopedic surgeons and 22% of cardiologists are female. Geriatric specialists take the lead with female specialists making up 70%.(Capaciteitsorgaan, 2016) The gender gap is also visible in academia and management. In the Netherlands, the number of female professors has increased over the past years to approximately 19% and women make up around 20% of academic management boards.(Science Guide, 2017)

While in most departments the gender gap is slowly becoming smaller, the number of women pursuing a PhD and the number of women on academic management boards have shown a declining trend over the past five years.(Science Guide, 2017) This is worrisome, as it contradicts the common belief that time is the key to achieving true gender diversity. It supports the idea that in order to close the gender gap in medicine, a more active approach is required.

THE ADDED VALUE OF GENDER DIVERSITY FOR CLINICAL OUTCOMES AND ORGANIZATIONAL HEALTH

Pursuing gender diversity is about much more than simply wanting to give women the same opportunities as men because we believe them to be just as capable and deserving. While this is a good starting point, it is well worth our effort to take a look at the different qualities that men and women have. When we move away from the concept that women and men have identical skills and look at how they actually complement one another, we will discover that we should actively pursue the advancement of female doctors.

The Need For Female Gendered Traits In Medicine

First, it is important to realize that recent studies have established that clinical performance by female physicians is equal to their male counterparts. For example, laparoscopic skills of female and male surgical trainees are similar.(White et al., 2012) One study even shows that patients treated by female physicians have lower mortality rates and lower readmission rates.(Tsugawa et al., 2017). Knowing that women are capable and skilled physicians, no less than men, focus can shift to the differences in clinical care that do exist, and learn how to benefit from them.

When considering how women and men practice medicine differently, it is important to understand that this distinction is not a black and white concept but a fluid one. Gendered skills can be displayed by any sex. However, these skills are considered gendered because either the female or male sex displays them more frequently. As illustrated in figure 1, both men and women, as identified by their biological sex, can find themselves anywhere on a fluid spectrum of masculine and feminine traits.

One example of a gendered skill in medicine is the way men and women interact with patients. During a consultation, female physicians spend, on average, more time on psychosocial counseling, engage more in participatory decision making and show more empathy.(Roter et al., 2004) Psychosocial counseling means taking time to explain how an illness will impact different areas of a patients' life and providing coping tools. Participatory decision-making means actively involving a patient in medical decisions. By doing so, the doctor shares the responsibility for the patients' well-being with the patient in question. Showing empathy is a part of non-verbal communication, and commonly believed to be an essential skill for a medical professional. Again, this does not mean that male physicians never display the above-mentioned skills but that these skills are more often expressed by females and are thus considered feminine traits.

These forms of interaction, in particular participatory decision making, have gained great popularity within the medical world over the past years. It is believed to take into account patient' autonomy, an important concept in medical ethics. In light of respect for autonomy, it has become a vital goal to include the individual patients' wishes in medical decisions. It is believed to contribute to patients' satisfaction and to therapeutic adherence (Cooper-Patrick et al, 1999; Kaplan et al, 1996). Furthermore, the modern

Figure 1. A fluid spectrum of feminine and masculine traits

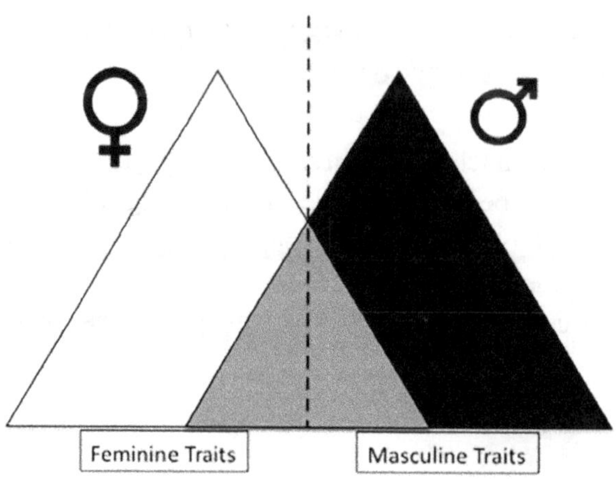

patient is more informed than ever, with an abundance of medical information at their disposal on the Internet. The result is that patients have more demands and increasingly propose their own ideas and reflections on what would be the best diagnostic tools or therapeutic interventions. Engaging with the patient as an equal partner and autonomous entity is often a fitting and successful approach.

In regards to clinical care, research has shown that women provide more preventative care and adhere more precisely to clinical guidelines.(Kim et al., 2005. Baumhäkel et al., 2009). In addition, one can reason that spending time during a consultation to discuss preventive care options such as lifestyle interventions, elaborating on how an illness will affect different areas of a patients' life and actively involving the patient in decision making, can especially improve the prevention and management of chronic disease. Chronic diseases have been identified as the main contributors to the Global Burden of Disease and are predicted to become even more prevalent over the next decades. In 2017, 73% of all global deaths were due to chronic disease and the majority could be accounted for by risk factors such as high blood pressure, smoking, high blood glucose and high body-mass index.(GBD, 2018) Each of these risk factors can in theory be reduced greatly by preventive care and lifestyle interventions. When we look at care for the chronically ill, the physician with female gendered traits might be of great value. Any hospital should want to benefit from these female assets in care, and actively integrate the qualities of female gendered practice in their groups of physicians.

The Need for Female Gendered Traits in Leadership

In addition to the differences observed in clinical care, it is of interest to look how women and men function differently in leadership positions and the consequences for organizational health.

McKinsey & Company, a well-recognized management-consulting firm, has thoroughly researched the impact of gender diversity on the organizational performance of companies worldwide.(McKinsey & Company, 2017) McKinsey measures organization performance by their diagnostic tool the 'Organization Health Index' (OHI). Using this tool, they determined that the presence of women in leadership positions leads to better performance of the company. The OHI comprises nine criteria such as: the quality of the leadership team, the company's ability to communicate a vision and a clear direction, the work environment and its level of innovation. A report called 'Women Matter' highlights that executive committees with three or more women on board outperformed those committees with no women at the top on each of the nine dimensions. They continued to establish that OHI is positively correlated with financial outcome of an organization. This is supported by their research that found that the presence of women in management positions leads to better financial results for companies.

McKinsey & Company continued to identify how women and men display different leadership behaviors. Women leaders tend more to people development, expressing expectations and rewarding success, role-modeling, inspiring and, as we have seen in clinical care, in participatory decision making. Women and men equally apply intellectual stimulation and efficient communication. Men typically show more control and corrective action, as well as individualistic decision-making. All of the above-mentioned leadership qualities are considered positive leadership behaviors but are gendered in nature. So, an organization with an executive committee that includes both men and women is bound to be more successful. McKinsey & Company show that through the positive leadership behaviors that are specific to women, women contribute to the accountability of the executive committee, work environment and values. To this date, there is no research that evaluates how gender diversity influences executive boards of hospitals specifically.

Women have more than proven to be capable physicians and leaders. It is time to reap the benefits from the differences in approach when handling clinical and organizational challenges. The only way that this can be achieved is when the value of gender diversity is recognized, and organizations choose to prioritize this.

IMPORTANT BARRIERS TO FEMALE PHYSICIANS' CAREER ADVANCEMENT

As previously said, women are attracted to the medical profession in large numbers. Yet we don't see an equal representation of males and females in the top clinical and academic positions. A common narrative is that women simply choose not to aim for these positions. Many believe that, when women reach a certain age ambition disappears, as motherhood becomes the main or only priority. This causes women to opt out of those positions that are too demanding or time consuming. While this is a familiar perspective, it is one of the most prevalent examples of gender bias, which we will explore later in this chapter. Research performed in corporate organizations, and the medical world, shows that women and men have equal drive to acclaim top positions and are equally willing to sacrifice their personal lives. (AAMC, 2016. McKinsey & Company, 2017) An important difference between men and women, however, is that women don't feel confident that they are able to succeed in their ambitions in the current environment and culture of organizations such as hospitals.(AAMC, 2016. McKinsey & Company, 2017) There are a number of barriers that are rooted in modern culture, and organizational culture of hospitals specifically, that stand in the way of gender equity. Figure 2 illustrates three important barriers that will be discussed: the double-burden syndrome, sexism and sexual harassment, and gender bias.

Double-Burden Syndrome

A major issue that has been well recognized is the *double-burden syndrome*. This syndrome is used to describe the fact that women, next to their professional responsibilities, carry most of the weight of domestic responsibilities as well. Decades ago, when women entered the workforce en masse, society

Figure 2. Barriers that female physicians face in the workplace

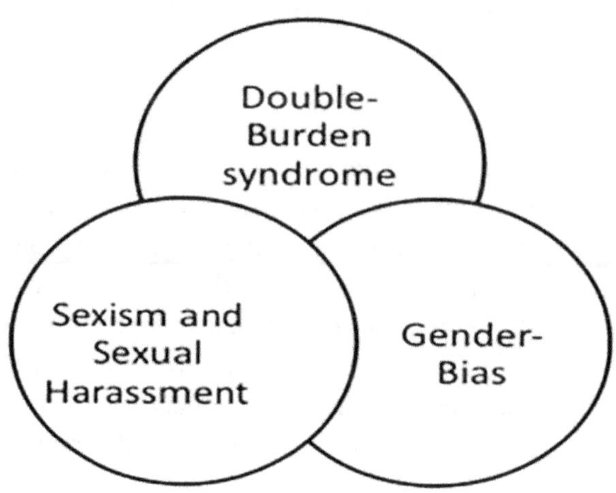

had to get used to the idea of women suddenly performing and succeeding at traditionally male tasks. Naturally, a similar shift had to take place at home. Domestic duties that were traditionally a women's responsibility, now needed to be shared. It deserves recognition that society has come a long way, but unfortunately true equality has not been reached. In Western Europe, women devote twice the amount of time to domestic care such as household tasks and care for children and elderly. On average, women spend 4 hours and 20 minutes a day on domestic duties, compared to their male counterparts who dedicate 2 hours and 16 minutes of their time to these tasks.(ILO, 2016)

During the years when doctors are completing their residency training, residents are assumed to be readily available at any time. Hours are often unpredictable, as shifts can run late. Working long hours is the norm: a survey among internal medicine residents in the Netherlands showed that they spend approximately 9,5 hours in the hospital and continue to do administrative tasks at home for another hour. Schuurman et al., 2018) Combine this with the fact that women still carry most of the weight of domestic duties as well, and work-family is inevitable. Female physicians identify work-family conflict as a major stressor and report the unequal division of domestic labor as an important limiting factor to their career.(Guille et al., 2017)

Sexism and Sexual Harassment

Another barrier that women face that has received a lot of intention in the wake of the *me too* movement is sexism and sexual harassment. Recent literature has revealed sexual harassment to be prominent across the spectrum of academic and professional institutions. The medical world is no exception. In two separate colleges in the United States, nearly half of female medical students reported sexual harassment by faculty or staff members.(Krupat et al., 2000) In the Netherlands, a recent survey revealed that amongst physicians, residents and medical students, 73% report having experienced sexual harassment in the form of jokes and comments, another 60% report inappropriate touching.(Paauw et al., 2018) Most women believe that objecting to sexual harassment or reporting this is a personal and professional liability. Almost 70% of medical students that experience sexual harassment do not take any action.(Paauw et al., 2018)

Research shows that organizations that have a strong hierarchical structure, such as hospitals, are prone to sexual harassment.(Binder et al., 2018) This is reflected by the fact that the majority of sexual harassment that occurs in the medical profession affects female medical students during their clinical rotations, i.e. when they are lowest in rank.(Paauw et al., 2018) In the survey performed in the Netherlands, over 60% of the cases described sexual harassment by a medical specialist.(Paauw et al., 2018) Another factor that can contribute to a culture where sexual harassment is prevalent is the perception that the organization will not take these complaints seriously.(Dzau et al., 2018) The medical world can be a tough and competitive environment, in which medical students and residents are hesitant to show weakness. Working long hours, powering through grueling night shifts and skipping meals in order to get more work done are all part of the routine. Reporting inappropriate behavior is avoided in order not to seem difficult or weak. One woman eloquently describes the shame and fear that came from the sexual harassment that she experienced during her residency:

If any women ever tell you that they had any experience like mine, please tell them to get out of there. Please tell them not to worry about the red flag it might be to transfer residencies, not to worry about potential damage to their reputation, not to worry about ' who would believe [them] anyway', not to worry about appearing weak, not to worry about the old boys' club that lets men cover for each other and makes the woman 'sound crazy,' the opportunities that they may miss in going to a smaller program, unwanted attention that would impinge on their privacy." Although she had not reported the harassment to her mentors – "They judge me based on my work. I don't want them to change the way they perceive me" – she said she "would advise any woman who came to me for advice to do something different from what I actually did. (Jagsi, 2018, paragraph 7)

Lastly, it is important to shed a light on ambient sexual harassment. This is a common phenomenon in male-dominated workspaces or leadership[(Dzau et al, 2018)]. It is a form of sexual harassment that is not directed at a specific person but describes a situation where sexist or crude remarks are made. It is something that rarely receives attention but can prevent women from feeling comfortable in their professional working space. Men openly making derogatory comments about women in general, despite it not being directed to the women present in the room, is a form of exclusion and sexual harassment. It can directly lead to female physicians not choosing for a certain specialization or other opportunities simply because ambient sexual harassment is part of the culture and they do not feel welcome.

Sexism and sexual harassment have great consequences for the person involved. Research has shown that people who have experienced sexual harassment are more likely to leave their field of work, let opportunities pass them by and experience burn-out.(Dzau et al., 2018) The astounding numbers of sexual harassment in the medical field ask for a cultural change.

Gender Bias

A far less visible form of sexism, and often an unconscious one, is gender bias. Gender biases are commonplace ideas that negatively affect women. To this day, stereotypes of whether females or males are supposed to fill a certain profession persist. Female physicians often have to clarify that they are in fact the attending physician and not the nurse, social worker or dietician. Even among colleagues, women are given less recognition for their successes. A recent study at internal medicine grand rounds revealed that significantly fewer females were introduced by their formal titles compared to their male peers.(Files et al, 2017) This implies that female achievements are somehow taken less seriously. Use of language can be a powerful tool in keeping gender bias alive. Omitting a woman's professional title and not doing so when referring to a man, only reinforces the traditional idea that men are more successful in the professional environment.

Amongst the different specialization in the medical field, there are some that are considered more masculine professions than others as reflected by the persistent gender gap. A study conducted amongst surgical trainees, asked participants to rate the prototypical surgeon on masculine traits. Next, they had to rate themselves on the same traits. The study showed that females disidentify with the prototypical surgeon along gender lines. This disidentification has serious consequences. It leads to surgical trainees not identifying with the profession, and increases their desire to leave.

Another gender bias that women face is the competency-likability tradeoff. A well-known case study presented a group of both male and female participants with two candidates who were applying for a job. Both candidates were venture capitalists, former entrepreneurs and networkers. They each joined the board of directors of several prestigious companies. In fact, there was only one difference: one candidate was called Howard and the other called Heidi. The participants judged both candidates as very competent and effective. Howard was also rated as likeable and someone the participants wanted to work with or hire as an employee. Heidi, on the other hand, was not likeable and not someone they wanted to work with. Gender was the only variable in the 'Howard vs. Heidi' case study and clearly showed that high-achieving women are not considered likeable. Instead, they are thought of as self-promoting and arrogant.(Bohnet, 2016) This competency-likeability tradeoff seems to increase as jobs are considered 'typically male', of which there are plenty in the medical profession.

Many identify second-generation gender bias as one of the more important factors that is preventing women from truly advancing to senior positions.(Rifkin, 2015) Second-generation gender bias follows first-generation gender bias, when women were deliberately excluded from the workplace. Second-generation gender biases are unintentional and often unconscious practices. They are a reflection of the values of men who have been in these professional positions from the start and have created the organization culture. An example is the notion that a leader is available at any time of day and geographically mobile. This is a pro-male, pro-childless assumption that only reinforces the status quo. It is the root cause of maternal bias: when women choose to have a family, many assume that they are now less committed to their career.(McKinsey & Company, 2017) A working mother is the opposite image of the traditional concept of a leader, at the time when these organizations were shaped. Organizations or practice groups that are male-dominated at the top are likely to continue to celebrate and promote male definitions of leadership and practice. By doing so, they reinforce second-generation gender bias.

WHAT NEEDS TO CHANGE

In order to truly pursue gender equity, we need to quit relying on time. The fact that more than half of medical students are female, unfortunately does not mean that over time the senior positions in the hospital and in academia will reach the same diversity. It does not mean that female medical students and physicians find themselves in a culture that truly allows them to flourish. Instead they find themselves in an organization where, due to second-generation gender bias, there is an 'anywhere, anytime' mentality that leads to work-family conflict. Due to male-dominant leadership and hierarchical structure of the organization, ambient sexual harassment as well as direct sexual harassment is very common. And yet, research shows that female physicians as well as female leaders are assets to an organization. It is therefore our societal responsibility to make a change in the organizational culture.

Due the nature of the job, medical students and physicians experience a certain degree of personal discomfort. Many accept high levels of stress, periods of little sleep or emotional distress due to suffering of patients or conflicts in care, all for the sake of contributing to good care. These are sometimes small but continuous personal sacrifices that physicians make on a daily basis. Combined with the competitiveness of the medical world, there is a danger that these personal sacrifices become too big in order not to show weakness. It is, therefore, very important that there is a cultural shift within medical organizations where there is room to have conversations about the personal experiences of students, residents and physicians. There needs to be given recognition by the leaders of medical organizations that the culture indeed is male-dominated and that there are barriers in place that pose difficulties for females to advance to top positions. There is a need for leaders to show that issues such as ambient sexual harassment or work-family conflict are legitimate concerns that need to be addressed and changed. The emphasis should not lie on women trying to fit into the mold of the traditional concept of leadership but should shift towards making organizational changes that will allow women to flourish. Offering childcare facilities and incorporating a degree of flexibility in working hours and availability are ways in which organizations can start this movement.

To this day, the medical world has not made gender diversity a true priority. This becomes evident through the vision document as drawn up by the Dutch Association of Medical Specialists, an organization that is made up by representatives of all medical specializations. They have formulated their vision and goals for 2025, including how medical professionals should execute care as well as how medical organizations should move forward. This vision document does not mention gender diversity as part of their agenda. It does, however, engage in gender bias. As they state their vision for the 'modern medical specialist', they consequently refer to the specialist as 'he', 'him', etc.(Dutch Association of Medical Specialists, 2017) There is a complete lack of gender-neutral language. This document illustrates not only a lack of priority, but also a lack of awareness.

A way to accelerate change is for organizations to formulate quotas for gender diversity, by their own initiative or through legislation. In 2015, all universities in the Netherlands stated that by 2020 at least 25% of professors need to be female.(Blik op nieuws, 2018) It is predicted that 10 out of 14 universities will reach this goal. In Europe, legislation passed by the European Parliament requires a certain number of female directors on corporate boards. For example, Norway and France require 40% of board directors to be female, the Netherlands and Italy have quotas set at 30%.(Rifkin, 2015) In the United States, where there is no such legislation, female representation on corporate boards is 17%.(Rifkin, 2015) Setting quotas prevents the pitfall of male leaders only recognizing and promoting masculine leadership behaviors. It is important to realize that legislation on the European or national level only reach larger companies and organizations such as academic hospitals, and will bypass smaller practice groups. Through legislation, smaller hospitals and practice groups should be pushed to strive for the same quotas.

What Women Can Do

One of the positive leadership qualities of females discussed previously in this chapter, is that women are role models. There are plenty of female physicians in place that inspire girls and young women to apply for medical school. However, role models in leadership positions are far scarcer. The women who do reach these positions, should embrace their potential to empower other women. Social media in particular provides an opportunity to easily create women networks and ways of mentoring other women. These networks are becoming prevalent in the United States, but are currently lacking in the Netherlands. Female leaders that talk openly about the barriers that they have overcome and how they have done this, have tremendous potential to help other women advance their careers.

REFERENCES

Association of American Medical Colleges (AAMC). (2016). The state of women in academic medicine: the pipeline and pathways to leadership, 2015-2016. Retrieved from (https:// www.aamc.org/members/gwims/statistics/)

Baumhäkel, M., Müller, U., & Böhm, M. (2009). Influence of gender of physicians and patients on guidelinerecommended treatment of chronic heart failure in a cross-sectional study. *European Journal of Heart Failure*, *11*(3), 299–303. doi:10.1093/eurjhf/hfn041 PMID:19158153

Binder, R., Garcia, P., Johnson, B., & Fuentes-Afflick, E. (2018). Sexual Harassment in Medical Schools. *Academic Medicine*, *93*(12), 1770–1773. doi:10.1097/ACM.0000000000002302 PMID:29794528

Blik op nieuws. (2018). Subsidie zorgt voor toename vrouwelijke hoogleraren. Retrieved from https://www.blikopnieuws.nl/nieuws/269428/subsidie-zorgt-voor-toename-vrouwelijke-hoogleraren.html

Bohnet, I. (2016). *What works: Gender equality by design*. Cambridge, MA: Belknap Press of Harvard University Press. doi:10.4159/9780674545991

Capaciteitsorgaan. (2016). Capaciteitsplan 2016. Retrieved from (https://capaciteitsorgaan.nl/app/uploads/2016/10/2016_10_21-Capaciteitsplan-2016-Deelrapport-4-SG-DEFINITIEF.pdf)

Cooper-Patrick, L., Gallo, J. J., Gonzales, J. J., Vu, H. T., Powe, N. R., Nelson, C., & Ford, D. E. (1999). Race, gender, and partnership in the patient-physician relationship. *Journal of the American Medical Association*, *282*(6), 583–589. doi:10.1001/jama.282.6.583 PMID:10450723

Dutch Association of Medical Specialists. (2017). Medical Specialist 2025. Retrieved from https://www.demedischspecialist.nl/sites/default/files/FMS_visiedoc_MS2025%28eng%29_2017_PL_v02%28lr%29.pdf)

Dzau, V. J., & Johnson, P. A. (2018). Ending Sexual Harassment in Academic Medicine. *The New England Journal of Medicine*, *379*(17), 17. doi:10.1056/NEJMp1809846 PMID:30207831

Files, J. A., Mayer, A. P., Ko, M. G., Friedrich, P., Jenkins, M., Bryan, M. J., ... Hayes, S. N. (2017). Speaker introductions at internal medicine grand rounds: Forms of address reveal gender bias. *Journal of Women's Health*, *26*(5), 413–419. doi:10.1089/jwh.2016.6044 PMID:28437214

GBD. (2017). A fragile world. (2018). *Lancet*, *329*, 1683. doi:10.1016/S0140-6736(18)32858-7

Guille, C., Frank, E., Zhao, Z., Kalmbach, D. A., Nietert, P. J., Mata, D. A., & Sen, S. (2017). Work-family conflict and the sex difference in depression among training physicians. *JAMA Internal Medicine*, *177*(12), 1766–1772. doi:10.1001/jamainternmed.2017.5138 PMID:29084311

International Labour Organization (ILO). (2016). Women at work. Retrieved from https://www.ilo.org/wcmsp5/groups/public/- --dgreports/---dcomm/---publ/documents/publication/wcms_457317.pdf

Jagsi, R. (2018). Sexual harassment in medicine - #MeToo. *The New England Journal of Medicine*, *378*(3), 209–211. doi:10.1056/NEJMp1715962 PMID:29236567

Kaplan, S. H., Greenfield, S., Gandek, B., Rogers, W. H., & Ware, J. E. (1996). Characteristics of Physicians with Participatory Decision-Making Styles. *Annals of Internal Medicine*, *124*(5), 497–504. doi:10.7326/0003-4819-124-5-199603010-00007 PMID:8602709

Kim, C., McEwen, L. N., Gerzoff, R. B., Merrero, D. G., Mangione, C. M., Selby, J. V., & Herman, W. H. (2005). Is physician gender associated with the quality of diabetes care? *Diabetes Care*, *28*(7), 1594–1598. doi:10.2337/diacare.28.7.1594 PMID:15983306

Krupat, E., Rosenkranz, S. L., Yeager, C. M., Barnard, K., Putnam, S. M., & Inui, T. S. (2000). The practice orientations of physicians and patients: The effect of doctor-patient congruence on satisfaction. *Patient Education and Counseling*, *39*(1), 49–59. doi:10.1016/S0738-3991(99)00090-7 PMID:11013547

McKinsey & Company. (2017). Women Matter. Retrieved from (https://www.mckinsey.com/~/media/McKinsey/Featured%20Insights/Women%20matter/Women%20Matter%20Ten%20years%20of%20insights%20on%20the%20importance%20of%20gender%20diversity/Women-Matter-Time-to-accelerate-Ten-years-of-insights-into-gender-diversity.ashx)

Paauw, S. & Kneepkens, E. (2018). #MeToo artsen gaan niet vrijuit. Retrieved from https://www.medischcontact.nl/nieuws/laatste-nieuws/artikel/metoo-artsen-gaan-niet-vrijuit.htm

Paauw, S. & Kneepkens, E. (2018). En hoe zit het eigenlijk met #MeToo bij medici? Retrieved from https://www.medischcontact.nl/arts-in-spe/nieuws/ais-artikel/en-hoe-zit-het-eigenlijk-met-metoo-bij-medici.htm

Peters, K., Ryan, M. K., Haslam, S. A., & Fernandes, H. (2012). To Belong or Not to Belong. Evidence That Women's Occupational Disidentification Is Promoted by Lack of Fit With Masculine Occupational Prototypes. *Journal of Personnel Psychology*, *11*(3), 148–158. doi:10.1027/1866-5888/a000067

Rifkin, G. (2015). Second-generation gender bias. Retrieved from https://www.kornferry.com/institute/second-generation-gender-bias

Roter, D. L., & Hall, J. A. (2004). Physician gender and patient-centered communication: A critical review of empirical research. *Annual Review of Public Health*, *25*(1), 497–519. doi:10.1146/annurev.publhealth.25.101802.123134 PMID:15015932

Schuurman, A., Bos, S., de Wit, K., & de Graaf, R. (2018). Een dag het uit het leven van de zaalarts interne geneeskunde. *Nederlands Tijdschrift voor Geneeskunde*, 162.

Science Guide. (2017). Monitor vrouwen in academie: aantal hougleraren stijgt, aantal bestuurders dealt. Retrieved from https://www.scienceguide.nl/2017/12/monitor-vrouwen-academie/

Tsugawa, Y., Jena, A. B., Figueroa, J. F., Oray, E. J., Blumenthal, D. M., & Jha, A. J. (2017). Comparison of Hospital Mortality and Readmission Rates for Medicare Patients Treated by Male vs Female Physicians. *JAMA Internal Medicine*, *177*(2), 206–213. doi:10.1001/jamainternmed.2016.7875 PMID:27992617

White, M. T., & Welch, K. (2012). Does gender predict performance of novices undergoing Fundamentals of Laparoscopic Surgery (FLS) training? *American Journal of Surgery*, *203*(3), 397–400. doi:10.1016/j.amjsurg.2011.09.020 PMID:22364906

Chapter 6
Sexism in Medical Communication

Yasmin Grant
Imperial College Healthcare NHS Trust, UK

ABSTRACT

Communication is one of the most essential skills of the medical profession, however, it is a tool through which sexism and gender discrimination are promoted and reproduced. There is often the perception in medicine and surgery that gender inequity centres on lifestyle, family responsibilities, and childcare issues. However, this chapter highlights that deeply engrained biases in medical communication still exist, and are perpetrated by institutions and individuals, women included. Awareness of gendered language must be raised and highlighted in order to make a change. It is achievable to speak in gender-neutral ways that are inclusive and precise as to not conjure biased attitudes towards women in medicine. Social change must be pursued at the level of the institution, the cultural structure, and at the interactional level of gender.

INTRODUCTION

Communication is an essential component of medical practice and occurs between doctors, patients and other healthcare professionals. Awareness of its importance has led to incorporation of communication skills assessments as part of medical school curriculums. However, gender bias is one of the obstacles to equity in medical career progression for females and has been shown to be reinforced through gender-subordinating language.

BACKGROUND

The study of gendered language in sociolinguistics is thought to have commenced in the Language and Woman's Place, a paper written by Robin Lakoff in 1973. In this text, Lakoff (1973) states: "Our use of language embodies attitudes as well as referential meanings. The marginality and powerlessness of women is reflected in both ways women are expected to speak, and the ways in which women are spoken of. In

DOI: 10.4018/978-1-5225-9599-1.ch006

appropriate women's speech, strong expression of feeling is avoided (and) expression of uncertainty is favoured. The personal identity of women thus is linguistically submerged; the language works against treatment of women, as serious persons with individual views."

Lakoff's paper was an attempt to provide diagnostic evidence from language use for the inequity between the roles of men and women that had been claimed to exist in society. Nearly 45 years on, women in medicine can relate and identify to this sociological phenomena through the use of language in the workplace. Language and communication is a very powerful system that offers clinicians and patients beliefs in which they can present their attitude to gender.

MAIN FOCUS OF THE CHAPTER

Types of Sexism in Medical Communication

History of Gendered Language

Discrimination of women through language has been present through mechanisms that are deeply embedded in Western culture to sever them from power. The first recorded example of gender inequity through language is at the start of Homer's Odyssey, written almost 3000 years ago. Throughout the epic poem, Telemachus, the son of Odyssey and Penelope is growing up and maturing from boy to man. This is best described by Mary Beard, a well-known British classicist, in her reflection on the gender agenda in Women & Power:

"The process starts in the first book of the poem when Penelope comes down from her private quarters into the great hall of the palace to find a bard performing to throngs of her suitors; he is singing about the difficulties the greek heroes are having in reaching home. She isn't amused, and in front of everyone she asks him to choose another, happier number. At which point young Telemachus intervenes: 'Mother' he says, 'go back into your quarters, and take up your own work, the loom and the distaff... speech will be the business of men, all men, and of me most of all; for mine is the power in this household.' And off she goes, back upstairs."

Beard (2017) comments further upon the significance of the actual words Telemachus uses "When he says speech is 'men's business, the word is muthos – not in the sense that it has come down to us of 'myth'. In Homeric Greek it signals authoritative public speech, not the kind of chatting, prattling or gossip that anyone – women included, or especially women – could do." (p7). This relationship between classic Homeric moment of silencing a women and some of the ways in which women's voices in contemporary medicine are not publicly heard is interesting. Beard (2017) states "Telemachus outburst was just the first case in a long line of largely successful attempts stretching throughout Greek and Roman antiquity, not only to exclude women from public speech but also to parade that exclusion." (p9). Repeated stress throughout ancient literature on the authority of the male voice in contrast to the female was placed. Beard (2017) postulates that this 'muteness' was not just a reflection of women's general disempowerment throughout the classical world such as the absence of the right to vote and limited legal and economic freedom. Moreover, it was a more active and loaded exclusion of women' voices in that public speaking and oratory were merely things that ancient women didn't do: they were exclusive practices and skills that defined masculinity as a gender. Beard adds 'public speech was a – if not the – defining attribute of maleness. Or to quote a well-known Roman slogan, the elite male citizen could be summed up as vir bonus dicendi peritus, 'a good man, skilled in speaking'. A woman speaking in public, was in most circumstances, by definition not a woman'. (p17) This can be represented in modern day medicine, as studies have shown that women are less likely to be invited to give grand rounds in hospital, particularly as an outside speaker (Boiko, 2017). Although these accounts may be distant in time, this representation is not a peculiar ideology in an alienated land. The classical tradition of gendered language has provided us with a powerful template for thinking about oratory in positions of privilege as a medical professional and is an important part of that debate of gender inequity in medicine.

The Development of Sociolinguistics

It is clear that sexism in communication in medicine is also linked to social and political history of feminism and changing attitudes to women. A chronological summary of these movements is first-wave feminism, second-wave feminism and post-modern feminism. First-wave feminism is the movement that focused on getting the right for women to vote, to have property rights and the right to an education. Second-wave feminism is the movement that focused on women's roles and rights within the workplace and in reproductive, sexuality and family issues. Post-modern feminism is the movement that covers different views and beliefs about women's rights and sees women as individuals as well as part of a group. Within post-modern feminism in sociolinguistics, the deficit approach sees male language as the norm and women's language is viewed as deficient to men (Titjen, 2018).

Two other 'Ds' define and judge women's language against that used by men in sociolinguistics, which the authors will explore more fully in this chapter. Dominance theory of language is the belief that the language differences between men and women can be explained by the hierarchical dominances of men in society. Difference theory of language is the belief that men and women have innate differences in the style and function of their speech and writing. Of late, the spotlight has moved to focus on how society influences the language we use and whether individuals 'perform' our gender by demonstrating lexicon and ways of speaking associated with being male or female in a social constructivist approach. (Titjen, 2018)

As discussed previously, Lakoff (1973) adopted an observational approach to linguistic focus on gender in 'Language and Women's Place' looking at a very specific group of women – American, white, middle class and educated – but interpreted her findings as relating to all women. Lakoff labelled women's spoken language as more polite with absences of expressions of strong statements, in an almost complete dissimilarity from men's language. She believed that women's prejudiced the case against themselves by use of language, highlighting their own uncertainty and powerlessness suggestive of inferiority to men. For example, she postulated that women used 'empty' adjectives, a questioning intonating on statements and hedges in their spoken interactions. The use of these choices was all declared to be undermining the authority of women and the content of their speech.

Non-Reciprocal Address

This is of note as perhaps instinctually or due to the way that society has traditionally received females, women doctors may shy away from their title. In settings where professional titles convey expertise and competence, failure to acknowledge the title may influence the perceived expertise and authority of the referenced individual (Files, 2017). In an NY Times article, Dr Julia Baird commented upon the criticism and taunting academics have received for using their titles, while many men who had not received such criticism were baffled (Baird, 2018). Ideally in a professional setting, occupational/professional titles and informal names should be used equally among men and women. Indeed, the manner in which individuals refer to a fellow professional may influence a linguistic expectancy bias, whereby subtle systematic variations in language, such as the use of a professional title or not, can reinforce a lack of equity in the workplace. In fact, a 2017 analysis of introductions of speakers at medical gatherings found that about half of the time a man introduced a woman to the group, he did not use her title, but used it for men more than 70% of the time (Files, 2017). Failure to use a woman's professional title may be a subtle reinforcement that women are of lower status and may be one of the factors contributing to the consistent finding that female physicians are paid less than their male counterparts and more likely to pursue career tracks with historically fewer career opportunities for academic promotion (Carnes et al., 2007; Jagsi et al., 2013; Jena et al., 2016; Mayer et al., 2014; Wright, 2007).

Within popular literature, there are also several anecdotal examples of professional women in medical spheres encountering non-reciprocal address practices, occurring in mixed-gender, professional workplace interaction (Berry, 2014; Grady, 2014; Post, 2015). This echoes Lakoff's (1973) findings of asymmetry used in labels for men and women, creating a power imbalance through the unequal way they address each other. Moreover, at a recent Women in Medicine summit hosted at the University of Calgary, a speaker found that nearly every women in the room had been unprofessionally introduced when speaking at an event – excluding professional titles, roles and expertise (Brown & Ruzycki, 2018). Within professional environments such as hospital-based practice, individuals may assume shared norms of a particular linguistic network or community of practice. Therefore, differences in formality can signal intentional, subconscious and/or institutionalised behaviour (Morand, 1996). At times, our patients can also project their own biases due to historical lack of females in medical and leadership roles. Many of us will be familiar with 'politely correcting our patients when we are mistaken for a nurse, which may chip away at our self-identity and lead us to question whether we really belong 'in the club'. Professor Claire Hopkins of Ear Nose & Throat Surgery in London recounts; 'If I had a pound for every time a patient had asked me (after I had examined the patient, explained the proposed treatment and gone through the consent process for surgery) 'So, will I ever get the meet the Professor Hopkins – is he here?', I would have retired a long time ago.' When undertaking rounds, if there is a man on the team (no matter how junior), the patient will often assume that he is in charge and address questions directly to him.' (Hopkins, 2018).

Lakoff (1973) expands upon these language discrepancies stating 'the ultimate effect of these discrepancies is that women are systematically denied access to power, on the grounds that they are not capable of holding it as demonstrated by their linguistic behaviour'. It could be argued that this reflection written in the 1970's is no longer relevant to today's medical world with the number of women outnumbering men in medical school recruitment. However, it appears that the same issues of voice and gender are still present in medical and surgical communities. In the medical profession, choice of word and forms of address continue reflect conscious or unconscious assumptions about gender roles (Kaatz, Magua, Zimmerman, & Carnes, 2015; Siegling, Eskritt, & Delaney, 2014). In an October 2018 Royal College of Surgeons of England Bulletin article, Professor Claire Hopkins of Ear, Nose & Throat Surgery comments upon the unconscious bias in address received whilst attending an international conference as one of the keynote speakers: 'On the first morning of the meeting, I sat at a conference table with one of the three invited speakers (a man), and I was introduced to others at the table as 'Professor Claire Hopkins, ENT surgeon from London' and identified as one of the guest speakers. I had been sitting next to a senior figure in ENT for most of the morning and he asked where my husband had gone. I was confused – I had left him back home in London looking after the kids. Then the penny dropped; I explained that I was actually attending as a speaker. 'I'm so sorry, I just assumed that as you were sitting next to X, you must be his wife' came the reply. There must have been about 100 other women in the room, many of whom were also sitting next to a man. I'm pretty sure that the vast majority of these women were ENT surgeons. 'So, are you an allergist?' followed. Once the assumption that my role as a wife had been dismissed, my colleague still couldn't entertain the possibility that a woman attending a conference on ENT surgery was most likely to be a surgeon' (Hopkins, 2018). Classicist Mary Beard believes these attitudes, assumptions and prejudices are hardwired into society: not neurologically or genetically but through our culture, language and millennia of our history. It is time to adopt a practice of self-awareness to uncover paradoxical conflicts and pertinent questions about the construction of women's voices in medicine. (Beard, 2017)

Gendered Pronouns and Forms

In Dale Spender's work entitled Man Made Language (1980), language is portrayed as male-centric, encompassing the historical dominance of men in public and private life. Spender's evidence for this is the language rules incorporated in the sixteenth to the eighteenth century by English grammarians. Syntactical regulations have been built in a way that feminine terms derive from the corresponding masculine forms. These rules embodied the ideas that the male pronoun should always come before the female one and the male term should be the generic one used to refer to all people regardless of gender and used as the 'norm'. This perpetuates gender inequity as the influence of language on thought is obligatory or at least habitual; thought is always, or under most circumstances, guided by language' (Harris, 2017). The first 'rule' centres on the custom in English that males tend to be mentioned first. In social terms, perhaps at a conference, convention says that the speaker introduces 'Mr' and 'Miss' in that order. Even now, if you search for address writing advice on the internet, it will offer this version as traditional (and by implication correct) form of English social etiquette. The second 'rule' represents that the male term should be used to represent all human beings regardless of their gender, for example 'That's one small step for man, one giant step for mankind.' (US astronaut Neil Armstrong's speech on landing on the moon in 1969). The masculine nouns and pronouns are often used with a generic function to refer to both sexes (Titjen, 2018). The result is that these lexical forms have compromising effects of making women absent from mental representations, causing readers and speakers to imagine men (Menegatti, 2017). Language therefore has a powerful effect on molding individuals attitudes toward gender and occupation, which has real and measurable consequences for individuals within medicine and society at large.

However, this type of grammatical formatting relating to gender is specific to certain languages. It does not frequent in other European languages such as Hungarian or Turkish (Titjen, 2018). Interestingly, there is a substantial and increasing body of evidence suggesting that societies with gendered language display deeper gender inequality than societies with neutral language. For example, a study of Russian/Spanish speakers conversing in languages with inherent has grammatical gender classifications for objects as masculine/feminine, a higher degree of sexism was displayed compared to English-speaking counterparts. (Thompson, 2014). Moreover, a study by Prewitt-Freilino et al. (2012) illustrated that nations where >70% spoke a gendered language ranked less on Global Gender Gap Index which 'benchmarks national gender gaps on economic, political, education- and health-based criteria' and further economic subscales. This demonstrates that linguistic relativity shapes cultural norms and can reinforce inequality.

Gender Specific Compounding

One way to signify gender lexically is through gender specific compounding. In compounding, two words are put together commonly without being 'male/man' or 'female/woman'. Here two words are put together, most commonly without being 'male/man' or 'female/woman'. It could be suggested that the highlighting of gender may signal circumstances or roles where women are either inferior to their male counterpart, or it is not the norm in society for women to perform this role. It is anecdotally common in medicine that job titles like 'doctor' or 'surgeon might often be preceded by 'lady', therein identifying this role as performed mainly by men (Titjen, 2018). In 2007, Oxford language professor Deborah Cameron published her article 'What Language Barrier?' in The Guardian, exploring the 'difference model' previously mentioned which is still a widespread view (Cameron, 2007). Cameron discusses Simon Baron-Cohen's argument in his book the Essential Difference (2003, 287) that people with a female brain 'make for the most wonderful counsellors, primary school teachers, nurses, carers, therapists, social workers, mediators, group facilitators or personnel staff'. This, he says, is because they have empathy, an attribute he clearly associates with women. It therefore must be questioned by 'doctor' or 'surgeon' is so commonly prefixed with 'lady' in anecdotal circumstances in the field of medicine, a vocation associating with caring and compassion. Lakoff (1973, 59-60) wittily recounts 'To say lady doctor is to be very condescending, it constitutes an insult. For men, there is no such dichotomy. Garbage man or salesman is the only possibility, never garbage gentleman. And of course, since in the professions the male is unmarked, we never have *man (male) doctor." Even Professor Claire Hopkins (2018) of Ear, Nose & Throat surgery states that her own son once requested to be seen by a 'proper doctor' because 'Mummy you're a girl so you must be a nurse' (RCS). Moreover, Dr Sherene Shalhub (2018), a vascular surgeon argues 'the qualifier "female" for a woman who is a surgeon reduces her status. None of my male colleagues aspire to be a male surgeon – everyone simply aspires to be a surgeon. If you are not convinced that using the word "female" before surgeon connotes "less than", consider how language shapes our gender biases. When we refer to a surgeon as a "female surgeon", we are not equating her to "surgeon" – even if only on a subconscious level. Rather, the implication is that she is inferior to other surgeons, who are by default men'.

Gender-specific compounding can also be used to mock or make fun of. The well-known colloquial term 'man flu' is a key example that foregrounds the stereotype of men exaggerating any illness they come down with (Titjen, 2018). However, it is not uncommon for women in the surgical field to receive comments whilst operating such as 'that was a bit of girly cut' when making a conservative incision. Furthermore, it reproduces the content of gender stereotypes according to which women should only display collaborative traits such as warmth, passivity and generosity (Lakoff, 1973). Ideas can also be associated about masculine and feminine qualities with particular words. Corpus linguistics as a research tool has allowed researchers to identify repeated patterns between real-life language examples. In a small-scale study of words, feminine ideas were associated with words such as 'nurturing, 'patience', 'tenderness' and masculine ideas were associated with words such as 'logic', 'focus', 'control' (Beard, 2017). Due to this ambivalence, prejudices against women therefore differ from prejudice against other groups and may appear as implicit and unintentional. Formal recommendations often commend female physicians for 'being part of a team', highlight women's teaching abilities, and refer to 'her training'. Comparatively, male physicians are referenced for 'decisiveness', their research and their 'career' (Chelsea, 2017).

Wood & Eagly (2002) highlighted that favourable collegiate traits describing women are also traits of defense that place a person in a subordinate position (Eagly, 1994). Two forms of sexual prejudice were further elaborated by Glicke and Fiske (1996); hostile and subjectively benevolent. Hostile sexism is demonstrated by a negative interpretation in order to justify male social power and traditional gender roles. Benevolent sexism is more understated, as it depicts women as gentle, in need of men's protection, therefore justifying male superiority and women's subordination. Thus, the favourable traits used to describe women may perpetuate their lower status and strengthen gender inequity (Eagly, 1987). By using these subtle linguistic biases and a different set of characteristics to depict valued masculine (ambitious, assertive) and female (warm, collaborative) behaviours, we predispose 'female surgeons' to face conflicts between their gender roles and professional advancement (Chelsea, 2017).

In an article from the Daily Telegraph, British Journalist Radhika Sanghani (2017) listed 25 words she believed were only ever applied to women. She cites examples of their use in political contexts, campaigns by celebrities and research done by Fortune magazine including abrasive, hormonal, and bolshy. It is worthwhile to reflect upon the conclusions that can be drawn about societal views of women's characteristics and the expression of attitudes to women's traits in medicine through language. In a qualitative study of residents in the US who left their general surgery training programs, the importance of gendered language was emphasised. Former residents recalled being described as 'weak' amidst a culture in surgery where 'strength' is personified as being able to handle anything under any circumstances. In this study a former surgical resident described this as "You cannot be seen as weak in a surgery residency, especially as a woman because they will chew you up and spit you out". (Bongiovanni et al., 2015).

Gender Stereotypes in Language

Again, historical influences can insidiously play a role in this discourse. Deborah Cameron in her book Verbal Hygiene (Cameron, 1995) explained why women's move from domestic roles to the workplace from the 1970s onwards caused a stir. There were long-standing typecasts about the desirable feminine qualities of women's speech and the problem in the workplace, she identified that women's logical and lexical semantics were seen as too feminine to be given due regard. She accounted for this by the fact that through the decades and centuries before, women had not been socialised into speaking in public contexts. She surveyed some of the advice given to women using the myth of Pygmalion – and its dramatic presentation in George Bernard Shaw's play to explore the ways that people seek to 'improve' women. (in the play the main character Professor Higgins, who is a phonetician, bets that he can turn an ordinary London flower girl into a 'lady' by teaching her to speak "properly"). Similarities can be drawn again to sexism in medical mentorship. Shannon Ruzycki in a 2018 article entitled 'The idea that medicine is above sexism is false – and destructive anecdotal comments received by a senior resident who was told she was clinically very good but there was 'just something he couldn't put his finger on' about her that made her 'rough around the edges'. (Brown & Ruzycki, 2018)

However, our understanding of informal collegial interactions of women in medicine remain poorly understood because there is a paucity of research examining their significance. Nevertheless, it has been shown that the evolution of productive professional relationships in the healthcare sphere can positively affect professional development and improve overall employment satisfaction (Sullivan et al., 2012). Furthermore among residents and junior faculty, successful mentorship is associated with improved academic productivity and more confidence for clinical practice, which may reduce the rate of attrition (Palepu et al., 1998; Lis, Wood, Petkova & Shatkin, 2009; McCord et al., 2009).

It follows that the lexical choices of everyday communication reflect the asymmetries of power and status in favour of males, which are attached to their occupational roles. It could be interpreted that women in medicine are still perceived as belonging outside of leadership positions. The system may genuinely want them to get to the inside of the 'club' or may, by various often unconscious biases, cast women as impostors when they make it. Professor Hopkins recounts attending the Royal College of Surgeons after passing her Membership of the Royal College of Surgeons (MRCS) exam; "I remember feeling great pride in walking up the staircase, past all the paintings of former presidents, wondering just for a moment whether I'd ever get my portrait hanging there. As we reached the top of the staircase, the president reached out his hand, extended it to my husband (who was dressed in a pinstriped suit) and congratulated him. His wife shook my hand and said 'You must be very proud of him, dear.' (Hopkins, 2018). Gargiulo et al., female sex was associated with the perception of surgery as an 'old boys club'. (Gargiulo, Hyman & Herbert, 2006). Moreover, Saalwachter et al found that female surgical residents were more likely to concur with the statement "female residents are treated in an inferior manner compared with male residents". (Saalwachter, Freischlag, Sawyer & Sanfey, 2005).

Stereotypes about genders are belief systems that produce expectations about the attributes of men and women in terms of their role and behaviour in society. Historically, male and females have held different social roles (Eagly, Wood, & Diekman, 2000) and women were not admitted to medical school until the 19th century (Bellini et al., 2019). Outside of the medical context, men have been more likely to be involved in tasks that require strength and the possibility of being away from the home, whereas women have been more likely to engage in homemaking and family responsibilities such as raising children. This results in the perception of males to be agentic, specifically active, independent and firm, whereas women are expected to communal, namely warm, kind and benevolent. It can be deduced that the content of gender stereotypes has been established by the characteristics and activities required by individuals of each sex in their sex-typical occupations and family roles: Women are expected to engage in a feminine gender role that reflects communal qualities but not agentic ones (Wood & Eagly, 2002).

Sexism in Written Communication

Of note, written forms of communication in medicine also demonstrate clear gender bias. A study performed in 2003 examined over 3000 letters of recommendation for medical faculty at a large American medical school in the mid-1990s were found to systematically differ between male and female applicants. Using methods from corpus and discourse analysis, discrepancies in the percentages with doubt raisers (an extended category of negative language, often associated with apparent commendation, and in frequency of mention of status terms. Moreover, the most common semantically grouped possessive phrases referring to female and male applicants ('her teaching', 'his research') reinforced gender schema that tended to portray women as teachers and students, and men as researchers and professionals (Trix & Psenka, 2004). Interestingly, a BMJ article entitled 'sexism in medical writing' recounted a reader who wrote to complain about a published article that used he for consultants and she for secretaries. However, by no means are all consultants men and all secretaries female. The staff editor, Sue Burkhart, provided further examples of sexist written language published in the medical sphere including "Research scientists often neglect their wives and children" and "It's the great secret of doctors, known only to their wives… that most things get better by themselves". (Burkhart,1987). In the attempt to neutralise gender biased language, Burkhart offers advice given in the American Psychological Association's Publication Manual: "Help the reader focus on the content of your paper by avoiding language that may cause irritation, flights of thought, or even momentary interruptions… [such as] linguistic devices and constructions that might imply sexual, ethnic or other kinds of bias… Language that reinforces sexism can spring from subtle errors in research design, inaccurate interpretation or imprecise word choices." (as cited in Burkhart, 1987).

Gendered Metaphors

Moreover, there must be cognisance that the use of shared metaphors of female access to medicine, for example 'pull their weight like a man', underlines female exteriority (Bellini et al., 2019). An audit published in 1992 of sex bias in the BMJ identified all medical staffing issues described as problems of medical 'manpower'. It further comments upon the strongly argued view that sexist language tends to ascribe more in power to men than women and contributes to inequalities of opportunity between the sexes (Usherwood, 1992). Women in surgery are seen as breaking down barriers, or alternatively as taking something to which they are not quite entitled and 'it is through language that we [women] come to know our subordinate place in the world' (Cameron, 1985). Accounts in a women's surgery working group stated 'Patients are often shocked that I will be doing their operation, and I have led ward rounds where the patients have talked to my tall male (foundation doctor) and not me'. Another respondent reported 'Patients are extraordinarily sexist for example, patients have walked into a consulting room and said to me 'I thought I would be seeing a doctor at least' before I had time to introduce myself. I am 34 and been a doctor for 10 years'. (Bellini et al., 2019). This gender bias is also reflected in other professional jobs as captured by a headline in The Times in early 2017. Above an article reporting on the possibility that women might soon gain the positions of the Metropolitan Police commissioner, chair of the BBC Unitary Board and bishop of London, it read: 'Women Prepare for a Power Grab in Church, Police and BBC' (Simpson & Zeffman, 2017). Interestingly, it was only Cressida Dick, the commissioner of the Met, that was appointed to a leadership position. Medical professionals must create the change needed to look a lot more carefully at our cultural assumptions and ingrained social prejudices against women's places in this profession.

Gendered Style of Language

The aforementioned dominance approach took place within the historical and political context of second-wave feminism, which had a central goal of eradicating gender inequality. This approach understands men as considered to be positioned above women because of their social and political ability to achieve their purpose. From a language perspective, men were seen as using syntax as a means of reinforcing or maintaining their power in conversations, and women were viewed as asserting their lack of power through their language choices (Titjen, 2018). Differences in interpersonal language style of women compared with men are well documented outside of medicine. One of the most famous of studies was Don Zimmerman's and Candace West's(1987) college campus study, which found that men were responsible for 96% of the interruptions in conversations occurring between men and women. Men's dominance seems from these to lie in their conversational management – i.e. speaking more, having longer turns and, in conversations with women, being interrupted less and interrupting more. Dale Spender (1980), in Man Made Language, drew further regard to this verbal dominance by interpreting women's silence as a form of oppression. However, linguists also saw other semantic rules as asserting dominance, which were more nuanced than men interrupting women in conversation. Of note, Deborah Tannen (1992) was one of the most influential linguistic academics whose work represented the difference view. She argued that male-female conversation could be viewed as a form of miscommunication in which women were more inclined to be obliging in conversation, and men as more competitive. Tannen coined the term ‘genderlect’ to describe the different language use of men and women.

Judith Baxter’s (2014) concept of double-voicing explores further the concept of gender identity in the workplace. It is suggested that women are more conscious than men that the people they are interacting with may have differing agendas and accordingly alter their own language to reflect this language. Real-life examples from her research include ‘I realise I am being over-simplistic as usual but….’ and ‘I am no expert like the rest of you but….’. Baxter expands by offering categories to describe the various forms that double-voicing which might take place including anticipatory and mitigating. With anticipatory double-voicing a speaker demonstrates in their language that they have anticipated the response others and attempts to dilute or deflect the criticism they expect. With mitigating double-voicing an individual efforts to build solidarity but may come across as hesitant or defensive. Baxter’s workplace research shows that women are more prone to double-voice than their male counterparts and she concludes that women use this as a method of gaining approval.

However, positive effects of female communication have been demonstrated in patient-physician relationships. A meta-analysis of physician gender effects in medical communication in 2002 found that female physicians were found to engage in communication relating to the broader realm of psychosocial issues, greater use of emotional language and more active enlistment of patient input. As female physicians ask more psychosocial questions, it may be that this communication approach promotes higher disclosure of both psychosocial and biomedical information (Roter, Hall, & Aoki, 2002). Moreover, an analysis by Henderson and Weisman of the Commonwealth Survey of patient-reported screening and counseling services concluded that female physicians provided more preventive counseling to both their male and female patients (Henderson & Weisman, 2001). This represents a positive benefit in the fostering of the patient-clinician relationship and medical dialogue (Hall, Irish, Roter, Ehrlich, & Miller, 1994).

Lastly, bias is not at the discretion of men alone. Women also display gender biases towards other women, a phenomenon called internalised misogyny, whilst holding other women to a double standard. This discrimination leads to further isolation of women in leadership positions (Shalhub, 2018). Gender inequity also affects our ability to work with other healthcare professionals. Dr Andrea Christopher, a physician in Boise, Idaho noted that nurses were more likely to assist male colleagues saying, ‘I would put in orders, and the male residents would put in orders, and theirs would be done and mine not’ (Badham, 2018). Moreover, a study in a Canadian hospital found that in simulated settings nurses were more willing to defer to male physicians and were more hostile to female clinicians (Zelek & Phillips, 2003). The insidious consequence is that people perceive gender bias in language from women and men as normative and enact gender discrimination by simply following communication rules (Ng, 2007). However, it is time to shift our narrative from the pervasive gendered language in professional conversation, casual discourse and social media.

SOLUTIONS AND RECOMMENDATIONS

More recently, sociolinguistics distanced themselves from the ‘three Ds’ of gender study (deficit, dominance and difference) by taking a different approach of social constructivism which acknowledges the importance of individual differences amongst men and women. This had a profound influence of ways of thinking about gender in contemporary linguistics, rather than simply setting the genders against each other. One of the key research focuses has been on how people within groups use language, calling upon social network theory and the concept of communities of practice. This approach focuses on an interpreted identity that is socially constructed by the shared nature of our interactions which are not fixed. The medical workplace is therefore an important social environment to explore gender. (Titjen, 2018).

Language Neutralization

Lesley Milroy characterised a theory called 'a web of ties' in which a social network is formed by formal and informal relationships, which can be applied to medical practice, Patterns of linguistic use emerge and evolve characterising the speech behaviour of this group as highlighted above. Jean Lave's and Etienne Wenger's (1991) community of practice model described how people come together for a particular purpose or passion to establish ways of doing things and ways of interacting to achieve their shared purpose as seen in world of medicine. Wenger further developed this idea into three crucial areas of mutual engagement, a joint negotiated enterprise and a shared repertoire (Wenger, 2000). From a gender point of view, other researchers such as Penelope Eckhert and Sally McConnel-Ginet (1992) took the idea of a community of practice to investigate how the language-gender interface is produced and reproduced within different communities. They suggested that the individuals belong to multiple communities of practice but that speakers develop vernacular patterns as they engage in activity in various communities that they are a part of. However, they argued that our gender may also inform which groups we become members of as communities of practice also produce gender arrangements and gender language differentiation. They also proposed that participation levels with the community of practice might be impacted by the different roles and status given to women and men within the group. As women have moved into medicine and occupational choices have grown within the profession, it is clear that language is adapting however perhaps not at the necessary rate. There is still more scope for change in terms of the words that we associated with gender and the meanings and beliefs behind these. The fact that there have not significant shifts in usage may suggest that changes to social reality are not reflected in the language we use. There needs to be more awareness of the production of sex biased language behaviours in communities of practice, with shifts to ensure there is no longer a male superiority whilst recognising the modern complexities of gender identity. This is supported by sociolinguist Judith Butler's book (2006) Gender Trouble which raises the argument of gender as a performance. She argues that we are constantly engaged in constructing gender. Here, Butler declares that gender is something we do and is not what we are. Professional societies should enact a policy of ensuring gender neutral language is used in all communications in the wider health sector in all nations to ensure masculine forms are removed altogether.

Gender Equality Charters

Medicine has now been a career path for women in the western world for over a century, with women entering the profession in equal numbers for many years. However, many women fail to progress and earn the same recognition or renumeration as their male counterparts in the US (Poorman, 2018). A study in 2016 found that only 16% of deans and interim deans are women in 136 US medical schools are female (Schor, 2018). An Association of American Medical Colleges report in 2013-2014 found that women in academic medicine have received only 30% of new tenured positions. The slowly shrinking gender disparity of women in leadership positions in medicine is held up as a marker of success however, more emphasis is required to be placed on linguistic habits. As stated by Dr Julie Silver, associate professor at Harvard Medical School, "medicine should be leading the way" in gender equity (Poorman, 2018). The Athena SWAN is one such initiative which has tackled the unequal representation of women in science, technology, medicine and mathematics (STEMM). It aims to address the high loss rate of women in science and to foster commitment and action from all levels of an organisation to address gender inequalities. The charter received a significant boost in 2011 when the UK Chief Medical Officer, Professor Dame Sally Davies, announced that the National Institute for Health Research (NIHR) would only shortlist medical schools for Biomedical Research Centre (BRC) and Unit (BRU) funding if the associate academic school holds a Silver Athena SWAN award. This was later expanded to include Patient Safety Research Centre funding in 2012. In 2016, in the first round of funding to be awarded since the Chief Medical Officer's announcement, the Department of Health awarded £816 million to 20 BRC's, all of which are associated with a Silver Athena SWAN award-holding academic unit (Department of Health and Social Care UK, 2016). In a recent event attended by the author at the Imperial College Department of Surgery and Cancer annual Athena Swan lecture, Professor Dame Sally Davies commented on the extreme resistance received from senior male academics in high institutions in the UK to the introduction of this charter. Similar international health research funding associations and bodies should aspire to support equality for women in science and release action plans to ensure the inclusion of women in science tackling attitudes and cultures across the organisation. However, diversity at management and policy-making levels may be required to institute this change.

Self-Awareness and Mentorship

Thus modifications to address biases in medical educators that facilitate collegial professional relationships which inherently involve language behaviours should be encouraged. Examples may include the creation of formalized mentorship programs for junior registrars/residents and consultants/attendings. Pairing residents with a mentor of shared female sex may promote an environment of comfort and assist in the identification of residents' professional and personal needs. Establishing this program may be difficult for female or minority residents given the relative paucity of female and minority faculty in surgery. Among junior and senior residents, mentorship may provide an opportunity to receive experience-based advice in a non-threatening setting. In addition, scheduled social activities are suggested. Such informal events assist in neutralising the power differential among registrars of different sexes and between residents and attendings. Speciality-specific team events at the conclusion of resident rotations may develop working relationships and promote a cohesive team dynamic. (Sullivan et al., 2012). Female leaders such as Dr Julie Silver and Dr Luanne Thorndyke at the University of Massachusetts Medical School are tackling discrimination by promoting and mentoring women and minorities in medicine. This requires institutional support and Massachussets Medical School now have a female faculty of 26%, compared to 17% at Harvard Medical School (Poorman, 2018). A national initiative by the Royal College of Surgeons of England is also dedicated to encouraging and enabling women to fulfill their surgical career ambitions to facilitate changes in attitudes and practices. The collaboration also endeavors to ensure female surgeons are represented positively in the media and to as wide an audience as possible (Women in Surgery, n.d.).

It has been demonstrated that biases find their way into our language. The language we speak and hear physically alters our neural connections including the areas related to how we experience reality and link words to ideas. As such, our language not only articulates our world-view, it also influences our perception of the world. Because culture is grounded in language, discerning our language can affect our culture. Although the use of gender-fair linguistic expressions can effectively prevent these negative consequences and promote gender equality, there are even more implicit forms of gender bias in language that are difficult to suppress. By choosing terms of abstraction, people can affect the designations of the receiver in a way that is consistent with their stereotypical beliefs. Linguistic abstraction, thus, is a resource used to represent women in a subtle, less advantageous way and promotes gender discrimination without meaning to discriminate or even the awareness that this linguistic habit has discriminatory results. In order to reduce gender bias, it is therefore necessary to change people's linguistic habits by increasing mindfulness of the advantages of gender-fair expressions in medicine as a whole. (Menegatti, 2017)

CONCLUSION

There is often the perception in surgery and medicine as a whole that gender inequity centres on lifestyle, family responsibilities and childcare issues. However, this chapter highlights that verbal communication is one of the most powerful tools through which gender inequity can be perpetrated throughout the medical profession. The insidious consequence of sexism in medical communication is that people perceive gender bias in language as normative and enact gender discrimination by following historically ordained communication rules (Ng, 2007). In the current climate, it is unlikely that faculty or patients intentionally and consciously undertake linguistic sexism. Public discussion opens a forum for gender bias awareness supported by objective and subjective data which will benefit the profession as a whole.

Mentoring schemes are significantly enabling, however, they form only part of the solution to tackling gender biases. If women wish to be empowered in medicine as a gender, and not just in the form of a few single-minded individuals, systems and institutions must think authentically about how we speak and the words that are used. Mary Beard (2017, 70) states in her book on Woman & Power; "The point is simple but important: as far back as we can see in Western history there is a radical separation – real, cultural and imaginary – between women and power."

It is clear that deeply engrained biases in medical communication still exist, and are perpetrated by institutions and individuals, women included. of gendered language must be raised and highlighted in order to make a change. In this day and age, medicine celebrates autonomy and empathy in medicine and both clinical and research outcomes are "patient-centered." These were unfamiliar concepts when first introduced into our vocabulary and are now deeply embedded in our professional conduct. This signals that we can confront and exploit the status quo of gender inequity in medical language.

Women in medicine have come so far with the number of female medical graduates equaling if not outnumbering men, but nonetheless those affected by sexism in medical communication should continue to share these experiences to remind us how far we still have to go. Doctors who are female should be encouraged that the battle is not yet won and must work hard at their specialty to ensure that all females who enter it are given equitable access and respect through appropriate communication. It is achievable to speak in gender-neutral ways that are inclusive and precise as to not conjure biased attitudes towards women in medicine. Social change must be pursued at the level of the institution, the cultural structure and at the interactional level of gender.

REFERENCES

Association of American Medical Colleges. (2013-2014). The State of Women in Academic Medicine. The Pipeline and Pathways to Leadership. Retrieved from https://members.aamc.org/eweb/upload/The%20 State%20of%20Women%20in%20Academic%20Medicine%202013-2014%20FINAL.pdf

Badham, V. (2018). Think sexism in medicine is unique to Japan? Think again. *The Guardian.* Retrieved from https://www.theguardian.com/commentisfree/2018/aug/13/think-sexism-in-medicine-is-unique-to-japan-think-again

Baird, J. (2018). Women, Own Your 'Dr' Titles. The New York Times. Retrieved from https://www.nytimes.com/2018/06/28/opinion/women-dont-back-down-online.html

Baron-Cohen, S. (2012). *The Essential Difference: men, women and extreme male brain*. London, UK: Penguin.

Baxter, J. (2014). *Double-voicing at work. Power, gender and linguistic expertise*. Basingstoke, UK: Palgrave Macmillan. doi:10.1057/9781137348531

Beard, M. (2017). *Women and Power*. London, UK: Profile Books.

Bellini, M. I., Graham, Y., Hayes, C., Zakeri, R., Parks, R., & Papalois, V. (2019). A woman's place is in theatre: Women's perceptions and experiences of working in surgery from the Association of Surgeons of Great Britain and Ireland women in surgery working group. *BMJ Open*, *9*(1). doi:10.1136/bmjopen-2018-024349 PMID:30617103

Berry, C. A. (2014). They Call Me Dr. Berry. *New York Times.* Retrieved from https://www.nytimes.com/2014/11/02/opinion/sunday/they-call-me-doctor-berry.html

Boiko, J. R., Anderson, A. J. M., & Gordon, R. A. (2017). Representation of women among academic grand rounds speaker. *JAMA Internal Medicine*, *177*(5), 722–724. doi:10.1001/jamainternmed.2016.9646 PMID:28264094

Bongiovanni, T., Yeo, H., Sosa, J. A., Yoo, P. S., Long, T., Rosenthal, M., ... Nunez-Smith, M. (2015). Attrition from surgical residency training: Perspectives from those who left. *American Journal of Surgery*, *210*(4), 648–654. doi:10.1016/j.amjsurg.2015.05.014 PMID:26238074

Brown, A. & Ruzycki, S. (2018). The idea that medicine is above sexism is false – and destructive. Healthy Debate. Retrieved from https://healthydebate.ca/opinions/sexism-in-medicine

Burkhart, S. (1987). Sexism in medical writing. *British Medical Journal, 295,* 19-26. Retrieved from https://www.ncbi.nlm.nih.gov/pmc/articles/PMC1257479/

Butler, J. (2006). *Gender Trouble*. London, UK: Routledge.

Cameron, D. (1985). *Feminism and linguistic theory*. London, UK: Macmillan. doi:10.1007/978-1-349-17727-1

Cameron, D. (1995). *Verbal Hygiene*. London, UK: Routledge.

Cameron, D. (2007) What language barrier? *The Guardian*. Retrieved from https://www.theguardian.com/world/2007/oct/01/gender.books

Carnes, M., & Bland, C. (2007). Viewpoint: A challenge to academic health centers and the National Institutes of Health to prevent unintended gender bias in the selection of clinical and translational science award leaders. *Academic Medicine*, *82*(2), 202–206. doi:10.1097/ACM.0b013e31802d939f PMID:17264704

Department of Health and Social Care UK. (2016). New £816 million investment in health research. Retrieved from https://www.gov.uk/government/news/new-816-million-investment-in-health-research on 22/07/2019

Eagly, A. (1987). *Sex differences in social behaviour: A social-role interpretation*. Hillsdale, NJ: Lawrence Erlbaum.

Eagly, A., & Mladinic, A. (1994). Are people prejudiced against women? Some answers from research on attitudes, gender stereotypes, and judgments of competence. *European Review of Social Psychology*, *5*(1), 1–35. doi:10.1080/14792779543000002

Eagly, A., Wood, W., & Diekman, A. B. (2000). Social role theory of sex differences and similarities: A current appraisal. In T. Eckes & H. M. Traunter (Eds.), *The developmental social psychology of gender*. Mahwah, NJ: Lawrence Erlbaum.

Eckert, P. & McConnell-Ginet, S. (1992). Communities of practice: where language, gender and power all live. In K. Hall, M. Bucholtz, & B. Moonwoman (Eds.), *Locating Power, Proceedings of the 1992 Berkeley Women and Language Conference*. Berkeley, CA: Berkeley Woman and Language Group. Retrieved from https://web.stanford.edu/~eckert/PDF/Communitiesof.pdf

<eref>Siegling, A., Eskritt, M., & Delaney, M. (2014). A Preliminary Investigation into Effects of Linguistic Abstraction on the Perception of Gender in Spoken Language. Current Psychology, 33, 479–500. doi:10.100712144-014-9224-

Files, J. A., Mayer, A. P., Ko, M. G., Jenkins, M., Bryan, M. J., & Vegunta, S. (2017). Speaker Introductions at Internal Medicine Grand Rounds: Forms of Address Reveal Gender Bias. *Journal of Women's Health*, *26*(5), 413–419. doi:10.1089/jwh.2016.6044 PMID:28437214

Gargiulo, D. A., Hyman, N. H., & Hebert, J. C. (2006). Women in surgery: Do we really understand the deterrents? *Archives of Surgery*, *141*(4), 405–408. doi:10.1001/archsurg.141.4.405 PMID:16618901

Glick, P. & Fiske, S. T. (1996). The ambivalent sexism inventory: differentiating hostile and benevolent sexism. *Personality and social psychology, 70*(3), 491-512. doi:10.1037/0022-3514.70.3.491

Grady, D. (2014). Carolyn Kaelin, Breast Cancer Surgeon Patient Advocate and Patient, Dies at 54. *New York Times*. Retrieved from https://www.nytimes.com/2015/08/10/us/carolyn-kaelin-breast-cancer-surgeon-dies-at-54.html

Hall, J. A., Irish, J. T., Roter, D. L., Ehrlich, C. M., & Miller, L. H. (1994). Gender in medical encounters: an analysis of physician and patient communication in a primary care setting. *Health Psychology,* 13, 384-293. Retrieved from https://www.ncbi.nlm.nih.gov/pubmed/7805632

Harris, C. A., Blencowe, N., & Telem, D. A. (2017). What is in a pronoun?: Why Gender-Fair Language Matters. *Annals of Surgery, 266*(6), 932–933. doi:10.1097/SLA.0000000000002505 PMID:28902666

Henderson, J. T. & Weisman, C. S. (2001). Physician gender effects on preventive screening and counseling: an analysis of male and female patients' health care experience. *Medical Care, 39,* 1281-1292. Retrieved from https://www.ncbi.nlm.nih.gov/pubmed/11717570

Hopkins, C. (2018). Confronting unconscious bias. *Royal College of Surgeons Bulletin, 100*(8), 321–323. doi:10.1308/rcsbull.2018.321

Jagsi, R., Griffith, K. A., Stewart, A., Sambuco, D., DeCastro, R., & Ubel, P. A. (2013). Gender differences in salary in a recent cohort of earlycareer physician-researchers. *Academic Medicine, 88*(11), 1689–1699. doi:10.1097/ACM.0b013e3182a71519 PMID:24072109

Jena, A. B., Olenski, A. R., & Blumenthal, D. M. (2016). Differences in Physician Salary in US Public Medical Schools. *Journal of the American Medical Association Internal Medicine, 176,* 1294–1304. doi:10.1001/jamainternmed.2016.3284 PMID:27400435

Kaatz, A., Magua, W., Zimmerman, D. R., & Carnes, M. (2015). A quantitative linguistic analysis of National Institutes of Health R01 application critiques from investigators at one institution. *Academic Medicine, 90*(1), 69–75. doi:10.1097/ACM.0000000000000442 PMID:25140529

Lakoff, R. (1963). Language and Woman's Place. *Language in Society, 2*(1), 45–80. doi:10.1017/S0047404500000051

Lave, J., & Wenger, E. (1991). *Situated learning legitimate peripheral participation.* Cambridge, UK: Cambridge University Press. doi:10.1017/CBO9780511815355

Lis, L. D., Wood, W. C., Petkova, E., & Shatkin, J. (2009). Mentoring in psychiatric residency programs: A survey of chief residents. *Academic Psychiatry, 33*(4), 307–312. doi:10.1176/appi.ap.33.4.307 PMID:19690111

Mayer, A. P., Blair, J. E., Ko, M. G., Hayes, S. N., Chang, Y. H., Caubet, S. L., & Files, J. A. (2014). Gender distribution of U.S. medical school faculty by academic track type. *Academic Medicine, 89*(2), 312–317. doi:10.1097/ACM.0000000000000089 PMID:24362384

McCord, J. H., McDonald, R., Sippel, R. S., Leverson, G., Mahvi, D. M., & Weber, S. M. (2009). Surgical career choices: The vital impact of mentoring. *The Journal of Surgical Research, 155*(1), 136–141. doi:10.1016/j.jss.2008.06.048 PMID:19041099

Menegatti, M., & Rubini, M. (2017). *Gender bias and sexism in language.* Oxford Research Encyclopaedias. doi:10.1093/acrefore/9780190228613.013.470

Milroy, L. (1980). Language and social networks. Oxford, UK: Basil Blackwell, University Park Press.

Morand, D. A. (1996). What's in a name? An Exploration of the Social Dynamics of Form of Address in Organizations. *Management Communication Quarterly, 9*(4), 422–451. doi:10.1177/0893318996009004003

Ng, S. H. (2007). Language-based discrimination: Blatant and subtle forms. *Journal of Language and Social Psychology, 26*(2), 106–122. doi:10.1177/0261927X07300074

Palepu, A., Friedman, R. H., Barnett, R. C., Carr, P. L., Ash, A. S., Szalacha, L., & Moskowitz, M. A. (1998). Junior faculty members' mentoring relationships and their professional development in U.S. medical schools. *Academic Medicine, 73*(3), 318-323. Retrieved from https://www.ncbi.nlm.nih.gov/pubmed/9526459

Poorman, E. (2018). Why does America still have so few female doctors? *The Guardian*. Retrieved from https://www.theguardian.com/commentisfree/2018/jan/14/why-are-there-still-so-few-female-doctors

Post, E. (2015). Professional Titles. *Emily Post Etipedia*. Retrieved from www.emilypost.com/communication-andtechnology/ social-names-and-titles/774-professional-titles

Prewitt-Freilino, J. L., Caswell, T. A., & Laakso, E. K. (2012). The gendering of language. A comparison of gender equality in countries with gendered, natural gender, and genderless languages. *Sex Roles*, *66*(3-4), 268–281. doi:10.100711199-011-0083-5

Roter, D. L., Hall, J. A., & Aoki, T. (2002). Physician gender effects in medical communication. *Journal of the American Medical Association*, *288*(6), 7–756. doi:10.1001/jama.288.6.756 PMID:12169083

Saalwachter, A. R., Freischlag, J. A., Sawyer, R. G., & Sanfey, H. A. (2005). The training needs and priorities of male and female surgeons and their trainees. *Journal of the American College of Surgeons*, *201*(2), 199–205. doi:10.1016/j.jamcollsurg.2005.03.016 PMID:16038816

Sanghani, R. (2017). Feisty, frigid and frump: 25 words we only use to describe women. *The Telegraph*. Retrieved from https://www.telegraph.co.uk/women/life/ambitious-frigid-and-frumpy-25-words-we-only-use-to-describe-wom/

Schor, N. F. (2018). The Decanal Divide: Women in Decanal Roles at US Medical Schools. *Academic Medicine*, *93*(2), 237–240. doi:10.1097/ACM.0000000000001863 PMID:28834842

Shalhub, S. (2018). Stop calling me a "female" surgeon. *Op-Med*. Retrieved from https://opmed.doximity.com/articles/stop-calling-me-a-female-surgeon-a2c87f9749f3

Simpson, J., & Zeffman, H. (2017). Women prepare for a power grab in church, police and BBC. The Times. Retrieved from https://www.thetimes.co.uk/article/women-prepare-for-a-power-grab-in-church-police-and-bbc-cwgsrwtwm</eref>

Spender, D. (1980). *Man Made Language*. London, UK: Pandora Press.

Sullivan, M. C., Bucholz, E. M., Yeo, H., Roman, S. A., Bell, R. H., & Sosa, J. A. (2012). "Join the Club" Effect of resident and attending social interactions on overall satisfaction among 4390 general surgery residents. *Archives of Surgery*, *147*(5), 408–414. doi:10.1001/archsurg.2012.27 PMID:22785631

Tannen, D. (1992). *You Just Don't Understand: Women and Men in Conversation*. London, UK: Virago.

Thompson, A. J. (2014). Linguistic relativity: Can gendered languages present sexist atttitudes? *Linguistics*.

Titjen, F. (2018). *Language and Gender*. Cambridge, UK: Cambridge University Press.

Trix, F., & Psenka, C. (2003). Exploring the color of glass: Letters of recommendation for female and male medical faculty. *Discourse & Society*, *14*(2), 191–220. doi:10.1177/0957926503014002277

Usherwood, T. (1992). Sex bias in the BMJ: an audit. *BMJ,* 304, 880-1. Retrieved from https://www.bmj.com/content/304/6831/880

Wenger, E. (2000). *Communities of practice: learning, meaning and identity*. Cambridge, UK: Cambridge University Press.

West, C. & Zimmerman, D. (1987). Doing Gender. *Gender & Society, 1*(2), 125-151. Retrieved from https://www.jstor.org/stable/189945?seq=1#page_scan_tab_contents

Women in Surgery. (n.d.). Royal College of Surgeons. Retrieved from https://www.rcseng.ac.uk/careers-in-surgery/women-in-surgery/

Wood, W. & Eagly, A. (2002). A cross-cultural analysis of the behavior of women and men: implications for the origins of sex differences. *Psychological bulletin, 128*(5), 699-727. Retrieved from https://www.ncbi.nlm.nih.gov/pubmed/12206191

Wright, A. L., Ryan, K., St Germain, P., Schwindt, L., Sager, R., & Reed, K. L. (2007). Compensation in academic medicine: Progress toward gender equity. *Journal of General Internal Medicine, 22*, 1398–1402. doi:10.100711606-007-0329-7 PMID:17694417

Zelek, B., & Phillips, S. (2003). Gender and power: Nurses and doctors in Canada. *International Journal for Equity in Health, 2*(1), 1–11. doi:10.1186/1475-9276-2-1 PMID:12605720

ADDITIONAL READING

Bruckmüller, S., Hegarty, P., & Abele, A. E. (2012). Framing gender differences: Linguistic normativity affects perceptions of power and gender stereotypes. *European Journal of Social Psychology, 42*(2), 210–218. doi:10.1002/ejsp.858

Douglas, K. M., & Sutton, R. M. (2003). Effects of communication goals and expectancies on language abstraction. *Journal of Personality and Social Psychology, 84*(4), 682–696. doi:10.1037/0022-3514.84.4.682 PMID:12703643

Gaucher, D., Friesen, J., & Kay, A. C. (2011). Evidence that gendered wording in job advertisements exists and sustains gender inequality. *Journal of Personality and Social Psychology, 101*(1), 109–128. doi:10.1037/a0022530 PMID:21381851

Heilman, M. E., & Eagly, A. H. (2008). Gender stereotypes are alive, well, and busy producing workplace discrimination. *Industrial and Organizational Psychology: Perspectives on Science and Practice, 1*(4), 393–398. doi:10.1111/j.1754-9434.2008.00072.x

Maass, A., Suitner, C., & Merkel, E. (2013). Does political correctness make (social) sense? In J. P. Forgas, J. Laszlo, & O. Vincze (Eds.), *Social cognition and communication* (pp. 331–346). New York: Psychology Press.

Madera, J. M., Hebl, M. R., & Martin, R. C. (2009). Gender and letters of recommendation for academia: Agentic and communal differences. *The Journal of Applied Psychology*, *94*(6), 1591–1599. doi:10.1037/a0016539 PMID:19916666

Silveira, K. (1980). Generic masculine words and thinking. In C. Kramarae (Ed.), *The voices and words of women and men* (pp. 165–178). Oxford, United Kingdom: Pergamon.

Stahlberg, D., Braun, F., Irmen, L., & Sczesny, S. (2007). Representation of the sexes in language. In K. Fiedler (Ed.), *Social communication* (pp. 163–187). New York, US: Psychology Press.

KEY TERMS AND DEFINITIONS

Feminism: The promotion of female rights and advocacy of equality of the sexes.

Gender Bias: Prejudice towards one gender.

Gendered Language: Language that has a bias towards a particular gender.

Gender Inequity: The unequal treatment of women and men.

Medicine: The occupation of the practice of promoting and restoring health through identification and treatment of illness.

Sociolinguistics: Study of the language differences between two sexes.

Surgery: The occupation of the treatment of tissues of the body by incision or manipulation.

Chapter 7
Gender Equity in Medical Leadership

Lizzie Chandra
Health Education England Yorkshire and the Humber, UK

Candice L. Downey
University of Leeds, UK

Hafdis S. Svavarsdottir
University of Leeds, UK

Helen Skinner
Health Education England Yorkshire and the Humber, UK

Alastair L. Young
Leeds Teaching Hospitals Trust, UK

ABSTRACT

Female representation in medicine is increasing, however women make up only a small percentage of senior roles in the NHS. Only 36% of consultants are female with wide variation between specialties ranging from 12% of surgeons to over half of paediatricians, gynaecologists, and directors of public health. Women comprise 77% of the NHS workforce and account for 44% of chief executives of all NHS Trusts and 47% of executive directors. This chapter analyses the role of women as leaders within the medical world and compares the representation of women in senior leadership roles within medicine and other parallel, male-dominated working environments. Alternative forms of leadership such as mentoring, coaching, and sponsorship are also considered.

DOI: 10.4018/978-1-5225-9599-1.ch007

INTRODUCTION

If you reflect back on your career you can most likely think of an individual that inspired you with their vision, elevated your confidence in your abilities and had a positive impact on your work. These individuals are the great leaders with whom we cross paths and they are invaluable to organisations, uniting the individuals within them to work towards a common vision. This chapter aims to outline the importance of leadership in healthcare, and in particular the value of diversity in leadership roles and the barriers and facilitators to improved gender equity in leadership.

What is a Leader?

Most of us intuitively know what the term leadership entails; however, when faced with defining leadership in clear terms we come to realise that the concept is quite vague and has a variety of meanings to different individuals. Academic literature contains countless different definitions of leadership and an abundance of theories on the lack of consensus. Nevertheless, the common principles are best represented by these definitions:

- Leadership is the principal dynamic force that motivates and coordinates the organisation in the accomplishment of its objective(Bass, Bass and Bass, 2009).
- Leadership is the art of influencing people by persuasion or example to follow a line of action(DuBrin, 2016).
- Leadership is a psychosocial influencing dynamic(Western, 2013).

In 2006, academics at the Regent University carried out a systematic literature review which aimed to propose an integrative definition of leadership.

A leader is one or more people who selects, equips, trains and influences followers that have diverse gifts, abilities and skills andfocuses the followers to the organisation's mission and objectives causing the followers to willingly and enthusiastically extend spiritual, emotional andphysical energy in a concerted coordinated effort to achieve the organisational mission and objectives (Winston and Patterson, 2006).

A key aspect of understanding the nature of leadership is to recognise the characteristics of a great leader. Defining key characteristics of leaders has been of great interest to leadership researchers with multiple comprehensive analyses of key traits. These definitions have faced some criticism about their simplicity from academics, but they are an accessible way to expand our understanding of leadership. The most widely used lists of character traits are the Stogdill "Traits and Skills of Leaders" from 1974(Stogdill, 1974) and more recently the Pew Research Centres analysis of leadership traits from 2015 (see Figure 1)(Parker *et al.*, 2015).

An important concept to recognise about leadership is that although you will find many great leaders in management and high-level positions, leadership is not dependent on the possession of a position of authority or rank. Great leaders may often find themselves in management positions as a result of their leadership skills, but those skills can be applied effectively at any rank. It is important to have leaders in all levels of an organisation to create a united vision. Individuals in lower level positions that possess

Table 1. Stogdill's traits and skills of leaders(Stogdill, 1974)

Traits	Skills
Adaptable to situations	Clever
Alert to social environment	Conceptually skilled
Ambitious and achievement-oriented	Creative
Assertive	Diplomatic and tactful
Cooperative	Fluent in speaking
Decisive	Organised
Dependable	Persuasive
Dominant	Socially skilled
Energetic	
Persistent	
Self-confident	
Tolerant to stress	
Willing to assume responsibility	

Figure 1. Pew research centres leadership traits (Parker et al., 2015)

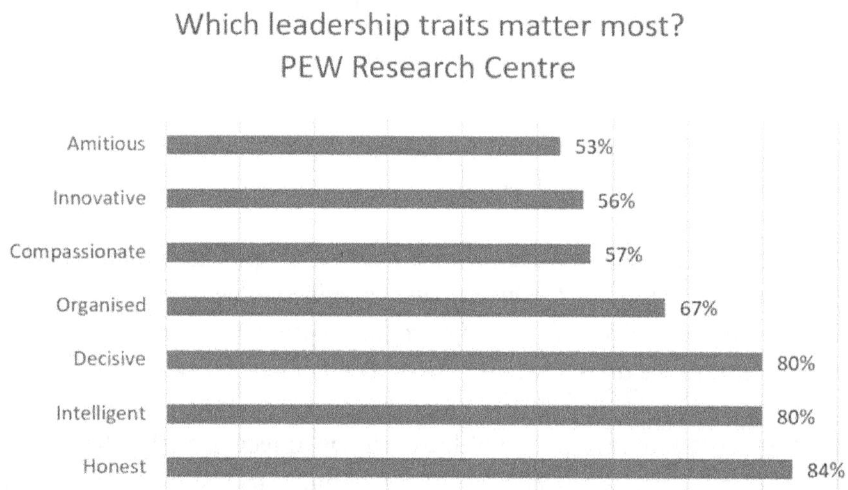

the characteristics of a leader and have a clear vision can be impactful leaders within an organisation. These types of leaders are invaluable to organisations because of their understanding of ground level work and because they often approach challenges from a different perspective to high-level leaders.

The Importance of Leadership in Healthcare

The importance of effective leadership is well recognised in the business sector. Studies have shown that leadership determines between 15-45% of an organisation's performance(Kaiser, Hogan and Craig, 2008). In addition, the leadership of an organisation is the single most important factor in shaping the organisation's values and culture(West *et al.*, 2015). Organisational culture has a profound impact on individual sense of membership, shared responsibility and work satisfaction, all of which ultimately translate into improved organisational outcomes(Western, 2013).

Similarly in the healthcare sector, effective leadership is an essential component of ensuring the delivery of safe, high quality and compassionate care, which is the key goal of all NHS facilities(West *et al.*, 2015). The Francis report into the failures of patient care at Mid Staffordshire hospitals concluded that "leadership was lacking at every level" and that this "had directly impacted the quality of care provided to patients"(Francis, 2013). With this in mind the Department for Health and NHS England have committed to supporting the development of leadership within the NHS. The NHS now recognises that cultivating leadership skills in NHS staff is essential for the delivery of progressive and high-quality service.

It is important that clinicians are willing and able to step into leadership roles. A report by Lord Darzi in 2008 found that a recent increase in dependence on non-clinical managers had fostered a culture of clinicians vs. managers in many NHS facilities(Darzi, 2008). Clinician leaders are essential at every level, and is a model that has been successfully adopted in other countries including the US(Swanwick and McKimm, 2011).

The Importance of Diversity in Leadership Roles

In the business sector, evidence shows that greater diversity of leadership teams is directly related to improved outcomes(Angier and Axelrod, 2014). Companies that have gender and ethnic diversity at senior management and board level have been shown to improve organisational and financial performance. Companies in the top quartile for gender diversity are 15% more likely to have financial performance above the national industry mean than companies in the lowest quartile(Devillard et al., 2013).

This knowledge is transferable to the healthcare sector where diversity in leadership offers many advantages. Research on the effects of gender in healthcare leadership has demonstrated that trusts with female Chairs or Chief Executives have reduced rates of negative social outcomes, and consequently lower clinical negligence costs(Ellwood and Garcia-Lacalle, 2015). Female presence in general executive roles has however, not been shown to result in a significant difference in service quality(Manner, 2010; Boulouta, 2013; Hafsi and Turgut, 2013; Ellwood and Garcia-Lacalle, 2015).

In addition to effects on workforce dynamics and social outcomes, diversity is beneficial for our patients. A service that is representative of its users is better equipped to understand the health barriers of different groups, including social and cultural health beliefs. This ultimately leads to improved quality of health service provision with fewer access barriers. Service evaluations demonstrate that increased diversity in health care teams results in improved patient satisfaction scores (West et al., 2011). A recent report of NHS staff management noted a number of important correlations which support the drive for diversity within the medical work force. In this report, trusts with perceived equal opportunities for career progression received better scores from the Care Quality Commission on the quality of care provided. Additionally, decreased workplace discrimination based on ethnicity was correlated with improved patient satisfaction scores(West et al., 2011).

Representation of Women in Formal Leadership Roles

It has long been recognised that work force diversity decreases as seniority increases. Men and women enter the global workforce in roughly equal numbers every year (Thornton, 2018); however, according to Europe, Middle East and Africa (UMEA) data, in 2018, women occupied 24% of senior management positions and 25% of companies had no women in senior management positions (Devillard et al., 2013). In the United Kingdom these figures are similar (Thornton International Ltd, 2018). In 2018, 96% of FTSE 250 companies had at least one female director, but at only 23% of FTSE 250 companies did females represent at least a third of directorships (Vinnicombe, Doldor and Sealy, 2018). Even accounting for the time taken to achieve senior positions, there is a disproportionate lag in the observed number of women in senior roles (Devillard et al., 2013).

In contrast, the overall NHS workforce is 77% female, with 47% of senior roles being held by women (Skinner et al, 2019). However, the expected increase in women in senior medical roles has not been observed. Women outnumber men as newly qualified doctors; 58% of doctors in training in 2017 in the UK were female(Britain, 2017). In 2018, women accounted for 36% of the medical consultant workforce; this has increased from 30% in 2009[20]. In surgery, only 12% of consultants are women, a figure that is increasing slowly (Royal-College-of-Surgeons, 2019). With the length of training from graduation to consultant for hospital based specialties ranging from 5 years (e.g. emergency medicine) to 10 years (e.g. neurosurgery) greater change in these figures would be expected, even accounting for some lag as a result of more women taking time out to have children and working less than full time (Royal-College-of-Surgeons, 2019).

It has also been shown there are a lack of females in leadership roles in surgical specialty organisations. Despite women making up 47% of the medical workforce and 27% of the surgical workforce, women make up only 15% of committee members of surgical specialty organisations and 8% of presidents(Skinner et al., 2019). Underrepresentation of women in surgical specialty leadership positions-likely contributes to the lower numbers of women entering these specialties. This helps maintain the status quo in imbalanced gender representation in leadership and slows resolution of the multiple barriers to women achieving the most senior positions(Skinner *et al.*, 2019).

In the last decade, the NHS has placed increasing focus on measures to improve gender imbalance and good progress has been made towards equal gender representation in senior, executive and management roles. An NHS Digital analysis of women in the NHS workforce demonstrated that in 2018 44% of chief executives in the NHS were women, compared to 38% in 2009(NHS-Digital, 2018). However, a more in-depth analysis by the University of Exeter in 2017 revealed that only 21% of medical directors across the NHS are women and that women held 41% of board positions in the NHS overall(Sealy, 2017). In contrast, women are much more likely to hold mid- and lower-level management positions; women occupy 61% of these positions. This figure has remained unchanged since 2009(NHS-Digital, 2018).

Women as Leaders

One of the barriers to women progressing to leadership roles is the belief that women's leadership styles do not fit the pervasive leadership model in most businesses(Devillard et al., 2013). Traditionally men have generally used a 'command and control' style of leadership, and most of the pioneering women who were early leaders followed this model. Within this leadership strategy is a heavy reliance on rank, and leadership is delivered by a series of 'transactions'(Devillard et al., 2013). As leadership development has become more popular, this has changed for both men and women. Women have demonstrated enhanced ability and confidence to display leadership styles that do not fit the traditional model and still progress in some environments; however, the traditional model still prevails in many workplaces(Rosener, 2011).

The leadership behaviours more commonly employed by women can be seen in Table 2. These behaviours are thought to be linked to the improvement in organisational performance observed when gender diversity increases(Devillard et al., 2013). Unfortunately, they are still often seen as weakness. For instance, women are more likely to use participative decision-making (use of evidence as well as experience and opinion within the team) but in male dominated environments this can be seen as indecisiveness and inability to make decisions independently(Devillard et al., 2013).

Female leaders are more likely to cultivate a culture of striving for a common goal(Rosener, 2011). It has been shown that teams who 'buy in' to a common goal are more productive and have better staff retention as people are invested in their work and feel accomplished and energised by what they are doing(Rosener, 2011). Having a shared mental model and involving people in decisions is also more commonly seen in women leaders(Eagly, Johannesen-Schmidt and Van Engen, 2003). This can give employees a sense of worth and encourages information to flow easily in both directions meaning issues are more likely to be tackled before they become problems(Eagly, Johannesen-Schmidt and Van Engen, 2003). The drawback of many female leadership styles is the time and energy required to maintain them. There are also times when difficult decisions have to be made quickly and the ability to adjust strategies and use less collaborative techniques is needed.

Barriers and Facilitators to Gender Equity in Leadership

The barriers to women's ascension to leadership and high level positions are often collectively described as the 'glass ceiling'(Cook and Glass, 2014). This phrase originated in the business sector, where women remain under-represented in high level positions. In 2018, there were just 30 women in full-time executive roles at FTSE 250 firms, amounting to 6.4% of the total(Vinnicombe, Doldor, and Sealy, 2018). The 'glass ceiling' poses several barriers that can be personal, societal and institutional. Although most of the research surrounding these barriers and potential solutions has been undertaken in the business sector, many of the themes are common to medicine and provide opportunities to understand the mechanisms that can lead to increased likelihood of women being appointed to top positions in healthcare.

Table 2. Leadership behaviours according to gender(Rosener, 2011)

Women apply more	Expectations and rewards
	Role model
Women apply slightly more	Inspiration
	Participative decision making
Women and men apply equally	Intellectual stimulation
	Efficient communication
Men apply more	Individualistic decision making
	Control and corrective action

Gender Bias

As explicit discrimination and sexual harassment have become less common(Greenberg, 2017), current research on gender bias is now mostly focussed on investigating 'second-generation' forms of gender bias as the primary cause of women's persistent underrepresentation in leadership roles(Ibarra, Ely, and Kolb, 2013). Among women in academic medicine, 70% report facing gender-specific bias and 30% report personally experiencing harassment compared with only 4% of men(Delisle and Wirtzfeld, no date). This bias erects powerful but often invisible barriers for women that arise from cultural assumptions, organisational structures and work practices that were designed to fit men's lives at a time when women made up only a small proportion of the workforce. Organisational culture is the main determinant of women's perception of their chances of successful career progression(Devillard et al., 2013). Amongst organisations that did not champion gender diversity only 12% of women reported feeling they had an equal chance of successful progression to senior positions, compared to 45% of women where organisational culture was more favourable, despite these women having similar levels of individual drive and dedication(Devillard et al., 2013).

Career-enhancing international posts, for example, often assume a 'trailing spouse' who has no career and can easily move; this family situation is more common for men than for women and, even if woman can offer this, assumptions are usually made that they cannot(Ibarra, Ely and Kolb, 2013; Angier and Axelrod, 2014). The value attributed to different types of work may also hinder women. Research indicates that many organisations undervalue 'behind-the-scenes' work, such as team-building or conflict avoidance, which women are more likely to do(Devillard et al., 2013). The cumulative effect of these practices disadvantages women, leading to the perception that men are more suited to leadership roles, propelling more men, and fewer women, to seek and attain top positions(Ibarra, Ely, and Kolb, 2013).

The accumulation of these factors facilitates the development of unconscious cognitive biases that systematically disadvantage women(Ibarra, Ely, and Kolb, 2013). Individuals that do not 'fit the mould' are often seen as having less valuable assets and this must be challenged if progress is to be made(Ibarra, Ely, and Kolb, 2013). Human nature is to approach difference and change with caution. Cognitively we are able to reconcile that change may bring benefit, but this pushes people out of their comfort zones as new skills and new ways of working may be required. Within a diverse organisation such as the NHS, conflicts often arise on the basis of differences and having diverse leaders is essential to resolve such issues successfully and reduce negative impacts of any conflict(Sealy, 2017). Excellent leadership is crucial to ensure that organisational diversity results in a positive impact. Leadership should model inclusivity, tolerance and encourage challenge and feedback(Ibarra, Ely, and Kolb, 2013).

Networking, Role Models and Mentors

Informal networks are a precious resource for potential leaders, and have a tremendous influence on success in achieving top positions(Schueller-Weidekamm and Kautzky-Willer, 2012). Men's networks are more efficient compared with those of women(Pololi and Jones, 2010). Differences in men's and women's roles and career prospects, along with their proclivity to interact with others of the same gender, result in weaker networks for women, and women consequentially lack access to influential colleagues(Ibarra, Ely, and Kolb, 2013).

An important aspect of networking is the formation of mentoring relationships. Men are more likely to have mentors who help them get promoted(Greenberg, 2017). The majority of female leaders in surgery (90%) had a mentor or mentors during their career(Kass, Souba, and Thorndyke, 2006). Half of the women, however, admit that they had never been effectively mentored and 60% used mainly male mentors because of the lack of females in the profession(Kass, Souba, and Thorndyke, 2006). Aspiring leaders need visible role models whose personal and professional experiences reflect their own(Ibarra, Ely, and Kolb, 2013). Fewer female leaders meaning fewer female role models may also discourage junior staff from viewing senior women as credible sources of advice and support(Ibarra, Ely, and Kolb, 2013).

Feminine Qualities

It has been suggested that female personality traits can hinder the path to leadership positions. In most cultures, men are expected to be assertive, instrumental, task-oriented and competitive(Greenberg, 2017). Conventionally feminine qualities, such as caretaking and selflessness, are undervalued. A classic example is Babcock and Laschever's *Women Don't Ask*, which suggests that women in the business sector are much less likely than their male peers to ask for promotions(Babcock and Laschever, 2009). More recently, Sheryl Sandberg, Chief Operating Officer of Facebook, urged women to 'have the confidence to reach for opportunities'(Sandberg, 2011). A study of female surgical leaders found that the most critical success factors are perseverance and drive(Kass, Souba, and Thorndyke, 2006).

However, behaviours that suggest self-confidence or assertiveness in women have been shown to be perceived negatively. A number of studies show that both men and women assign lower status and salaries to women who engage in self-promotion, have task-oriented speaking styles, have an authoritative leadership style, administer discipline, and initiate salary negotiations(Greenberg, 2017). Women are especially punished for power-seeking behaviour, whereas men who seek power are viewed as more competent. Meanwhile, women in positions of authority who enact a conventionally feminine style may be liked but are not respected. They are deemed too emotional to make tough decisions and too soft to be strong leaders(Ibarra, Ely, and Kolb, 2013). These are entrenched beliefs that may take decades to overcome.

Children and Work-Life Balance

A study of women in medical leadership positions found that children were cited as the most important obstacle on the way to the top(Schueller-Weidekamm and Kautzky-Willer, 2012). Family life, childcare, and child education is time-consuming and requires copious energy. In most cultures, the predominant responsibility for child care is still borne by the woman, as demonstrated by the fact that women exhibit significantly higher rates of emotional exhaustion compared with men after having children(Delisle and Wirtzfeld, no date). The 'maternal wall' is described as the barrier for career progression for women after having children(Mangurian et al., 2018). This is largely due to having insufficient time to devote to opportunities that might otherwise enhance promotion prospects.

Established attitudes see parental status as a more significant barrier to women in career progression than men(Devillard et al., 2013). This may be because the time when some women wish to start a family coincides with the time in career life when men make their mark and begin their career progression. An example of how this can affect career progression would be to use that of clinical academia. An employee who has taken parental leave or a career break may have fewer publications overall, and therefore less chance of funding, promotion or tenure. However, it is important to note that not all women have children; 40% of female surgeons do not have children(Dyrbye et al., 2011). Organisations must recognise that parenting and other issues of work-life balance are critical for everyone, regardless of gender or parental status(Greenberg, 2017).

Facilitators to Improve Gender Equity in Leadership

In order for gender parity to become reality in medical leadership a culture change is required. Experience from the business sector shows that individual policies with piecemeal tokenism do not lead to the differences sufficient to gain parity(Devillard et al., 2013). It is common for companies and health care organisations to have policies in place but these are often not well implemented or embedded into the culture of the organisation, resulting in many companies making little progress with diversity(Devillard et al., 2013). This is true of medical leadership where measures exist to improve equity but whole scale culture change is lacking. There is a drive to improve the publishable statistics, but culture change is required for lasting improvement and to reap the rewards that diversity can bring.

Pervasive culture change requires top level buy-in and activism, with measurement and reporting of progress. Employees take their cues from those above them; if senior level executives and board members are not invested in change it is unlikely to happen(Angier and Axelrod, 2014). Clear aims and objectives should be set and the progress data reviewed regularly and presented transparently(Angier and Axelrod, 2014). Visibility of all types of female leader encourages acceptance and normalises female traits in top positions(Cook and Glass, 2014). Crucially, the integration of women amongst decision-makers promotes women's ability to overcome the barriers posed by the glass ceiling and engrains the culture change. Institutional diversity significantly impacts women's mobility and tenure at all levels in Fortune 500 companies(Cook and Glass, 2014). Organisations committed to women's representation would do well to focus their efforts on promoting gender diversity among top leadership positions.

It is necessary to level the playing field and offer equal opportunities. Equal opportunity ensures people from minority groups with different characteristics who show relevant skills and potential have the same chance of progressing in their career as those considered conventional candidates(Devillard et al., 2013; Krivkovich et al., 2017). It is necessary to recognise that different people need different conditions in which to thrive(Devillard et al., 2013). Open-minded reviews of working practices by a diverse team are valuable. For the sake of all staff, there should be flexible and family-friendly work policies in place(Devillard et al., 2013). These could include paid parental leave, provision for breastfeeding, on-site childcare services and emergency back-up care for sick children at home at competitive rates. Meetings should be held within normal working hours, and staff should not be penalised for teleconferencing into meetings(Angier and Axelrod, 2014).

Although measures to improve diversity have been shown to improve working conditions for all employees, introducing gender equity measures in workplaces can be perceived as positive discrimination, especially to those who have unconscious bias or fail to recognise the barriers for women(Devillard et al., 2013). Those who firmly believe they hold do not unconscious biases are likely to score more highly on unconscious bias assessments(Devillard et al., 2013). Organisations should therefore ensure that unconscious bias training is delivered globally with focus on those in appointing positions. This is best done in face to face sessions but e-learning is an alternative method(Devillard et al., 2013; Krivkovich et al., 2017).

Bias is closely related to common social assumptions. Women have traditionally suffered from being dismissed as candidates for promotion when it is presumed that they won't want to progress and take on extra responsibility when their children are young or when they may want to start a family(Angier and Axelrod, 2014). Career planning is a valuable tool that prevents assumptions being made about individual's career aspirations and life plans. To facilitate meaningful career planning a meeting template can be valuable(Angier and Axelrod, 2014). This recognises the effect of topics that are difficult for women to raise and may be difficult for predominantly male senior leaders to address for fear of being considered discriminatory(Angier and Axelrod, 2014).

Networking is an important element of leadership in business and health(Devillard et al., 2013). Formal and informal networking opportunities within the working day lead to a culture of inclusivity and do not disadvantage colleagues who have family commitments(Angier and Axelrod, 2014; Krivkovich et al., 2017). This may allow women to identify and access appropriate mentors, an important resource that some women may otherwise struggle to access. Formalising networking and mentoring opportunities with published lists of willing mentors or organised mentorship programs will benefit all but crucially ensure women do not miss out. The Academy of Medical Sciences' one-to-one mentoring programme is a good example of formal pairing of leaders and mentees that bridges gender gaps(The-Academy-of-Medical-Sciences, 2019). It is not essential for women to be mentored by women but having some women available to fulfil this role is desirable.

There are several companies where strategies have been implemented leading to successful improvement in female representation in high-level and executive roles. For example GlaxoSmithKline (GSK) and eBay. GSK are in the top 10 of the FTSE 100. Their mean gender pay gap is 2.8%, 45% of the board are women, including the CEO(Vinnicombe, Doldor, and Sealy, 2018). Their strategy has been to focus on equity at every level and support all minority groups including women, LGBTQ, minority ethnic groups and people with disability to progress(GlaxoSmithKline, 2019). They have a strong focus on: flexible working models, job share and part time working, coaching for emerging talent and addressing attitudes that may create barriers to equity(GlaxoSmithKline, 2019).

Many of the strategies described above have been embraced by eBay in their drive to increase diversity(Angier and Axelrod, 2014). Although they acknowledge they have further progress to make, they have a strong programme in place. They have incorporated many of the elements which are deemed in the literature to be essential to success, namely a whole culture shift within the organisation with transparent policies and a sustained effort to improve figures, see case study below.

Case Study: eBay (Angier & Axelrod, 2014)

eBay have committed to improving gender parity in senior positions. The drive for change has been led by their CEO, John Donahoe, whose strategy was to:

- Hold personal responsibility for progress
- Ensure clear goals and objectives
- Measure progress and review data at board level
- Make the data available and transparent within the company

Specific objectives included:

- Commitment to ensuring diverse candidates and interview panels for all positions
- Opportunities for mentoring from top level managers
- Ensuring top talent women at all levels have career development plans drawn up and discussed with their manager.

Both these companies provide evidence that these strategies can be successful in driving change and improving equity as long as there is buy in at all levels, support from the top and sustained effort.

NHS Strategies and Leadership Development Opportunities

The NHS has sought to address diversity across all staff groups; as with many organisations there has been partial success. At the most basic level the NHS ensures all legislative requirements for equality are met through the Equality Delivery System(NHS-England, 2013). This is a framework for promoting diversity for both staff and patients and its implementation is a requirement of all NHS contracts. In addition, NHS Employers have launched the Diversity and Inclusion Partners Programme(NHS-Employers, 2019). This aims to work with Trusts to improve their equality performance over 12 months; part of this is focused on gender equity. This work does not specifically focus on medical leadership and, as previously discussed, there is a greater problem in gender equity in medical leadership than in the NHS as a whole. Nevertheless, it is an indication that work is ongoing to improve the representation of minority characteristics at senior levels and represents a desired culture change which is essential for improving gender equity(Angier and Axelrod, 2014; NHS-Employers, 2019).

As the value of good leadership has been recognised by the wider world, medical leadership has also seen an evolution and meaningful promotion in recent years(Sandberg, 2011). Formal leadership development schemes that have emerged are not gender directed but they hold valuable opportunities for women to progress in leadership roles (see below for examples). Women find it easier to progress when their skills are evidenced and validated(Devillard et al., 2013). Making the most of the leadership development opportunities available is one obvious way to do this.

The NHS Leadership Academy is a good place to start when looking to develop leadership skills. This national organisation is part of NHS England and is working towards 'great leadership across the NHS'. The Academy has drawn up a health care leadership model, which has been developed from validated leadership models used in other sectors but has been made specific to health care in the NHS(NHS-Leadership-Academy, 2013). This is essential reading for those wishing to progress in medical leadership. The Academy also offers structured leadership development programmes, such as the Edward Jenner Programme, which is free of charge to NHS staff fulfilling the relevant criteria. The entry level program is an online distance learning course which can be tailored to individual needs and time constraints.

The King's Fund has been instrumental in developing both gender equity and leadership guidance. It is a charitable organisation working to improve health care in England. Their document, 'Leadership and leadership development in health care', sets out an evidence base for effective leadership behaviours at all levels(West *et al.*, 2015). Shared vision, clear objectives, supportive and enabling management and an embedded culture of quality improvement are all stated as important features of effective medical leadership. This plays to the strengths of most women's natural tendencies and should give confidence to women wishing to progress in medical leadership(West *et al.*, 2015).

Other opportunities are available, some of which are specifically available to women in certain roles or fields. The Athena SWAN Charter aims to support the progression and retention of women in STEMM subjects of academia (science, technology, engineering, mathematics and medicine) and has been successful in supporting clinical academics to progress their careers and take on senior academic roles(HE-Advance, 2018). The Royal College of Surgeons of England runs The Lady Estelle Wolfson Emerging Leaders Fellowship; this offers female surgeons the opportunity to be involved in college activities and develop leadership skills(Wynn-Mackenzie, 2016). The Royal College of Physicians runs the Emerging Women Leaders Programme for consultants within 10 years of completion of training(Royal-College-of-Physicians, 2019). Data on the success of these programmes is not published. Although they are positive developments they do not represent the deep-seated culture change drivers that are needed.

It is essential to have medical leaders at all levels, and attention to the development of leadership skills for doctors in training has also received attention. The postgraduate medical curriculum, for all specialities, now includes leadership domains. This is based on a competency framework and supports the notion that, although some leadership characteristics are innate, the skills needed to lead can be learned. This is being used to ensure all medical trainees develop leadership competencies and are able to lead teams, large or small, as part of their daily jobs(NHS Institute for Innovation and Improvement and Academy of Medical Royal Colleges, 2010). A framework developed skillfully and by a diverse team clearly has the potential to have a positive impact on acceptance of differing leadership styles that may benefit women aspiring to leadership roles in medicine.

SUMMARY

Leadership has been shown to be essential in healthcare for the delivery of safe, high quality, compassionate care. It is essential to have leaders in all levels of an organisation, irrespective of rank, to create a united vision. Improvement of leadership has become a priority issue within the NHS, with emphasis on empowering clinicians to step into leadership roles.

Diversity in leadership roles has been shown to improve both quality of care and patient satisfaction. In light of this, current persistent underrepresentation of women in formal leadership roles is of concern. Gender differences in leadership styles are thought to be one of the main barriers to women progressing in leadership roles. Female leaders are more likely to use what some consider unconventional leadership styles such as participative decision making and active role modeling, which can be perceived negatively despite their proven effectiveness. Other barriers include conscious or unconscious gender bias, unequal access to career progression opportunities and system structures that are unaccommodating to women with children. Some ways to overcome these barriers are suggested in Table 3.

Table 3. Ways to access leadership opportunities

Identify a mentor to support and advise on career progression.
Find a sponsor who can represent your interests and create pathways to progression.
Join local and national networks which can facilitate access to leadership opportunities.
Exploit current leadership programmes such as those provided by the Royal College of Surgeons and the NHS Leadership Academy.
Apply for leadership roles and accept the potential for knock-backs.
Realise that the desirable attributes on any job description are not a necessity for application.

Gender equality in medical leadership can only become a reality with implementation of systematic interventions in addition to culture change that must be role-modeled by top-level leaders. The NHS has actively implemented measures to improve gender equity in clinical leadership; however, these measures have so far failed to become embedded in NHS culture and have had limited effect. Visibility of a variety of female leaders encourages a more accepting organisational culture and normalises female traits in top positions. Some of the most important factors that facilitate cultural change for equality in leadership are unconscious bias training sessions, inclusive formal networking opportunities, career progression planning tools and systematic flexibility for all employees. Formal leadership training schemes that have emerged in the last decade have the potential to influence progression of women into leadership roles.

Targeted measures to improve diversity in clinical leadership are vital to enhance the experiences of healthcare workers and improve the quality of care received by patients and service users. Increasing diversity in leadership roles results in greater variety of working styles and patterns which allows flexibility to become a new norm. This benefits all employees and can results in better work life balance and more positive and productive working environments; these influence the positive outcomes that have been reported as attributable to increased diversity.

REFERENCES

Angier, M., & Axelrod, B. (2014). Realizing the power of talented women. *The McKinsey Quarterly.*

Babcock, L., & Laschever, S. (2009). *Women don't ask: Negotiation and the gender divide.* Princeton, NJ: Princeton University Press.

Bass, B. M., Bass, R., & Bass, B. M. (2009). *The Bass handbook of leadership: theory, research, and managerial applications.* Simon and Schuster.

Boulouta, I. (2013). Hidden Connections: The Link Between Board Gender Diversity and Corporate Social Performance. *Journal of Business Ethics. Springer Netherlands, 113*(2), 185–197. doi:10.100710551-012-1293-7

Cook, A. & Glass, C. (2014) Women and Top Leadership Positions: Towards an Institutional Analysis. *Gender, Work & Organization.* Hoboken, NJ: John Wiley & Sons. 21(1), pp. 91–103. doi:10.1111/gwao.12018

Darzi, A. (2008). *A high quality workforce: NHS Next Stage Review.* London, UK: Department of Health.

Delisle, M. & Wirtzfeld, D. (n.d.). Why do we lack gender diversity in academic medical leadership. *Are we there yet?*

DuBrin, A. J. (2016). *Leadership: research findings, practice, and skills. Eighth.* Boston, MA: Cengage Learning.

Dyrbye, L. N., Shanafelt, T. D., Balch, C. M., Satele, D., Sloan, J., & Freischlag, J. (2011). Relationship between work-home conflicts and burnout among American surgeons: a comparison by sex. *Archives of surgery. American Medical Association, 146*(2), pp. 211–217.

Eagly, A. H., Johannesen-Schmidt, M. C., & Van Engen, M. L. (2003) Transformational, transactional, and laissez-faire leadership styles: a meta-analysis comparing women and men. *Psychological bulletin. American Psychological Association, 129*(4), p. 569.

Ellwood, S., & Garcia-Lacalle, J. (2015). The Influence of Presence and Position of Women on the Boards of Directors: The Case of NHS Foundation Trusts. *Journal of Business Ethics. Springer Netherlands, 130*(1), 69–84. doi:10.100710551-014-2206-8

Francis, R. (2013) Report of the Mid Staffordshire NHS foundation trust public inquiry: executive summary. The Stationery Office, 947.

G. M. C. (Great Britain). (2017) *The State of Medical Education and Practice in the UK: 2017*. General Medical Council.

Devillard, S., Sancier, S., Werner, C., Maller, I., & Kossoff, C. (2013). Gender diversity in top management: Moving corporate culture, moving boundaries. Women Matter.

GlaxoSmithKline. (2019) *Inclusion and diversity*. Retrieved from https://www.gsk.com/en-gb/responsibility/our-people/inclusion-and-diversity/

Greenberg, C. C. (2017). Association for Academic Surgery presidential address: Sticky floors and glass ceilings. *Journal of Surgical Research. Elsevier, 219*, ix–xviii. doi:10.1016/j.jss.2017.09.006 PMID:29078918

Hafsi, T., & Turgut, G. (2013). Boardroom Diversity and its Effect on Social Performance: Conceptualization and Empirical Evidence. *Journal of Business Ethics. Springer Netherlands, 112*(3), 463–479. doi:10.100710551-012-1272-z

HE-Advance. (2018). *Athena SWAN Charter, Equality Charters*. Available at https://www.ecu.ac.uk/equality-charters/athena-swan/

Ibarra, H., Ely, R., & Kolb, D. (2013). Women rising: The unseen barriers. *Harvard Business Review, 91*(9), 60–66. PMID:23593768

Kaiser, R. B., Hogan, R., & Craig, S. B. (2008). Leadership and the fate of organizations. *The American Psychologist, 63*(2), 96–110. doi:10.1037/0003-066X.63.2.96 PMID:18284278

Kass, R. B., Souba, W. W., & Thorndyke, L. E. (2006). Challenges Confronting Female Surgical Leaders: Overcoming the Barriers. *The Journal of Surgical Research, 132*(2), 179–187. doi:10.1016/j.jss.2006.02.009 PMID:16564542

Krivkovich, A., Robinson, K., Starikova, I., Valentino, R., & Yee, L. (2017). Women in the workplace 2017. McKinsey Report.

Manner, M. H. (2010). The Impact of CEO Characteristics on Corporate Social Performance. *Journal of Business Ethics. Springer Netherlands, 93*(S1), 53–72. doi:10.100710551-010-0626-7

NHS-Digital. (2018) *Analysis of the representation of women across the hospital and community health services workforce.*

NHS-Employers. (2019) *Diversity and Inclusion Partners Programme*. Available at https://www.nhs-employers.org/your-workforce/plan/diversity-and-inclusion/partners-programme

NHS-England. (2013). *A refreshed Equality Delivery System for the NHS*. London, UK: NHS England.

NHS Institute for Innovation and Improvement and Academy of Medical Royal Colleges. (2010). *Medical Leadership Competency Framework* (3rd ed.).

NHS-Leadership-Academy. (2013) *The Healthcare Leadership Model*. Retrieved from https://www.leadershipacademy.nhs.uk/resources/healthcare-leadership-model/

Mangurian, C., Linos, E., Sarkar, U., Rodriguez, C., & Jagsi, R. (2018). What's holding women in medicine back from leadership. *Harvard Business Review*, 24.

Parker, K., Horowitz, J. M., & Rohal, M. (2015). *Women and leadership: Public says women are equally qualified, but barriers persist*. Washington DC: Pew Research Center.

Pololi, L. H. & Jones, S. J. (2010). Women faculty: an analysis of their experiences in academic medicine and their coping strategies. *Gender medicine*. Elsevier, 7(5), pp. 438–450.

Rosener, J. B. (2011). Ways women lead. In *Leadership, Gender, and Organization* (pp. 19–29). Springer. doi:10.1007/978-90-481-9014-0_3

Royal-College-of-Physicians. (2019). *Emerging Women Leaders Programme*. Available at https://www.rcplondon.ac.uk/education-practice/courses/emerging-women-leaders-programme

Royal-College-of-Surgeons. (2019). *Women in Surgery*.

Sandberg, S. (2011). *Why we have too few women leaders, TED: Ideas Worth Spreading*. Retrieved from http://www.ted.com/talks/sheryl_sandberg_why_we_have_too_few_women_leaders.html

Schueller-Weidekamm, C., & Kautzky-Willer, A. (2012). Challenges of Work–Life Balance for Women Physicians/Mothers Working in Leadership Positions. *Gender Medicine*, *9*(4), 244–250. doi:10.1016/j.genm.2012.04.002 PMID:22626768

Sealy, R. (2017). Equal gender representation. *Nursing management*, *24*(3), p. 12. doi:10.7748/nm.24.3.12.s15

Skinner, H., Burke, J. R., Young, A. L., Adair, R. A., & Smith, A. M. (2019). Gender representation in leadership roles in UK surgical societies. *International Journal of Surgery*, *67*(1), 32–36. doi:10.1016/j.ijsu.2019.05.007 PMID:31121326

Stogdill, R. M. (1974). *Handbook of leadership: A survey of theory and research*. New York, NY: Free Press.

Swanwick, T., & McKimm, J. (2011). What is clinical leadership… and why is it important?. The clinical teacher. *Wiley Online Library*, *8*(1), 22–26. PMID:21324068

The-Academy-of-Medical-Sciences. (2019). *Mentoring*.

Thornton, G. (2018). *Women in business: beyond policy to progress*.

Thornton International Ltd, G. (2018) *Diversity snapshot – ethnicity, age and gender.*

Vinnicombe, S., Doldor, E., & Sealy, R. (2018) *The Female FTSE Board Report 2018: Busy going nowhere with the female executive pipeline.*

West, M., Armit, K., Loewenthal, L., Eckert, R., West, T., & Lee, A. (2015). Leadership and leadership development in healthcare: the evidence base. London, UK: The Kings Fund.

West, M., Dawson, J., Admasachew, L., & Topakas, A. (2011). NHS staff management and health service quality: results from the NHS staff survey and related data. London, UK: Department of Health.

Western, S. (2013). *Leadership: a critical text. Second.* London, UK: Sage.

Winston, B. E., & Patterson, K. (2006). An Integrative Definition of Leadership. *International Journal of Leadership Studies*, *1*(2), 6–66.

Wynn-Mackenzie, C. (2016). The Lady Estelle Wolfson Emerging Leaders Fellowships. *Medical Woman*, *35*(1), 23.

Chapter 8
The Gender Pay Gap in Medicine:
Causes and Solutions

Rebecca C. Grossman
Buckinghamshire Healthcare NHS Trust, UK

ABSTRACT

The gender pay gap is a symptom of the pervasive inequalities inherent in modern society. Among doctors, the gap has been increasing. The Gender Pay Gap in Medicine Review is exploring the scale of the problem and the reasons behind it. Although motherhood and flexible working both contribute to the salary discrepancy, the aetiology is complex and multifactorial, with important roles played by recruitment and representation of women at senior levels, as well as gender occupational segregation. Addressing the root causes of gender inequalities and shining a light on the pay gap data are both required in order to one day close the gap.

INTRODUCTION

The gender pay gap is paradigmatic of gender inequality in medicine and Science, Technology, Engineering and Mathematics (STEM), and a critical topic to consider when discussing such themes. This section will define the gender pay gap, and explain how it is researched. The implications of the pay gap will also be explored, including the effects on employee well-being. Up-to-date figures will be provided for the gender pay gap in medicine. These will be compared to the pay gap elsewhere in STEM, as well as to national and international averages. Putative causes will be outlined in order to combat prevalent myths on the topic. The chapter will end with potential solutions and reasons to be optimistic that the gap will improve.

DOI: 10.4018/978-1-5225-9599-1.ch008

BACKGROUND

The gender pay gap is the difference between the average hourly earnings of men and women (Topping & Barr, 2018). It is pervasive across different disciplines, and medicine is no exception. It is also not a new phenomenon. Women's work has been assigned a lower value than men's work throughout history (Griffin, 2018). This has allowed men to excel in their professional lives, while encouraging women to take on the greater share of domestic work.

The pay gap has persisted despite the Equal Pay Act 1970 and Equality Act 2010, which enshrined in law the entitlement for men and women to be paid equally for work of equal value. The UK currently ranks 20th in gender equality on the list of nations by the World Economic Forum (Chapman, 2017).

The Gender Pay Gap in Medicine Review

In July 2016, then-Secretary of State for Health Jeremy Hunt commissioned an independent report into the gender pay gap in medicine chaired by Professor Jane Dacre, which included an analysis of lifetime gender pay differences and the gender pensions gap (Medical Women's Federation, 2018b). The research – the largest examination of gender pay data conducted in the public sector – is led by Carol Woodhams at the University of Surrey (Medical Women's Federation, 2019; Rimmer, 2018). The approach to analysing the pay gap included performing quantitative analysis of existing data, circulating workforce surveys, and using mathematical modelling to determine the size of the overall gender pay gap and break it down into individual components. Interim results were published in early 2019, and the final report and recommendations are due to be published in September 2019 (Department of Health and Social Care, 2019).

The founding principle of the NHS is to treat everyone equally, yet women employed in the health service are still experiencing inequality. (Health Minister Stephen Hammond, 2019)

Women: Like Men, Only Cheaper?

'I should like to buy an egg, please,' she said timidly. 'How do you sell them?'

'Fivepence farthing for one — Twopence for two,' the Sheep replied.

'Then two are cheaper than one?' Alice said in a surprised tone. (Alice Through the Looking Glass, by Lewis Carroll, 1871)

Britain has one of the widest gaps in salary between men and women in Europe ("Forcing employers to reveal their gender pay gaps is making them think," 2018). In the UK, full-time male employees earned 9.4% more than female employees in 2016. This pay gap was the lowest on record, and down from 17.4% in 1997 (The Office For National Statistics, 2016). The gap for all employees (full-time and part-time) reduced from 27.5% in 1997 to 18.1% in 2016. Although this looks promising, it has been predicted that the gap will not close until 2069 (Codd, 2016). The hourly pay gap between full-time men and women is closing at a rate of only 2.5 pence per year in the UK. Globally, the gap is widening, as men's earnings are increasing more rapidly than women's (Harris, 2017).

In general, gaps in starting salary are less for individuals who have studied STEM subjects (Codd, 2016). The youngest female STEM respondents (25 to 34 years) to a survey performed by *New Scientist* with the science recruitment specialists SRG earned 2.5% less on average than their male counterparts (Fleming, 2018). But overall the average pay gap is still 20%, with men in STEM in the UK earning £41,200 on average in 2017, while women were paid £33,000. This peaks at 35% for women aged 55 and above.

The NHS is the largest single employer in Britain, with a workforce of 1.5 million (Appleby, 2018). Most NHS trusts employ over 250 staff, the threshold above which organisations have been required to publish their gender pay gap data since April 2018; 220 NHS organisations have already published their data. Over ninety per cent of these organisations revealed that men were paid more than women. This ranged from 0.1% of median hourly pay (Lancashire Teaching Hospitals) to 52.5% (Health Education England). Eight organisations reported no difference between male and female salaries, and 5% reported a pay gap in favour of women.

Among doctors, the pay gap has been increasing: in 2004, male doctors earned 21% more than women, but by 2016 this figure had risen to 34% (Brown et al., 2018; Dean, 2017; Rimmer, 2017). Full-time male doctors (average salary £120,890) earned £20,000 more than full-time female doctors (£99,833) when bonuses, overtime, and awards were included (Medical Women's Federation, 2018a). The gap remains even when examining basic pay, where a difference of £6,000 is found for full-time doctors (£87,327 *versus* £81,216). Latest figures from the 2019 Gender Pay Gap in Medicine Review show that there persists a 17% average gap among doctors (Campbell, 2019; Medical Women's Federation, 2019). The greatest disparity is experienced by female GPs, who earn an average £38,000 less than their male counterparts. Hospital doctors experience a £1,166 pay gap.

In the United States, data from The National Census Bureau in 2015 revealed that female doctors make 64-69 cents on the dollar compared with male doctors, or $62,497 less on average (Greenberg, 2017; Kuwick, 2018). A survey on Doximity in 2017 showed this average difference to be as high as $105,000 ("Doximity 2018 Physician Compensation Report," 2018; Kavilanz, 2018). To put it into perspective, female full professors make roughly the equivalent salary as male associate professors (Oaklander, 2016). Interestingly, the difference is even higher for dentists than doctors (Le, Lo Sasso, & Vujicic, 2017).

The inequality in the American medical profession is worsening: the pay gap between newly graduated male and female doctors at State University of New York, Albany more than doubled from $11,931 in 2010 to $26,367 in 2016 (Kuwick, 2018). Although the pay gap affects all doctors, it varies geographically and among specialties, e.g. higher in orthopaedic surgery and lower in geriatric medicine (Satyanarayana, 2017). The 2017 Medscape Physician Compensation Report showed that this gap is wider for specialists ($95,000) than for primary care physicians ($32,000) (Kuwick, 2018). Between male and female surgeons, there is a pay gap of $44,000-$83,000.

Inequality is of course not restricted to gender. The gender pay gap is compounded by intersectionality with the race pay gap. In the US, black female doctors make nearly $100,000 less than black male doctors, and black doctors earn an average of $50,000 less than white doctors (Hicks, 2018).

Why Does it Matter?

It is worth remembering that male and female doctors go through the same training and sit the same examinations (Dean, 2017). Most reasonable people would not dispute that individuals should be paid equally for work of equal value. A person's salary reflects the worth that is attributed to the work they are providing. With systematic inequality in pay throughout their careers, and a career-expansive difference in salary of $1.3-2.5 million, women suffer negative effects to their financial security, retirement, and pensions (Greenberg, 2017).

I also hadn't clocked just how professionally damaging it would feel. When you are paid less it's hard not to question your own ability and value to your employer. (BBC Radio 4 presenter Sarah Montague, 2018)

There are also implications for recruitment and retention of the best candidates. According to Professor Ruth Sealy, gender parity and diversity are used in the private sector by investors as a marker of quality (Grossman, 2018). There is abundant research that shows how diversity acts as a competitive indicator; companies that rank more highly in terms of racial or gender diversity are more likely to have financial returns above the national industry medians. In the UK, for every 10 per cent increase in gender diversity, there was a 3.5% increase in earnings before interest and taxes – the highest performance uplift in a study by the McKinsey Group (Hunt, Layton, & Prince, 2015). In the Nordic countries, which are often found at the top of the World Economic Forum's annual Global Gender Gap Report, the Organisation for Economic Co-operation and Development has reported that higher female employment rates have resulted in an increase of 10 to 20% in per capita GDP (Organisation for Economic Co-operation and Development, 2018; Zalis, 2018).

The pay gap isn't the choice of women. It is both a cause and consequence of gender inequality. In many respects it is more important than pay discrimination because it shines a light on the deep structural inequalities in every part of our society and economy. (Presenter and political activist Sandi Toksvig, 2018)

In the NHS, staff surveys have shown that the percentage of staff believing their trust provides equal opportunities for career progression or promotion is an important predictor of patient satisfaction (Appleby, 2018). A 10% decrease in staff believing that this is the case is associated with a 0.2 point drop in patient satisfaction scores (Dawson, 2018).

Common Myths

If I had £1 every time someone asked if we still need a women's network, I would have a lot of 85p's. (Professor Ruth Sealey, 2018)

According to a poll conducted by Time magazine in March 2019, nearly half of American men believe that the gender pay gap is "made up to serve a political purpose", and a quarter of men aged between 18 and 34 years do not believe media reports on the subject (Steinmetz, 2019).

If you're not living it, maybe you're blissfully unaware. (Hired CEO Mehul Patel, 2019)

Men were also more likely to explain the gap by saying that women choose to work fewer hours, and are "generally in careers that don't pay as much," while women were more likely to report unconscious bias and sexism as likely causes (Steinmetz, 2019). Over half (58%) of men claimed that obstacles that may have previously barred women's career progression are now "largely gone."

One explanation for the gender wage gap is that men typically gravitate towards higher paying jobs like doctor, engineer, CEO... While women tend to gravitate towards lower paying jobs like female doctor, female engineer and female CEO. (Comedian Jeremy McLellan, 2016)

Other myths include that women choose lower-paying work, and jobs with flexibility over high pay in order to prioritise childcare. In addition, a common statement is that women are attaining more higher degrees than men, with the erroneous conclusion that the pay gap will eventually close by itself (Posner, 2018).

The status quo is very good at defending the status quo. (Emily Martin, Vice President for Education and Workplace Justice at the National Women's Law Center, 2019)

PUTATIVE CAUSES OF THE PAY GAP

The Glass Ceiling

We have to start questioning whether business is built on a foundation of meritocracy when consistently we're appointing senior white men into all of our leadership jobs. That doesn't feel like it is a meritocracy, does it? That feels like a highly biased selection process. (Denise Wilson-White, CEO of the Hampton-Alexander Review, 2018)

A summary of the putative causes of the gender pay gap can be seen in Figure 1.

Previously, women's education and training corresponded to an increase in salary. This benefit now appears to be limited by the glass ceiling (Lam, 2017). It is an inescapable fact that there are fewer women than men in higher paid, more senior positions (Nawrockyi, 2016). The NHS workforce comprises 77% female staff. Despite women outnumbering men at each level, the proportion of women in the top pay quartiles is lower than in the bottom quartiles across the NHS (Appleby, 2018). This matches what is seen in other industries ("Forcing employers to reveal their gender pay gaps is making them think," 2018). There is inequality in the senior medical grades, with nearly 32,000 male consultants, and only 18,000

Figure 1. Putative causes of the gender pay gap

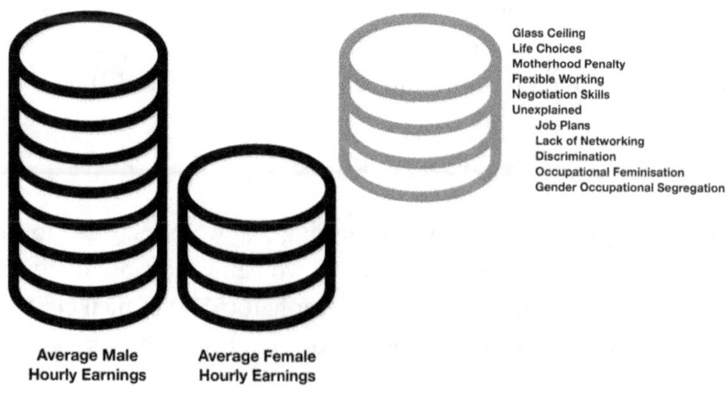

female consultants; i.e. women make up 36% of consultants in England (Medical Women's Federation, 2019). Just five out of the top 100 earning consultants in England are women, despite women making up more than a third of the workforce (Triggle, 2018). The highest salary earned by a man was nearly £740,000 – two-and-a-half times that of the highest-paid woman.

It also takes longer for women to reach the more senior roles, which results in a career-wide gender pay gap, particularly as they accrue fewer years at the top-banded consultant salaries (The British Medical Association, 2018). A cross-sectional study of surgical trainees by Brown et al. (2018) showed that overall attrition rates were similar between male and female trainees, but the authors found that time to completion of training was on average 16 months longer for women than men. There was no sex difference in the number of trainees who require additional training time due to inadequate progress. However, only six of the 38 women studied, compared with 31 of the 63 men, achieved higher degrees during their training, and men had a higher number of publications, a greater first-author role, and more citations than women. As the authors point out, new consultants who have higher degrees may receive an immediate salary increment of circa 3.2% (with compound interest, an additional £22,190 of salary over 6 years, or a 23% increase).

A detailed exploration of the reasons for the glass ceiling are beyond the scope of this chapter, but the most likely factors include traditional gender roles resulting in unconscious bias, and a lack of visible role models and mentors (Zhuge, Kaufman, Simeone, Chen, & Velazquez, 2011). Increasing attention has been paid to the lack of visibility of women in senior healthcare and STEM roles, even when women are reasonably well-represented in these fields (Silver, 2016; Silver et al., 2017). In addition, when trying to enter or advance in male-dominated fields, women may find themselves facing harassment or hostility (Steinmetz, 2019; Zhuge et al., 2011).

Life Choices

As mentioned above, many individuals put the gap down to personal choice; but how much freedom do individuals have to choose their circumstances (Lam, 2016)? Some women may want to pursue a job that happens to be paid less, or because they want flexibility or a less demanding career due to caring commitments. But it is difficult to tease this apart from the effects of early socialisation, and the expectation that women should bear a larger share of the burden of caring and home responsibilities, also known as "invisible labour" (Chakelian, 2018). It is also worth noting how little those roles are valued economically (Schieder & Gould, 2016). According to the Office of National Statistics, men in the UK enjoy nearly five more hours of leisure time per week than women, and this gap is increasing (Chakelian, 2018; *Men enjoy five hours more leisure time per week than women*, 2018). Men therefore have more free time, despite "choosing" to spend more time working to achieve higher-paying roles (Chakelian, 2018).

Women are also told from a young age that they will not excel in STEM subjects, either subliminally with the pervasive gender stereotyping among toys that are marketed to girls, or explicitly by misguided teachers and advisers at school (Blau & Kahn, 2017; Posner, 2018). This is compounded by a lack of role models in STEM subjects. Furthermore, the jobs that women choose often lack the flexibility that women are supposedly meant to prioritise (Posner, 2018).

It is often repeated that women do not put themselves forward for higher-earning positions. This is laying the blame at the feet of women. But, as stated by Chakelian (2018), it is men who have shaped the pay structures, the management, the hiring practices, and all other aspects of the workplace since time immemorial, creating a familiar and comfortable habitat in which men thrive. Men have not provided an environment that treats the sexes equally. Is it any wonder that this deters women from coming forward?

Motherhood Penalty and Flexible Working

The national full-time median pay gap is 2% among workers in their 30s, 14% in their 40s, and 16% in their 50s ("Forcing employers to reveal their gender pay gaps is making them think," 2018). As mentioned above, one of the most common reasons given for the pay gap is the *motherhood penalty*, where women's career progression is affected by having children and working part-time (Campbell, 2019). One in nine new mothers ends up leaving their employment due to the actions of her employer ("Forcing employers to reveal their gender pay gaps is making them think," 2018). Men are in effect rewarded for continuous service. There is indeed a motherhood penalty, and this penalty is also applied to women without children: the discrepancy persists at 12% between men and women without children (Dossa & Baxter, 2018; Trades Union Congress, 2016). This is often followed by the *good daughter penalty*, whereby women are charged with taking care of elderly relatives ("Forcing employers to reveal their gender pay gaps is making them think," 2018).

It is also true that women are more likely to work less than full time: 41% of UK women do so, compared with only 12% of men (The Office For National Statistics, 2016). It is well-known that employees are disproportionately disadvantaged for requesting flexibility (Blau & Kahn, 2017; Miller, 2016). Interestingly, female part-time employees earned 6% more than male part-time employees in 2016, suggesting that a bias may exist against part-time male employees.

It is important to note that women's decisions to take time out or work less than full time do not account for the whole pay gap.

Negotiation Skills

Medical students aren't taught how to negotiate salaries. But it's vital for them, especially for women, to learn this skill. (Dr Fatima Stanford, 2018)

In the UK medical profession, there are nationally agreed salary scales, which should in theory eliminate any effects of individuals negotiating their own pay. Certainly, the wage gap is higher when employer discretion is greater, i.e. in the private sector, than where wages are formally dictated, as in the public sector (Murphy & Oesch, 2016). In general, women are more likely to work in careers where it is not possible to negotiate one's salary (Uwagba, 2019).

Men are traditionally considered better at negotiating than women (Babcock & Laschever, 2008; Oaklander, 2016). Some argue that there is an "expectation gap", whereby women believe they are worth less despite objective evidence to the contrary (Steinmetz, 2019). This correlates with studies showing higher rates of impostor syndrome among women (Legassie, Zibrowski, & Goldszmidt, 2008; Oriel, Plane, & Mundt, 2004). Studies of pay disparities in the technology industry have shown that women tend to ask for less money than similarly-qualified male peers (Steinmetz, 2019). However, these studies generally do not control for industries where one gender dominates, which can skew the findings when investigating the overall numbers of employees negotiating salaries (Uwagba, 2019).

Nawrockyi (2016) argues that it is good performance and behaviour that should be rewarded, not the ability to ask for more money. Furthermore, when women are too aggressive in their requests for pay raises, they are perceived more negatively than men. Certainly research has shown that women face more backlash from asking for higher pay, which may act as a social barrier to asking again (Amanatullah & Morris, 2010; Amanatullah & Tinsley, 2013; Bowles, Babcock, & Lai, 2007).

Artz, Goodall, and Oswald (2018) used matched employer–employee data from the Australian Workplace Relations Survey, in which workers were questioned about their asking behaviour between 2013-2014, to investigate promotion and pay negotiation within current jobs, and levels of satisfaction. The authors concluded that male and female employees asked equally often for promotions and raises. This was after the study was controlled for hours worked, resulting in a direct comparison between full-time male and female employees. However, Artz et al. (2018) found that, while women asked for raises at the same rate as men, they were less likely to receive what they asked for (with the exception of the younger cohort). An interesting finding in the study was that there was no evidence that women were more concerned than men about possible deleterious effects on their relationships with managers when deciding whether to ask for a raise, despite the above studies demonstrating a backlash in such scenarios. Furthermore, other studies have actually shown women to negotiate pay at a slightly higher rate than men (31% *versus* 29% respectively) (Uwagba, 2019).

I hate the idea of putting the onus on women to overcome the gender pay gap, or somehow implying that they are the ones at fault. Instead, I prefer to see it this way: It's important to keep asking (…) Women are asking. It's high time we were heard. (Writer Otegha Uwagba, 2019)

Nevertheless, it is clear that female doctors do not demand good salaries and pay review as consultants, and that they put themselves forward for fewer clinical excellence awards (CEAs). This is mirrored by the statements that women and men put on their CEA forms and how they describe their achievements (Rimmer, 2014).

In England, more than half of hospital consultants (22,874 of 43,856) received a CEA of between £17,000 and £77,000 in 2015 (Donnelly, 2017). These bonuses are normally life-long, and are pensionable. In 2015, of those receiving awards for the first time, only 65 were women, while 252 were given to men. Success rates were equal at 26% for both men and women applying for CEAs. Women were more likely to be successful than men when applying for the highest level awards of £77,000, which are awarded nationally. However, six-and-a-half times fewer women applied: only five women compared with 31 men (Triggle, 2018).

Despite recommendations that CEA selection panels should be "gender balanced wherever possible" by Baroness Deech, chair of the National Working Group on Women in Medicine in 2009, there has been a significant discrepancy in the representation of women on these panels: in 2012, 29% of all committee members were female (Rimmer, 2014).

Remainder Unexplained

The pay gap in medicine persists when the above popular explanations are factored in – maternity leave, clinical excellence awards, fewer years of experience, etc. (Dean, 2017). The causes of up to 50% of the pay gap for trainees – and 40% for consultants – are unknown (Dean, 2017), and these unaccountable discrepancies have grown with time (Le et al., 2017).

One contributory factor for this unexplained gap could be that women focus more on service provision and caring for patients, rather than on activities that may further their careers, such as networking and joining committees (Rimmer, 2014), and research (Brown et al., 2018). Women often end up in more pastoral extracurricular positions, such as teaching, rather than the better-paid management positions (Lord, 2019).

It is thought that up to 38% of the wage gap may be caused by pure discrimination (Blau & Kahn, 2017; Miller, 2016; Oaklander, 2016). Female dominated fields are generally less well paid, as work performed by women is valued less than that done by men (Blau & Kahn, 2017; Miller, 2016). Part of the pay gap may therefore be explained by *gender occupational segregation* and *occupational feminisation*.

Gender Occupational Segregation and Occupational Feminisation

As has been established above, the pay gap is present between the sexes even in female-dominated fields, such as healthcare and teaching (Steinmetz, 2019), and it has widened over time in these fields.

The 2019 Gender Pay Gap in Medicine Review update showed that women were over-represented in the medical specialties that involve lower pay, such as public health and occupational health, while male-dominated specialties, e.g. urology, have wider pay gaps (Campbell, 2019). Within surgery in the UK, male-dominated specialities such as plastic surgery, orthopaedics, and neurosurgery are better paid. Paediatric surgery is the least well paid, for both best-paid and average earnings (Dean, 2017).

The difference between male and female-dominated fields accounts for more than half of the unexplained pay gap. Researchers call the distribution of men and women in different occupations *gender occupational segregation* (Lam, 2016). A cross-sectional example of wage discrepancies between different gendered jobs that require the same level of education, time investment, and job-specific skills can be found in information technology managers (mostly men), who earn 27% more than human resources managers (mostly women) (Miller, 2016). Within STEM, biotechnologists (mostly women) are paid less than engineers (mostly men) (Fleming, 2018).

As the proportion of women in a previously male-dominated field increases, so-called *occupational feminisation* (Levanon, England, & Allison, 2009; Murphy & Oesch, 2016; Schieder & Gould, 2016), the pay declines, for the exact same job previously performed by men (Figure 2). This has been demonstrated over time in recreational park employees, ticket agents, designers, housekeepers, and biologists, with wages falling by 18-58% as these jobs changed from male- to female-dominated (Miller, 2016). Conversely, as more men enter a field, the job becomes more desirable, and the pay increases. This is what happened in computer programming. In computing's infancy, hardware development was performed by men, and was considered far more prestigious than the womanly work of programming (Cohen, 2016). This role was increasingly masculinised through the 1950s and 1960s as recruitment became based on psychological profiles of the "antisocial" programmer. Wages and prestige increased as the number of women in the field declined.

In Britain, a shift from an entirely male to an entirely female occupation results in an individual wage penalty of 13% (Murphy & Oesch, 2016). The cut-off appears to be when occupations consist of more than 60% women.

POSSIBLE SOLUTIONS TO THE GENDER PAY GAP

Transparency

The advice from the business sector is to conduct wage audits to better understand the wage gap, and to make salaries for similar roles transparent (Newman, 2012; Rimmer, 2014; Zimmermann, 2018). As the economist Iris Bohnet has previously stated, this approach has been successful when awarding hygiene ratings to restaurants and putting energy-efficiency labels on white goods ("Forcing employers to reveal their gender pay gaps is making them think," 2018). Transparency may help employees better understand their true market value (Steinmetz, 2019). For example, Norway, which currently ranks third out of 144 countries regarding wage equality, allows employees to see the wages of colleagues, and it is not unusual for Norwegian jobs advertisements to specify the salary on offer. Abolishing negotiations for salary would also help to close the gap (Zimmermann, 2018).

Rosenfeld and Denice (2015) used the 2004 and 2011 series of the British Workplace Employment Relations Survey to examine the effect of transparency. They found that pay disclosure resulted in higher employee salaries, after adjusting for factors such as profit and productivity levels. Employees who reported that their managers were "very good" at sharing organisation financial information earned 8% to 12% more than those who said their managers were "very poor". The authors argued that transparency shifts power in the direction of employees.

As mentioned earlier, since April 2018, the UK has required organisations with 250 or more employees to publish their mean and median wages by gender (Topping & Barr, 2018). The median is usually more representative, as the mean can be skewed by small numbers of highly paid employees ("Forcing employers to reveal their gender pay gaps is making them think," 2018). Inequality at either end of the pay spectrum can be detected by large discrepancies between the two values. Companies that do not publish their pay gaps risk unspecified fines and sanctions by the Equalities and Human Rights Commission. Legally mandating these publications is necessary; a 2010 request for voluntary reports was, unsurprisingly, not successful.

Following these changes in 2018, the difference in salary between men and women was found to be much higher than expected, and higher than previously published. This may be due to the fact that the new law required a level of transparency that was previously evaded by presenting data within very narrow parameters (Suddath, 2018). As reported by Bloomberg, Microsoft Corp. published internal gender pay gap data in 2016 showing that women earned 99.8% of what men earned for the same role. It turns out that this figure was masking the fact that the multiple pay grades and salary scales did not reveal whether women were assigned to the correct role or pay grade in the first place, or whether they were promoted as often as men. Women may have been doing the same job as men, but at a different pay grade.

The government has not however required these companies to include the salaries of partners, who are paid a share of profits. Most partners are male, and the difference in the gap can be as high as 20% (Savage, 2018). Furthermore, incorporating discretionary bonuses widened the gender pay gap among UK Goldman Sachs employees from 56% to 72.2% (Finch & Hellier, 2018). The bonus pay gap, as high as 86% at HSBC, suggests that seniority may not be the real issue – men are just paid more (Chakelian, 2018).

It is also worth noting that transparency is only as effective as the data that are collected. In April 2019, it was revealed that up to 15% of submissions may have contained errors, with up to 1,000 reports considered suspicious (Narwan, 2019). The data were also not adjusted for different roles, so the highest paid positions were compared directly with the lowest ("Forcing employers to reveal their gender pay gaps is making them think," 2018). Enforcement of pay reporting has been sub-optimal. There are still, sadly, plenty of opportunities for companies to misrepresent the figures, and for the public to misinterpret them ("Forcing employers to reveal their gender pay gaps is making them think," 2018). The most useful information to come out of the pay gap reporting has actually been on female representation at different levels of industry, rather than the absolute salary figures.

What companies really need to find out is whether they are hiring equitably, paying equitably and are offering equitable opportunities to advance. (Brian Levine, Partner and Innovation Leader, Mercer, 2018)

Access to Childcare

An important step to closing the pay gap is to improve access to childcare, particularly for anti-social hours. Encouraging men to play a large role in childcare and other caring responsibilities may also go some way to reduce the gap. Shared parental leave is a start, but it remains to be seen how high the uptake will be. Perversely, men may be judged more harshly than women for taking time out for parental leave.

Recruitment and Career Progression

More should be done to encourage women into the higher-paid specialties, as well as of course improving the pay in the already female-dominated specialties. Initiatives such as Women in Surgery at the Royal College of Surgeons of England, the Association of Surgeons of Great Britain and Ireland Women in Surgery, and the Medical Women's Federation are all working to achieve these goals. In addition to improving the recruitment of women into higher-paid specialties, more work is needed to examine the factors affecting the career pathways of female doctors in training. The above organisations, among others, also contribute to leadership training, mentoring, and providing advice for flexible working (Triggle, 2018). It may also be helpful for women to receive coaching on salary negotiation techniques.

It is essential to examine the current systems of recruitment and promotion to assess for areas of bias and discrimination. For example, there is little chance a woman will be hired if she is the only female candidate on a shortlist, as the unconscious message is that the position is more suited to a man (Government Equalities Office, n.d.; Johnson, Hekman, & Chan, 2016; Samuelson & Zeckhauser, 2016). It also helps to maximise flexible working opportunities to signal that the organisation has an inclusive environment. Using structured interviews and skill-based assessment are other ways to reduce bias in the hiring process.

Targets and Quotas

Targets and quotas remain controversial, but some organisations such as Lloyds Banking Group have committed to having 40% of its senior roles filled by women by 2020 ("Nine ways to narrow the gender pay gap," 2018). In the public sector, NHS Employers have set the target of equal gender representation on boards by 2020 (Sealy, 2017). In Norway, a 40% quota for board members is mandatory, enforced by the threat of sanctions (Morgenroth & Ryan, 2018). Some studies have shown that quotas can raise the standard of competence of male employees where female representation is increased (Besley, Folke, Persson, & Rickne, 2017; Chapman, 2017). Morgenroth & Ryan (2018) argue that the use of quotas results in the increased availability and visibility of role models, and is effective in increasing representation of minority groups in senior positions, as well as increasing the pool of available applicants. They caution that this effect is mitigated by whether or not the quotas are voluntary, and by cultural factors.

Reasons for Optimism

The gender pay gap is one of the most demoralising areas of gender inequality. However, there are reasons to be optimistic. For example, members at the British Medical Association's 2017 annual conference voted to end the on-going gender pay gap in health and the consistent under-representation of women in leadership positions (Gallagher, 2017).

There is evidence that, when organisations are proactive at reducing the pay gap, it can be successfully abolished. Somerset Care, a care home provider, managed to reduce their mean pay gap to 2.44% and median gap to -0.96%. One of Australia's biggest energy companies managed to eliminate their gender wage penalties overnight, by providing 350 women, who had been paid less than their male counterparts, with a $1.2 million salary increase: $3,500 each (Morgan, 2018).

In medicine, interesting data were gleaned from a retrospective review of faculty total compensation within the surgical department at an American hospital between 2009 and 2017 (Hoops et al., 2018). After implementation of a university-wide objective compensation plan to bring salaries into alignment with Association of American Medical Colleges regional median salary, women's pay increased, and the gender pay gap disappeared. Encouragingly, this corresponded to equalised promotion rates among men and women, and higher retention among both genders.

Finally, Secretary of State for Health Matt Hancock recently published an article outlining the government's plan to promote women in the NHS and to narrow the pay gap (Hancock, 2019). Together with the upcoming publication of the Gender Pay Gap in Medicine Review, there is hope that things may change for the better.

The findings of the review will help us to work with government, employers and the profession to identify and understand the main contributors to the gap, and to explore ways to reduce it, based on our evidence. (Professor Jane Dacre, 2019)

CONCLUSION

The gender pay gap is a symptom of the pervasive inequalities that are inherent in modern society. By addressing the root causes of these inequalities, as well as shining a light on the pay gap data, it is possible that we can one day close the gap.

REFERENCES

Amanatullah, E. T., & Morris, M. W. (2010). Negotiating gender roles: Gender differences in assertive negotiating are mediated by women's fear of backlash and attenuated when negotiating on behalf of others. *Journal of Personality and Social Psychology, 98*(2), 256–267. doi:10.1037/a0017094 PMID:20085399

Amanatullah, E. T., & Tinsley, C. H. (2013). Punishing female negotiators for asserting too much…or not enough: Exploring why advocacy moderates backlash against assertive female negotiators. *Organizational Behavior and Human Decision Processes, 120*(1), 110–122. doi:10.1016/j.obhdp.2012.03.006

Appleby, J. (2018, April 5). The gender pay gap in the NHS: the story so far. Retrieved from https://www.nuffieldtrust.org.uk/news-item/the-gender-pay-gap-in-the-nhs-the-story-so-far

Artz, B., Goodall, A. H., & Oswald, A. J. (2018). Do Women Ask? *Industrial Relations, 57*(4), 611–636. doi:10.1111/irel.12214

Babcock, L., & Laschever, S. (2008). *Why Women Don't Ask: The high cost of avoiding negotiation - and positive strategies for change.* Princeton, NJ: Princeton University Press.

Besley, T., Folke, O., Persson, T., & Rickne, J. (2017). Gender Quotas and the Crisis of the Mediocre Man: Theory and Evidence from Sweden. *The American Economic Review, 107*(8), 2204–2242. doi:10.1257/aer.20160080

Blau, F. D. & Kahn, L. M. (2017). The Gender Wage Gap: Extent, Trends, and Explanations. *The New York Times, 55*(3), 789–865. doi:10.1257/jel.20160995

Bowles, H. R., Babcock, L., & Lai, L. (2007). Social incentives for gender differences in the propensity to initiate negotiations: Sometimes it does hurt to ask. *Organizational Behavior and Human Decision Processes, 103*(1), 84–103. doi:10.1016/j.obhdp.2006.09.001

Brown, C., Harries, R. L., Abdelrahman, T., Thomas, C., Pollitt, M. J., & Lewis, W. G. (2018). Surgical gender gap: A curriculum concordance and career vector perspective. *Postgraduate Medical Journal, 94*(1115), 483–488. doi:10.1136/postgradmedj-2017-135437 PMID:30355590

Campbell, D. (2019, March 29). Male NHS doctors earn 17% more than their female peers. *The Guardian.*

Chakelian, A. (2018, April 4). What to say when someone tries to mansplain away the gender pay gap. *New Statesman (London, England).*

Chapman, B. (2017, June 19). Workplace gender quotas weed out incompetent men and make businesses more efficient, study finds. *The Independent.*

Codd, E. (2016). *Women in STEM. Technology, career pathways and the gender pay gap* (pp. 1–24). Deloitte. Retrieved from https://www2.deloitte.com/uk/en/pages/growth/articles/technology-career-pathways-gender-pay-gap.html

Cohen, R. (2016, Sept. 7). What Programming's Past Reveals About Today's Gender-Pay Gap. *Atlantic (Boston, Mass.).*

Dawson, J. (2018). *Links between NHS staff experience and patient satisfaction: Analysis of surveys from 2014 and 2015.* nhsstaffsurveys.com.

Dean, E. (2017). The gender pay gap in surgery. *The Bulletin of the Royal College of Surgeons of England, 99*(1), 12–14. doi:10.1308/rcsbull.2017.12

Department of Health and Social Care. (2019, March 29). New data on gender pay gap in medicine. Retrieved from https://www.gov.uk/government/news/new-data-on-gender-pay-gap-in-medicine

Donnelly, L. (2017, July 29). Hospital consultants gender pay gap revealed: Four times as many men get bonuses than women. *The Telegraph.*

Dossa, F., & Baxter, N. N. (2018). Reducing gender bias in surgery. *British Journal of Surgery*, *105*(13), 1707–1709. doi:10.1002/bjs.11042 PMID:30462365

Doximity 2018 Physician Compensation Report. (2018). Doximity 2018 Physician Compensation Report. Retrieved from https://blog.doximity.com/articles/doximity-2018-physician-compensation-report

Finch, G. & Hellier, D. (2018, March 16). Goldman Sachs Pays Females in U.K. 56% Less Than Male Colleagues. Retrieved from https://www.bloomberg.com/news/articles/2018-03-16/goldman-sachs-pays-female-staff-56-less-than-male-colleagues

Fleming, N. (2018, Feb. 28). How the gender pay gap permeates science and engineering. *New Scientist*, *237*(3167), 22–23. doi:10.1016/S0262-4079(18)30389-0

Forcing employers to reveal their gender pay gaps is making them think. (2018, April 5). Forcing employers to reveal their gender pay gaps is making them think. *The Economist*.

Gallagher, P. (2017, June 28). Stop the increasing gender pay gap, doctors tell BMA conference. *I News*.

Government Equalities Office. (n.d.). *Reducing the gender pay gap and improving gender equality in organisations: Evidence-based actions for employers*. Retrieved from gender-pay-gap.service.gov.uk

Greenberg, C. C. (2017). Association for Academic Surgery presidential address: Sticky floors and glass ceilings. *The Journal of Surgical Research*, *219*, ix–xviii. doi:10.1016/j.jss.2017.09.006 PMID:29078918

Griffin, E. (2018, March 12). What's to blame for the gender pay gap? The housework myth. *The Guardian*.

Grossman, R. (2018, Nov. 1). Gender parity and diversity are being used in the private sector by investors as a quality marker. - @RuthSealy #LiftAsYouClimb @hcwomenleaders [Tweet]. Retrieved from https://twitter.com/rebgross/status/1057949609027399680

Hancock, M. (2019, April 25). The NHS is a huge employer of women – I want it to be one of the best as well. *The Guardian*.

Harris, B. (2017, Nov. 6). *What the pay gap between men and women really looks like*. Retrieved from https://www.weforum.org/agenda/2017/11/pay-equality-men-women-gender-gap-report-2017/

Hicks, J. (2018, April 11). Women and Black Doctors Still Make Far Less Than White Male Doctors. Retrieved from https://tonic.vice.com/en_us/article/bjp595/women-and-black-doctors-still-make-far-less-than-white-male-doctors

Hoops, H. E., Brasel, K. J., Dewey, E., Rodgers, S., Merrill, J., Hunter, J. G., & Azarow, K. S. (2018). Analysis of Gender-based Differences in Surgery Faculty Compensation, Promotion, and Retention. *Annals of Surgery*, *268*(3), 479–487. doi:10.1097/SLA.0000000000002920 PMID:30063494

Hunt, V., Layton, D., & Prince, S. (2015, February). Why diversity matters. Retrieved from https://www.mckinsey.com/business-functions/organization/our-insights/why-diversity-matters

Johnson, S. K., Hekman, D. R., & Chan, E. T. (2016, April 26). If There's Only One Woman in Your Candidate Pool, There's Statistically No Chance She'll Be Hired. *Harvard Business Review*.

Kavilanz, P. (2018, March 14). The gender pay gap for women doctors is big -- and getting worse. Retrieved from https://money.cnn.com/2018/03/14/news/economy/gender-pay-gap-doctors/index.html

Kuwick, L. (2018, March 7). Commit to a conversation about the gender pay gap. Retrieved from https://www.kevinmd.com/blog/2018/03/commit-conversation-gender-pay-gap.html

Lam, B. (2016, July 27). What Gender Pay-Gap Statistics Aren't Capturing. *Atlantic (Boston, Mass.).*

Lam, B. (2017, March 28). Education Doesn't Solve the Gender Pay Gap. *Atlantic (Boston, Mass.).*

Le, T. A. N., Lo Sasso, A. T., & Vujicic, M. (2017). Trends in the earnings gender gap among dentists, physicians, and lawyers. *The Journal of the American Dental Association*, *148*(4), 257–262.e2. doi:10.1016/j.adaj.2017.01.005 PMID:28238360

Legassie, J., Zibrowski, E. M., & Goldszmidt, M. A. (2008). Measuring Resident Well-Being: Impostorism and Burnout Syndrome in Residency. *Journal of General Internal Medicine*, *23*(7), 1090–1094. doi:10.100711606-008-0536-x PMID:18612750

Levanon, A., England, P., & Allison, P. (2009). Occupational Feminization and Pay: Assessing Causal Dynamics Using 1950-2000 U.S. Census Data. *Social Forces*, *88*(2), 865–891. doi:10.1353of.0.0264

Lord, A. (2019, April 15). Also perhaps women tend to choose other things (e.g. teaching) over research? Which is fine as long as they have equal opportunity to do either and it's a true choice! [Tweet]. Retrieved from https://twitter.com/AmyLord1/status/1117712428530315265

Medical Women's Federation. (2018b, May 28). Press Release: Gender Pay Gap Review in Medicine. Retrieved from medicalwomensfederation.org.uk

Medical Women's Federation. (2019, March 29). Press Release: MWF responds to Gender Pay Gap in Medicine Review interim findings. Retrieved from medicalwomensfederation.org.uk

Medical Women's Federation [medicalwomenuk]. (2018a, Feb. 16). On average full-time men earned £20,000 more than full-time women when you include bonuses, overtime and awards: £120,890 v £99,833 Even if you look at basic pay, there is a difference of £6,000 for full-time doctors: £87,327 v £81,216 #GenderPayGap [Tweet]. Retrieved from https://twitter.com/medicalwomenuk/status/964410742316220416

Men enjoy five hours more leisure time per week than women. (2018). Men enjoy five hours more leisure time per week than women. Retrieved from ons.gov.uk

Miller, C. C. (2016, March 18). As Women Take Over a Male-Dominated Field, the Pay Drops. *The New York Times*.

Morgan, E. (2018, March 7). Energy Australia closes gender pay gap overnight, literally. Retrieved from http://www.abc.net.au/news/2018-03-07/energy-australia-closes-gender-pay-gap-overnight/9524770

Morgenroth, T., & Ryan, M. K. (2018). Quotas and affirmative action: Understanding group-based outcomes and attitudes. *Social and Personality Psychology Compass*, *12*(3), e12374–e32. doi:10.1111pc3.12374

Murphy, E., & Oesch, D. (2016). The Feminization of Occupations and Change in Wages: A Panel Analysis of Britain, Germany, and Switzerland. *Social Forces*, *94*(3), 1221–1255. doi:10.1093fov099

Narwan, G. (2019, April 23). Hundreds of errors mar pay gap data. *The Times.*

Nawrockyi, K. (2016, Nov. 15). Closing the gender pay gap: Stop telling women they just need to negotiate harder. Retrieved from http://www.womanthology.co.uk/pdwti

Newman, P. (2012). *Releasing Potential: Women Doctors and Clinical Leadership.*

Nine ways to narrow the gender pay gap. (2018, April 5). Nine ways to narrow the gender pay gap. Retrieved from https://www.bbc.com/news/business-43643989

Oaklander, M. (2016, July 11). Women and Black Doctors Still Make Far Less Than White Male Doctors. *Time*. Retrieved from http://time.com/4398888/doctors-gender-wage-gap/

Organisation for Economic Co-operation and Development. (2018). *Is the last mile the longest? oecd.org.*

Oriel, K., Plane, M. B., & Mundt, M. (2004). Family medicine residents and the impostor phenomenon. *Family Medicine*, *36*(4), 248–252. PMID:15057614

Posner, L. (2018, March 13). 4 of the biggest myths about the gender pay gap. Retrieved from https://www.salon.com/2018/03/13/4-of-the-biggest-myths-about-the-gender-pay-gap_partner/

Rimmer, A. (2014). Why do female doctors earn less money for doing the same job? *BMJ (Clinical Research Ed.)*, *349*, g5604. doi:10.1136/bmj.g5604

Rimmer, A. (2017). The gender pay gap: female doctors still earn a third less than male doctors. *BMJ*, j1967. doi:10.1136/bmj.j1967

Rimmer, A. (2018). Medicine's gender pay gap: Five minutes with . . . Jane Dacre. *BMJ (Clinical Research Ed.)*, *363*, k4559. doi:10.1136/bmj.k4559 PMID:30377157

Rosenfeld, J., & Denice, P. (2015). The Power of Transparency: Evidence from a British Workplace Survey. *American Sociological Review*, *80*(5), 1045–1068. doi:10.1177/0003122415597019

Samuelson, W. & Zeckhauser, R. (2016, April 26). *Status quo bias in decision making.* doi:10.1007/BF00055564

Satyanarayana, M. (2017, April 27). *Female doctors earn less than men, even in the same specialty.* Retrieved from https://www.statnews.com/2017/04/27/gender-pay-gap-specialty-doctor/

Savage, M. (2018, March 10). Top-paid men outstrip women by 4 to 1, shock figures reveal. *The Guardian.*

Schieder, J., & Gould, E. (2016). *"Women's work" and the gender pay gap.* Economic Policy Institute.

Sealy, R. (2017). NHS Women on Boards: 50:50 by 2020. Retrieved from nhsemployers.org.

Silver, J. K. (2016, Oct. 24). Why are female doctors being hidden in plain sight? Retrieved from https://www.statnews.com/2016/10/24/female-doctors-invisible-women/

Silver, J. K., Slocum, C. S., Bank, A. M., Bhatnagar, S., Blauwet, C. A., Poorman, J. A., ... Parangi, S. (2017). Where Are the Women? The Underrepresentation of Women Physicians Among Recognition Award Recipients From Medical Specialty Societies. *PM & R*, *9*(8), 804–815. doi:10.1016/j.pmrj.2017.06.001 PMID:28606837

Steinmetz, K. (2019, April 2). Nearly Half of Men Believe the Pay Gap Is "Made Up," Survey Finds. *Time*.

Suddath, C. (2018, March 29). New Numbers Show the Gender Pay Gap Is Real. Retrieved from https://www.bloomberg.com/news/features/2018-03-29/the-gender-pay-gap-is-real-say-new-numbers-from-the-u-k

The British Medical Association. (2018, Dec. 6). Pay scales for consultants in England. Retrieved from https://www.bma.org.uk/advice/employment/pay/consultants-pay-england

The Office for National Statistics. (2016). *The gender pay gap - what is it and what affects it?* The Office for National Statistics. Retrieved from https://www.ons.gov.uk/employmentandlabourmarket/peopleinwork/earningsandworkinghours/articles/thegenderpaygapwhatisitandwhataffectsit/2016-10-26

Topping, A. & Barr, C. (2018, Feb. 28). What you need to know about gender pay gap reporting. *The Guardian*.

Trades Union Congress. (2016). (pp. 1–8). The Motherhood Pay Penalty.

Triggle, N. (2018, Feb. 16). Top women doctors earn less than men. Retrieved from https://www.bbc.com/news/health-43077465

Uwagba, O. (2019, March 8). *Actually, women do ask for money. They just don't get it.* Retrieved from https://www.thecut.com/2019/03/women-do-ask-money-work-salary-raise.html

Zalis, S. (2018, Oct. 30). Lessons from the world's most gender-equal countries. *Forbes*.

Zhuge, Y., Kaufman, J., Simeone, D. M., Chen, H., & Velazquez, O. C. (2011). Is There Still a Glass Ceiling for Women in Academic Surgery? *Annals of Surgery*, *253*(4), 637–643. doi:10.1097/SLA.0b013e3182111120 PMID:21475000

Zimmermann, A. (2018). *What can organisations do to close the gender pay gap?* LSE Business Review.

ADDITIONAL READING

Brown, C., Harries, R. L., Abdelrahman, T., Thomas, C., Pollitt, M. J., & Lewis, W. G. (2018). Surgical gender gap: A curriculum concordance and career vector perspective. *Postgraduate Medical Journal*, *94*(1115), 483–488. doi:10.1136/postgradmedj-2017-135437 PMID:30355590

Chakelian, A. (2018, April 4). What to say when someone tries to mansplain away the gender pay gap. *New Statesman (London, England)*.

Department of Health and Social Care. (2019, March 29). New data on gender pay gap in medicine. Retrieved April 14, 2019, from https://www.gov.uk/government/news/new-data-on-gender-pay-gap-in-medicine

Forcing employers to reveal their gender pay gaps is making them think. (2018, April 5). Forcing employers to reveal their gender pay gaps is making them think. *The Economist*.

Hoops, H. E., Brasel, K. J., Dewey, E., Rodgers, S., Merrill, J., Hunter, J. G., & Azarow, K. S. (2018). Analysis of Gender-based Differences in Surgery Faculty Compensation, Promotion, and Retention. *Annals of Surgery*, *268*(3), 479–487. doi:10.1097/SLA.0000000000002920 PMID:30063494

Lam, B. (2016, July 27). What Gender Pay-Gap Statistics Aren't Capturing. *Atlantic (Boston, Mass.)*.

Rimmer, A. (2018). Medicine's gender pay gap: Five minutes with . . . Jane Dacre. *BMJ (Clinical Research Ed.)*, *363*, k4559. doi:10.1136/bmj.k4559 PMID:30377157

Steinmetz, K. (2019, April 2). Nearly Half of Men Believe the Pay Gap Is "Made Up," Survey Finds. *Time*. doi:10.1177/0003122415597019

Uwagba, O. (2019, March 8). Actually, Women Do Ask for Money. They Just Don't Get It. Retrieved April 14, 2019, from https://www.thecut.com/2019/03/women-do-ask-money-work-salary-raise.html

KEY TERMS AND DEFINITIONS

Gender Occupational Segregation: The distribution of workers across and within occupations, based upon demographic characteristics, most often gender.

Gender Pay Gap: The difference between the average hourly earnings of men and women.

Glass Ceiling: An invisible barrier to advancement in a profession, especially affecting women and members of minorities.

Invisible Labour: The expectation that women should bear a larger share of the burden of caring and home responsibilities.

Motherhood Penalty: The systematic disadvantages experienced by working mothers.

Occupational Feminisation: The increase in the proportion of women in a previously male-dominated field.

Unconscious Bias: Learned stereotypes that are automatic, unintentional, and that influence behaviour and attitudes towards groups of people.

Chapter 9
Parallels Between Improving the Culture for Women in Surgery and a Surgical Approach to Improving Health for All

Scarlett A. McNally
East Sussex Healthcare NHS Trust, UK

ABSTRACT

Every person should be valued for their skills and potential, for every moment they are present. Training on Diversity and Unconscious bias is urgently needed. All staff must see themselves as role models, creating culture and reacting to another's name badge/role, with "fake it till you make it". Those with poor behaviour may lack insight. Zero tolerance involves others taking a poorly-behaving peer for 'a Vanderbilt cup of coffee'. Informal mentors should avoid gendered assumptions, e.g. all medical students need to scrub in. Leadership roles should have a clear application process. Inequality is not just a women's issue. Improvements must focus on the women themselves, the others around them, and the structures/processes. There are parallels with prevention in healthcare needing 3-pronged change: in individuals, society/culture, and organisations. More people being active can rapidly reduce the need for, and cost of, healthcare and social care by £Billions annually. The current paradigm of health is perhaps passive and paternalistic and a radical approach is needed.

SUMMARY

Having highly trained women in a role, equipped with knowledge and skills is not enough. Those around them and structures need to try harder. Information and training can help. Clear accessible information should be available to anyone who might give advice about pregnancy, childrearing, breastfeeding and part-time training/working for all genders. Performance management should be against defined job tasks.

DOI: 10.4018/978-1-5225-9599-1.ch009

Mandatory training on 'Equality & Diversity' currently only teaches that difference must not be mentioned at exams, interviews or summative assessments. Training on Diversity, Unconscious bias and dealing with difference is urgently needed. All staff need to see themselves as role models, creating culture and reacting to another's name badge rather than what they look like. We all need to try harder with "fake it till you make it" when someone does not seem to fit the image. Those with leadership roles need training in management skills, including Human Resources and how to chair a meeting inclusively. Those with poor behaviour may lack insight. Zero tolerance for poor behaviour involves others taking a peer with perceived poor behaviour for 'a Vanderbilt cup of coffee'. Informal mentors should avoid gendered assumptions, eg all medical students need to scrub in, not only those who look like future surgeons.

Leadership roles should have a person specification, fixed tenure and a clear application process. Each role should be analysed to ensure a realistic workload and admin or IT support. For example, Doctors in training spend 50% of their time doing admin or basic clinical tasks, whereas "Doctors' Assistants" can be trained from HealthCare Assistants and this frees up Doctors' time (McNally & Huber, 2018). Many staff are at risk of overwork and burnout, which can lead to poor behaviour; measures to improve wellbeing may mitigate this.

Educating and empowering women improves wider health and the economy. 70% of NHS spending is on long-term conditions that have a large preventable component. The patriarchal model of health focusses on interventions rather than holistic care. Empowering people to be physically active can rapidly reduce the need for, and cost of, social care by £Billions annually in the UK alone. Prevention in healthcare needs individuals, society/culture and organisations to change.

Opportunity for every individual helps everyone. Inequality must move away from being seen as an issue only for those in the underrepresented group to sort out. This chapter includes some context around women in surgery and detailed suggestions on how to improve the lot of women, by focussing on the women themselves, the others around them and the structures and processes that need to change.

A similar three-pronged approach is suggested to embed a massive change in the health of the population and reduce the need for social care. In a similar way to supporting women, health promotion and primary and secondary prevention should focus on the three areas of individual empowerment, society and organisations. The current paradigm of health could be argued to be passive and paternalistic and a radical approach is needed.

There have always been Margaret Thatchers. Us pioneering alpha women can give the impression there is no problem. It is only later that historical sleep-deprivation, miscarriages or discriminatory throw-away remarks get acknowledged (McNally, 2018a). In the UK NHS, after qualifying, doctors complete a two-year Foundation programme and those intending a surgical career have either one hurdle or two hurdles, depending on whether their chosen specialty is "run-through" (e.g. neurosurgery) or has 2-3 year Core Surgical Training, followed by a further selection into a 5-7 year Higher Surgical Training programme for their specialty. The establishment was reassured by my definitive 2012 analysis (McNally, 2012) of 12,000 applicants to UK surgical training that there no discrimination against women, and even that women doctors who applied to surgical training were statistically *more* likely to be appointed. That data also showed 30% of applicants to Core surgical training were women, dispelling the myth that women don't want to do surgery; yet only 10% of applicants to Higher Surgical training (typically following two years of Core) were female (McNally, 2012). Women were actively choosing not to continue. The Royal College of Surgeons of England (RCSEng) has done great work since early 1990s with 'Women in Surgical Training' (WIST) which changed to 'Women in Surgery' (WinS) in 2007 and now has over

6000 members. The problem is more than just encouraging the women to feel part of a community and supported. This is not purely a woman's issue. Women have proved that it is possible and that they want to do it, but barriers persist.

The barriers occur around appointment, doing a role, getting leadership roles and getting paid for work done. Work between WinS and Exeter university psychologists identified that those surgeons in training who did not "fit in" with their perception of their boss' personality were more likely to burn out and less likely to continue (Peters et al., 2013). Many surgeons at all levels have a different experience if they are female. Unconscious bias affects all humans, including other staff and patients (RCS, 2016a). Women surgeons recount being mistaken for nurses or other staff or being over-looked, talked over or expected to do a more menial task; vital opportunities can be lost, especially for those in training or starting a new role (McNally, 2017). Furthermore, the 'Glass Cliff' effect means that women who are promoted to leadership roles are more likely to be given impossible tasks and the gender pay gap means their work may feel less valued (Peters et al., 2013). The years of childbearing are a short time in a career and in surgery these years coincide with surgical training, but unless a woman gets through this phase she will never get to the great job at the end.

Barriers for women still exist because of individual behaviours, cultural attitudes, structures and historical budgets. All these areas are fruitful for improvement. NHS structures reward macho behaviour. Although an organisation's executive team may extol good values, its budget may have been devolved to middle managers who have the power to say no and an overwhelming workload. Bullying is commonplace as people suffer unrealistic deadlines and targets. Look carefully into a recent article on the gender pay gap in surgery (Dean, 2017), and you see I followed the macho path of going to the Executive to get my pay "corrected", essentially undermining the middle manager who had dutifully saved on the budget.

A career or role may have an outdated awe attached. Historically, surgery was viewed as all-encompassing requiring heroic nocturnal operating and sharp decision-making. The biggest change to improve work-life balance that might be overlooked is the 1999 report of the National Confidential Enquiry into Perioperative Outcome and Death (NCEPOD); this improved lifestyle for surgeons greatly in 1999 by reporting worse outcomes for the 60% of emergency patients undergoing surgery outside normal hours at that time (NCEPOD, 1999). Within months, day-time emergency lists were created, allowing surgeons to have a more humane diurnal lifestyle and to operate with a familiar team. The European Working Time Regulations (EWTR) limiting all workers to a maximum of 48 hours per week have applied to doctors in training since 2009. Before this time, 90-hour weeks were commonplace. Although doctors in training are now busier, time off is mandated and surgical specialties are no longer outliers.

Cohort studies provide data, but lag behind changes in rotas and hours and can only surmise an explanation; some suggest that historically women in surgery had to choose between having their career and a family, whereas men in surgery did not (Goldacre et al., 2012). Many doctors and educationalists are aged over 50 and in other specialties but currently giving advice to young doctors and medical students; they may not realise that since their own experience last century, surgical training has become focussed and diurnal with strict limits on hours of work and training. Their advice may be outdated. All those advising future surgeons should be very clear that all specialties have a legal limit of 48 hours per week, under the European Working Time Regulations (EWTR) and that Less Than Full Time Training (LTFT) is open to those in training in any specialty, of any gender, with a well-founded reason. Many good surgeons complete Less Than Full Time Training (LTFT) combining parenthood or other commitments with surgical training, although this can be difficult to plan. Paradoxically, legislation around age discrimination has enabled more senior surgeons to opt for part-time work. There are more senior surgeons working part-time than those in surgical training doing LTFT, and it is often easier to arrange for the senior surgeons. Amongst physicians, 23% of Consultants work LTFT, compared to 15% of those in training; the situation is likely to be similar in surgery (RCP, 2018). Sadly, those undertaking LTFT in surgery report that this is difficult to organise and over half experience negative comments or bullying as a perceived direct result of their LTFT from Consultants and colleagues (Harries et al., 2016). A greater visible diversity of the workforce can allow a discussion about what the minimum standards are and how to value each member of the team to be most productive. Although childbearing is exclusively female, childrearing can be undertaken irrespective of gender. It could be argued that improving the uptake of paternity leave, Shared Parental Leave and LTFT by male surgeons in training would aid understanding that child-rearing does not need to be the sole preserve of women. Unfortunately, the system of Shared Parental Leave has been set up so fewer than 2% take this up and a "use it or lose it" policy may encourage uptake (Norman & Fagan, 2017).

Over 50% of medical students have been women for over 25 years (BMA, 2009; Moberly, 2018). Women are being actively and passively discouraged from considering a surgical career from medical school. Different medical schools vary widely in the number of their graduates entering a surgical training programme; ranging from 3% to 12% for women and from 6% to 22% for men (Twigg et al., 2018). Cohort studies show a similar picture. The biggest impact on students' interest in surgery is how well they are treated in the operating theatre; conversely, many report poor experiences or remarks that makes them feel that they would not fit in (Sutton et al., 2014).

During training, doctors in the UK NHS spend around 50% of their time on tasks that do not require a medical degree (RCS, 2017). This contributes to burn-out and missing educational opportunities. Major initiatives are underway to increase the number and training of senior non-medical clinicians, but there is insufficient focus on supporting doctors on the wards with basic tasks, such as could be undertaken by un-Registered "Doctors' Assistants" with basic training (McNally & Huber 2018).

As women surgeons progress in their career, they are more likely to drop out, but numbers vary widely across different regions suggesting different mechanisms or levels of support involved (Hampton et al., 2018). An Australian analysis suggested the "tower of blocks" theory, that accumulation of multiple negative experiences can cause a final relatively minor event to precipitate leaving the specialty (Liang et al., 2019). The Royal College of Surgeons in Ireland (2017) has listed 25 recommendations to improve gender equity in surgeons, grouped as individual, cultural and structural changes, with data gathering. Other international comparisons should be viewed with caution since the UK training structure mandates a maximum of 48 hours per week, irrespective of specialty, which is very different from expectations in the US, and has a huge impact on the perception of work-life balance.

There are parallels with other programmes of change. Initiatives to tackle bullying in healthcare have a three-pronged approach on the individual, society/culture/department and structures (McNally, 2018). The Australasian surgical experience established that alleged bullies often had no idea how they were perceived (RACS, 2016). Unconscious bias means we form judgements and treat people differently (RCS, 2016a). Individuals can learn skills to show respect and to "fake it till you make it". The Royal Australasian College of Surgeons runs a very successful programme, with a suite of materials including training other senior staff to 'call it out' so that no episode of poor behaviour goes unchallenged (RACS, 2016). They recommend another senior colleague taking the initiative to go for 'a Vanderbilt cup of coffee' with the alleged perpetrator as a means of changing culture within a department (RACS, 2016).

There is impending failure of the UK NHS. The Western paradigm of healthcare could be argued as paternalistic and intervention-focussed, contributing to a view of care that is passive and even worsens health (AoMRC, 2015; McNally et al., 2017). Educating and empowering women is a 'best buy' to improve the health and economy of any nation (McNally, 2013). There are suggestions that women doctors consult in a different manner. A diversity of surgeons with varied consulting styles allows for a fuller discussion of risks, benefits, complications and putting the patient's immediate issue into perspective (Cooper et al., 2019). Many forget that most ill-health is related to lifestyle (AoMRC, 2015; McNally et al., 2017). 70% of NHS spending is on long-term conditions that have a large preventable component. This includes primary prevention (reduced risk of diagnosis of disease) and secondary prevention (reduced risk of complications and part of treatment for an established condition) and works rapidly. This includes surgical conditions where non-interventional disease management is given insufficient prominence in the traditional surgical model. Interventions to improve physical activity and nutrition would improve overall health and reduce the need for, and cost of, social care by several £Billion annually in the UK alone (McNally et al., 2017). As with other change initiatives, the struggle for prevention in healthcare needs individuals, society/culture and organisations to change (AoMRC, 2015; McNally et al., 2017). For individuals to change behaviour requires knowledge (eg that 20 minutes' daily exercise can reduce your risk of dementia by 30%) skills and a way of keeping going (eg training for a charity event) and fitting it into normal (eg cycling to work) (AoMRC, 2015; McNally et al., 2017). Training programmes such as www.movingmedicine.ac.uk teach healthcare professionals to broach the topic of exercise in a 1-minute consultation. The culture needs to change so that this behaviour becomes normal. At a structural level, processes and facilities need to support the new normal.

There are some clear targets where interventions may improve support for women in the workplace. Many focus on education.

Focussing on the under-represented group:

1. Knowledge and skills are key – giving us the right to be there. All four UK surgical Colleges contribute to formal surgical training programmes. In addition, the Royal College of Surgeons of England has resources for medical students and Foundation Doctors and those who teach them about being supported to scrub in, valuing clear principles, practicing practical skills and being active in the team, whatever their eventual specialty (RCS, 2016b; RCS, 2015). Although communication skills and empathy are highly valued, surgeons need exceptional knowledge and skills. I am forever grateful to the obstetrician with few words who pulled my first baby out.
2. Clear labels and name badges are needed for those likely to be mistaken for other staff. For example: stating Doctor (not junior doctor) or Surgeon for those who have the RCS Membership exam and who operate. Patients and other staff should be encouraged to react to the name badge. This helps reduce unconscious bias.

Focus on other staff and seniors to change culture:

3. Role models. All staff should realise that they act as role models for others. Medical students or the public may realise there is a diversity of people labelled 'Surgeon' (McNally, 2017). Other staff may realise that professional behaviour is expected.
4. Clear accessible information should be available about pregnancy, childrearing, breastfeeding, LTFT or part-time training and working (RCS, 2019). The rules and expectations should be clear.

5. An urgent change is needed in mandatory 'Equality and Diversity training'. This currently focusses on 'Equality' requesting that participants do not mention any difference at the point of a summative assessment, exam or interview. Allowing diversity is almost the opposite of this, in that if an individual may need more help to do a role, their supervisor/line-manager should explicitly ask the supervisee what else they need to get the most out of their placement.
6. Training on Unconscious bias and how to react to difference (RCS, 2016a). For rapid dissemination, this could be added to mandatory 'Equality and Diversity' training.
7. Those in leadership roles should be given formal training (RCS, 2016a) in management skills – including Human Resources, project management and how to Chair a meeting inclusively. There should be clear expectations or a code of conduct for managers.
8. Mentoring. Those able to act as mentors, either formally or informally need to be encouraged to "say what you'd say to a bloke". There are courses or guides simplifying the need to listen to the mentee's needs and work with them (RCS, 2016c).
9. Male staff and male surgeons in training who are parents should be encouraged to be active in their child(ren)'s upbringing.
10. There should be a Zero tolerance rule for poor behaviour. Each member of staff, especially established staff, should understand their role in creating culture and eliminating poor behaviour. Taking a peer for 'a Vanderbilt cup of coffee' is recommended and effective.

Focussing on structures:

11. Individuals need clear tasks and performance management against these tasks (RCS, 2016a).
12. Leadership roles should have a clear person specification and a fixed tenure to support new talent and allow succession planning (RCS, 2016a). The means of applying should be clear. For example, to get onto the Council of the Royal College of Surgeons of England requires a Member or Fellow to submit 100 words and be successful in a vote of the membership. Once you are in, you deserve to be there. Other roles should be advertised with sufficient time to apply and the role well defined.
13. Each role should be analysed to ensure the support is realistic, especially admin and IT support. For example, Doctors in training spend 50% of their time doing admin or basic clinical tasks; our pilot developing "Doctors' Assistants" from HealthCare Assistants proved successful in freeing up Doctors to get to their training opportunities and improving patient flow (McNally & Huber, 2018).
14. All organisations should have facilities to ensure staff wellbeing, including facilities to rest, active travel options, water fountains and positive social interactions. Health staff should be role models for good health (AoMRC, 2015; McNally et al., 2017). Many are at risk of burnout, which can lead to poor behaviour and measures to improve wellbeing may mitigate this. Inspection regimens should look for details to ensure compliance.
15. Structures for maternity leave and LTFT working and training should be clear.

Measures that improve the lot of women improve matters for all. With 1.5 million employees and a culture of regulation, the NHS could be a model employer with changes disseminating across other organisations. Creating a new normal, seeking data and identifying points to change should be an ongoing process. Each member of staff should be valued for what they contribute.

REFERENCES

Academy of Medical Royal Colleges. (2015). Exercise the miracle cure and the role of the doctor in promoting it. Retrieved from http://www.aomrc.org.uk/publications/reports-guidance/exercise-the-miracle-cure-0215/

BMA, British Medical Association Equal Opportunities Committee. (2009). Equality and diversity in UK medical schools. BMA.

Cooper, W. O., Spain, D. A., Guillamondegui, O., Kelz, R. R., Domenico, H. J., Hopkins, J., ... & Webb, L. E. (2019). Association of coworker reports about unprofessional behavior by surgeons with surgical complications in their patients. *JAMA surgery.* doi:10.1001/jamasurg.2019.1738

Dean, E. (2017) The gender pay gap in surgery. *Bulletin Royal College of Surgeons of England 99*(1), 12-14. Retrieved from https://publishing.rcseng.ac.uk/doi/full/10.1308/rcsbull.2017.12

(2012). <eref>Goldacre, M. J., Davidson, J. D., & Lambert, T. W. (2012). Doctors' age at domestic partnership and parenthood: Cohort studies. *Journal of the Royal Society of Medicine, 105*, 390–399. doi:10.1258/jrsm.2012.120016

Hampton, T., Greenhalgh, R., Ryan, D., & Das-Purkayastha, P. (2016) Female surgical trainee attrition. *Bulletin of Royal College of Surgeons, 98*(3), 134-137. doi:10.1308/rcsbull.2016.134

Harries, R. L., Gokani, V. J., & Smitham, P. F. (2016). JEF on behalf of the councils of the Association of Surgeons in Training and the British Orthopaedic Trainees Association. Less than full-time training in surgery: a cross-sectional study evaluating the accessibility and experiences of flexible training in the surgical trainee workforce. *BMJ Open 4*(6), 1-7. Retrieved from https://bmjopen.bmj.com/content/bmjopen/6/4/e010136.full.pdf

Liang, R., Dornan, T., & Nestel, D. (2019) Why do women leave surgical training? A qualitative and feminist study. *Lancet 393*(10171), 541-549. doi:10.1016/S0140-6736(18)32612-6

McNally, S. (2012). Surgical Training: Still Highly Competitive But Still Very Male. *Bulletin Royal College of Surgeons of England, 94*(2), 53–55. doi:10.1308/147363512X13189526438675

McNally, S. (2013). Global population explosion: Economic and health meltdown. *Journal of the Royal Society of Medicine, 106*(2), 38–39. doi:10.1258/jrsm.2012.120246 PMID:23401631

McNally, S. (2017). *A woman at a surgical conference: They thought I was the waitress.* Retrieved from https://www.bma.org.uk/connecting-doctors/b/work/posts/a-woman-at-a-surgical-conference-they-thought-i-was-the-waitress

McNally, S. (2018a). How I became a woman in surgery. *Association of Surgeons of Great Britain and Ireland.* Available at www.scarlettmcnally.co.uk

McNally, S. (2018b). Unconscious bias, bullying and behaviour change. *Royal College of Surgeons of Edinburgh event presentations.* Retrieved from https://www.rcsed.ac.uk/professional-support-development-resources/anti-bullying-and-undermining-campaign/resources-to-help-change-the-culture

McNally, S., & Huber, J. (2018). Award-winning new doctors' assistants freeing time in acute NHS hospitals *Health Management, 18*(1). Retrieved from https://healthmanagement.org/c/healthmanagement/issuearticle/award-winning-new-doctors-assistants-freeing-time-in-acute-nhs-hospitals

McNally, S., Nunan, D., Dixon, A., Maruthappu, M., Butler, K., & Gray, M. (2017). Focus on physical activity can help avoid unnecessary social care. *BMJ (Clinical Research Ed.), 359*(j4609), 108–110. doi:10.1136/bmj.j4609 PMID:29042359

Moberly, T. (2018, January). Number of women entering medical school rises after decade of decline. *BMJ (Clinical Research Ed.), 27*, 167. Retrieved from https://www.bmj.com/bmj/section-pdf/959692?path=/bmj/360/8138/Careers.full.pdf

National Confidential Enquiry into Patient Outcome and Death [NCEPOD]. (1999). *Who operates when?* Retrieved from http://www.ncepod.org.uk/1995_6.html

Norman, H. & Fagan, C. (2017). *Shared parental leave in the UK: is it working? Lessons from other countries.* Retrieved from https://www.workingfamilies.org.uk/workflex-blog/shared-parental-leave-in-the-uk-is-it-working-lessons-from-other-countries/

Peters, K., Ryan, M., Haslam, S. A., & Morgenroth, T. (2013). *The psychology and economics of women in leadership.* Retrieved from http://www.europarl.europa.eu/RegData/etudes/workshop/join/2013/474408/IPOL-FEMM_AT(2013)474408_EN.pdf

RCP, Royal College of Physicians of London. (2018). *Focus on physicians: 2017–18 census (UK consultants and higher specialty trainees).* Retrieved from https://www.rcplondon.ac.uk/projects/outputs/focus-physicians-2017-18-census-uk-consultants-and-higher-specialty-trainees

Royal Australasian College of Surgeons. (2016). *Discrimination, Harassment and Bullying.* Retrieved from www.surgeons.org/respect

Royal College of Surgeons of England. (2015). *National Undergraduate Surgical Curriculum.* Retrieved from www.rcseng.ac.uk/study

Royal College of Surgeons of England. (2016a). *Avoiding unconscious bias: a guide for surgeons.* Retrieved from www.rcseng.ac.uk/avoiding-unconscious-bias

Royal College of Surgeons of England. (2016b). *Learning in operating theatres.* Retrieved from www.rcseng.ac.uk/learning-in-operating-theatres

Royal College of Surgeons of England. (2016c). *Mentoring.* Retrieved from https://www.rcseng.ac.uk/-/media/files/rcs/library-and-publications/non-journal-publications/good-surgical-practice--mentoring.pdf

Royal College of Surgeons of England. (2017). *Improving surgical training.* Retrieved from https://www.rcseng.ac.uk/-/media/files/rcs/careers-in-surgery/improving_surgical_training_text.pdf

Royal College of Surgeons of England. (2019). *Careers.* Retrieved from www.rcseng.ac.uk/career

Royal College of Surgeons of Ireland. (2017) *Promoting gender equity in surgery. Report of a working group.* Retrieved from http://www.rcsi.ie/index.jsp?p=164&n=2790&a=10970

Sutton, P. A., Mason, J., Vimalachandran, D., & McNally, S. (2014). Attitudes, motivators, and barriers to a career in surgery: A national study of UK undergraduate medical students. *Journal of Surgical Education*, *71*(5), 662–667. doi:10.1016/j.jsurg.2014.03.005 PMID:24776853

Twigg, V., Aldridge, K., McNally, S. A., & Eardley, I. (2018). Does choice of medical school affect a student's likelihood of becoming a surgeon? *Bulletin of Royal College of Surgeons, 100*(2), 90-95. doi:10.1308/rcsbull.2018.90

Chapter 10
Impostor Syndrome as a Risk Factor in the Development of Psychiatric Symptoms in Female Doctors

Ángeles Martínez Hernanz
Hospital Universitario de Getafe, Spain

María Herrera de la Muela
Hospital Clínico San Carlos, Spain

Montserrat González-Estecha
Hospital Clínico San Carlos, Spain

ABSTRACT

Impostor syndrome is a psychological phenomenon in which an individual lacks self-esteem and confidence in their ability to perform well in positions of responsibility and tries to make up for this inadequacy with excess effort and workload. Although it can occur in men, it is most prevalent in women. The healthcare sector, specifically the medical profession, has a number of characteristics that facilitate the appearance of this phenomenon, for example: a high number of women in intermediate positions, high professional skills, and good educational qualifications. The symptoms of this affliction can negatively affect job performance and reduce the sufferer's quality of life.

INTRODUCTION

The aim of this chapter is to offer an overall view of impostor syndrome, which is less well-known but just as important as other conditions and can have serious repercussions for women in the medical profession, among others. As with all lesser-known clinical conditions (those not classified as disorders), it can be fairly difficult to identify. This lack of recognition and, therefore, treatment, can lead to a worse outcome and significant potential losses at both the personal and professional levels.

DOI: 10.4018/978-1-5225-9599-1.ch010

The importance of gender differences in this syndrome has been studied and validated and results from a society which, despite efforts in recent years, in some ways still perpetuates the gender roles that have led to the existence of this syndrome, even more so in professions traditionally linked to men. Individuals affected by this condition, which is not classified as a mental disorder, are unable to internalize their accomplishments and have a persistent fear of being revealed as a fraud despite the existence of objective evidence to support their competence. Although it is not a mental disorder as such, it does have a strong correlation with disorders such as anxiety and depression.

BACKGROUND

The term "impostor syndrome" was coined in 1978 by two American psychologists, Pauline Rose Clance and Suzanne Imes, to describe a phenomenon initially described in women. Clance defines it as a condition in which a high achiever experiences intense feelings of being a fraud or an intellectual phony (Clance & Imes, 1978). Clance and Imes' work was followed by others, such as *If I'm So Successful, Why Do I Feel Like a Fake: The Impostor Phenomenon*, published by Joan C. Harvey in 1985, which states that over 50% of successful people have experienced this syndrome. One of the reasons for the existence of this condition is that socially, men and women have always been, and continue to be, brought up to play different roles, as demonstrated by the existence of gender traits such as difficulty with delegation, self-denial and the role of nurturer and peacemaker as part of women's maternal role. Thus, although studies have shown that impostor syndrome exists in both sexes, it is far more prevalent in women.

Clance and Imes used the term "syndrome" in their first work (1978), and it was Harvey (Kats & Harvey, 1995) and Kolligian and Sternberg (2000) who suggested that it would be more scientifically accurate to define it as a construct of the subject's personality, since it is related to cognitive and affective personality traits (Ghorbanshirodi, S., 2012) (Holmes, Kertay, Adamson et al., 1993). However, no matter what point of view you look at it from (personality vs. syndrome), we are dealing with a concept in which gender differences marked by society are definitive, as these structure the subject's adult personality beyond any genetic aspects.

This syndrome was first identified last century and, despite important progress in women's rights, it continues to exist nowadays with the same degree, possibly even more so due to the amount of women who are gradually moving up to positions of greater responsibility. On the other hand, it is perhaps more silent due to the urgent need in today's workplace to hide any possible sign of weakness, leading us to consider whether this leads to greater emotional suffering and a higher possibility of suffering different psychiatric disorders, with the price that this entails in the loss of potential.

IMPOSTOR SYNDROME, THE MEDICAL PROFESSION, AND GENDER IDENTITY

Does the medical profession facilitate the appearance of impostor syndrome as much as other professions that are more clearly dominated by men? Medicine is sometimes cited as an example of the substantial progress made by women and is often used to illustrate the integration of women in the workplace, which is backed up by the exponential increase of female medical students and doctors (recalling that it was not so long ago that they were not even allowed access to this profession). However, even now, and in spite of the clear increase in female medical students over the years, the scarce number of women in hospital management and leadership positions is striking. This shows that the medical profession is a true reflection of the gender discrimination that still exists in society today, not just in positions of power but also in middle and upper management. The percentage of job insecurity is greater in women than in men, as evidenced by the fact that men progress more rapidly to an indefinite term employment contract while women take longer to earn these types of contracts. In fact, the percentage of indefinite term contracts among men and women does not become equal until the age of 45. The same occurs when analysing the number of workers with second jobs, with men coming out ahead, although this varies by specialty. This seems to reflect the way in which society puts a brake on advances in gender equality. (Pastor, Belzunegui & Pontón, 2012).

Hiring processes for management positions are often based more on trust than on academic merit; this is where women's tendency toward lower participation becomes more evident, sustaining their reduced possibilities of acceding to these positions and reinforcing their lack of incentives to compete for a managerial position, sometimes disguised an apparent lack of personal interest in achieving them. All this has a background of social constraint hidden under the appearance of a personal choice (Reed & Buddeberg-Fisher, 2001). Professional women are also influenced by society's expectations, according to which women must first meet the demands of their family or private life and then juggle their personal and professional lives, giving them less time to promote themselves professionally and perform activities that oftentimes require an extension of their working hours, overburdening them and causing them a great deal of stress in the event they try to take everything on.

Although the typical dominant male argument denies the existence of gender discrimination in the health sector, this is not borne out by an analysis of the true situation. While it is surprising that this argument is maintained by the professionals themselves, it can perhaps be explained by the fact that this discrimination is usually indirect, i.e., it is either less acknowledged or directly denied.

The same social factors prevail in the medical profession as in any other profession, and as we will see throughout this chapter, they act as risk factors for the appearance of impostor syndrome and other syndromes that present important gender differences.

The work environment in the medical profession is therefore no better than in other professions in terms of the achievement and maintenance of gender equality - gender discrimination persists in the same proportion as in any other work environment.

Among women, it fundamentally comes down to a lack of self-esteem when performing jobs in professions traditionally performed by men and the need to work more and better as a way of being entitled to this recognition, i.e., low self-esteem coupled with high self-demand. These constraints have been internalized throughout the life of women in their day to day experiences. As stated by Clance and Imes, "Despite outstanding academic and professional accomplishments, women who experience the impostor phenomenon persist in believing that they are really not bright and have fooled anyone who thinks otherwise. (...) (They feel) their success has been due to (…) luck (…and that) unless they go to gargantuan efforts to do so, success cannot be repeated." (Clance and Imes, 1985).

Sufferers of impostor syndrome do not allow themselves to enjoy their achievements because they believe they do not deserve them, thereby eliminating an important positive reinforcement that could break the vicious cycle of this syndrome. The sufferers do not enjoy their successes, instead experiencing them as one more source of anxiety. The feeling that one's identity is a sham shakes the affected person's ego, making her believe that she is not really the person she is pretending to be and that she is a fraud.

From the perspective of those affected, it is a lack of skills rather than a lack of preparation that makes them feel like they need to make an extra effort to perform well, and they then attribute their success almost exclusively to this extra effort, thereby perpetuating the symptoms. An implicit part of this, which has caught the attention of some researchers, is the doubt in one's own ability, the fear of failure and low expectations of success despite a history of prior professional accomplishments. Those who exhibit this syndrome internalise negative aspects or shortcomings and externalise facts that could reinforce higher self-esteem. They understand that this negative assessment of themselves is not so much due to a lack of preparation (a more easily modifiable external constraint) but rather to a lack of skills (an internal limitation that is more difficult to modify and keeps their feelings of incompetence alive) (Fernández & Bermúdez,2000). They believe this to the point that they even interpret constructive criticism negatively, seeing it as a clear indication of their lack of skills rather than as a way to increase their knowledge. Men, on the other hand, more often attribute their success to their own inherent attributes.

Other factors, such as gender differences and particularly their survival throughout the evolution of society, are involved in the aetiology of this syndrome. Historically, patriarchal culture has taught that women's professional skills are not as important as those of men, which limits the reinforcement of their self-esteem by the social environment. Female stereotypes make it easier for this syndrome to take root; reinforced by beliefs about the male-female dichotomy that have been perpetuated for centuries, such as the identification of power with masculinity, in such a way that women were not expected, and are still not expected, to reach positions of power and were seen as an exception when they did so. Another enduring dichotomy is the traditional division between public and private (professional life / home life), which assigns women to household tasks and reinforces what has been identified for centuries as the "good social order", which ensures the perpetuation of new men who guarantee the existence of the labour market (Bonilla,2010). This social aspect, kept alive by women, has historically been invisible and unvalued. All this has allowed the idea of women's inferiority and secondary social role to become firmly established. This idea still exists today, although probably to a lesser degree in Western countries. Added to this equation is the old-fashioned idea of women's supposedly lower abilities in tasks that require reasoning such as physics or mathematics, assigning them other qualities that throughout the centuries were considered second class, such as sensitivity and understanding.

Today's society is obsessed with appearances to the point that, especially in higher-level jobs, you not only have to be good, you have to look even better than you really are. But for people suffering from this syndrome, marketing themselves as better than they are is just an added difficulty. This can lead to them feeling less competent and not competing for higher positions, denying themselves the possibility of developing new ideas and proposing potentially valuable solutions to different problems because of the fear that this would expose their supposed ignorance to others, all of which just adds to the image of women as playing a supporting role in a society which even today is dominated by men.

We could ask ourselves why, despite a history of successes that prove otherwise, these women continue to believe they are impostors. A possible explanation can be found in family dynamics that are unconsciously shaped and perpetuated by society; dynamics in which children fall into one of two different groups in their families, even when they are too young to have verifiable qualities. One child will be the sensitive one and the other the intelligent one. These labels are given at a very early age and are kept alive over time, regardless of whether or not they are validated by reality. The first of them, the so-called sensitive child, will continue to doubt his/her intelligence and ability even when these characteristics have been proven beyond doubt. Traditionally, the role of intelligent child in the family unit is given to the son and the sensitive one to the daughter (Clance & Imes, 1978).

As if the above were not enough, women tend to handle guilt as something more personal, particularly as they have historically held the role of caretaker in the family and take for granted that they have to neglect this obligation in order to attend to work obligations that may at times go beyond the established schedule. The societal component thus acquires a special relevance, forming an interpersonal pattern in which one is open to others' scrutiny. McIntosh indicates that messages from society that reinforce gender stereotypes help this syndrome to appear in women (McIntosh,1989).

Within the family dynamics that survived throughout history and in spite of the changes in favour of gender equality, traditional family dynamics persist and become evident over time, even without one even being fully aware of it. For example, mothers can sometimes interfere in their own daughters' steps towards independence, teaching a pattern in which they deny their own needs in order to give to others (caretaker function) and they feel more comfortable satisfying others rather than themselves. This pattern predictably becomes even more intense when raising children, which usually coincides with the beginning of a medical professional's work life (Thompson, Davidson & Barber,1995; Leung & Kwan,1998; Ferrari & Olivette, 2000; Thompson, 2004; Want & Klietman, 2006).

Despite progress in recent years, successful professional women continue to be labelled as hostile and seen as a somewhat destructive component within society and their femininity is even called into question. They defy sexual stereotypes but have to pay a price for it. This price may perfectly well be anxiety, whereas if a professional woman believes that she is not brilliant and is really an impostor, she does not have to bear the weight of rupturing the traditional social structure (Oriel, 2004).

The existence of peers both by profession and couples, who do not measure the success of the woman or her dedication to work as a risk to the maintenance of the social structure, could help to decrease the appearance of this symptomatology.

All this helps to generate two characteristics of these women: pessimism and high self-criticism (Fernández & Bermúdez, 2000), leading them to use different standards to measure themselves and others.

Numerous authors have written about the easy-to-see relationship between the two, pointing out that, although these women are perfectionists in evaluating themselves, they not aware of doing so, meaning that they are also not aware that they are using different yardsticks to measure themselves and others. In this way they deny themselves positive reinforcement for their achievements and even attribute such achievements to reasons outside their control (Dudau, 2013).

Sufferers of impostor syndrome use different techniques when they have to present their work, achievements etc. to others, tending to compensate their fear of failure either with over-preparation and extreme effort or by using techniques that only manage to limit them due to the fear of being exposed, such as procrastination, followed by the need to make a gargantuan effort at the last minute.

Why it is so difficult to eradicate this vicious circle of negative thinking if the behaviours that lead to it have been identified? In order not to be exposed as an impostor, those affected work extra hard, which makes it easier to achieve good results but reinforces the belief that this extra effort is what led them to achieve their goals. This belief is also reinforced by praise for their achievements, which in their minds places the achievement of their objectives as due to this extra effort rather than to their personal characteristics such as intelligence.

Another reason is that they believe they are frauds, which will often lead them to not bring up their own ideas or discoveries but instead base themselves on those presented by other people. They conceal their own ideas, reinforcing the belief that, if they had presented them, they may have been shot down, but it is impossible to reveal this as a lie if they do not allow themselves to even think about presenting their ideas.

Social conditioning leads to another behaviour that helps keep impostor syndrome alive: women's use of charm and seduction to achieve the approval of their superiors, always volunteering and helping to perform their tasks, in an attempt, whether conscious or unconscious, to lead them to discover the woman's intellectual value, as this is the only way in which she would allow herself to believe it. However, this tactic does not make it any easier to change the feelings caused by impostor syndrome since, on the one hand, if the woman's capacity is recognized, or even if it is not, she will attribute this recognition to qualities other than her intellect. Moreover, if her superiors recognise her value, she experiences it as a failure to have faith in her own abilities, reinforcing her belief that her efforts in seeking recognition by others are further proof of her inadequacy, since the people who achieve great things do so without the need for recognition and sometimes even despite the disapproval of others. This is even more proof of her inability to achieve results and externalising of credit for any success she may obtain.

Although this is not the single cause of a very complex problem, it seems obvious that sufferers of impostor syndrome are unlikely to expose themselves to hiring processes for positions of power, and those that do may pay the emotional price of discomfort and even psychopathology when compared to unaffected people, both male and female. Women have the added burden of the idea that persists in today's society of incompatibility between a proper family life (which continues to be a woman's job) and professional success at high levels.

Sufferers repeatedly externalise their success and internalise their failures, a cycle that is not weakened by their consistent achievements. In fact, Clance and O'Toole (1987) highlight subjects' ingenuity in discrediting positive feedback received from others and negating objective external evidence of their skills. This is also based on their interest in not making an unfavourable impression on others (protective self-observation) since they expect to be unmasked as a fraud, and it becomes kind of self-fulfilling prophecy. These feelings can generate a mind-trap that causes those affected to not reach their full potential, due to their own efforts to avoid exposure and possible unmasking as a fraud. Consequently, when they do not reach their goals, they feel they have proved that they are frauds, without stopping to consider that the true reason is that they simply haven't tried. They never acknowledge any of their achievements as sufficient, and this causes them significant distress and chronic dissatisfaction, which can lead to greater psychopathological disorders.

In the medical profession, valid for both sexes, the low frequency of positive reinforcements is added along with the importance of negatives. Since college, we are constantly compared to others. n the medical work the comparative statistics between professionals, between specialties and between hospitals, are used at all times as a mode of evaluation, reaching to determine part of the supplements received at the economic level. In addition, society assumes that a medical act must be carried out to perfection. While in the event of any failure, inert fact to the human condition, the doctor will be faced with complaints, complaints from patients and recriminations that even end in legal convictions. However, it is uncommon to receive congratulations for a job well done. This determines a greater weight of negative reinforcements than of positive ones.

In spite of impostor syndrome not being recognized as a mental disorder, it acts as a risk factor for conditions such as depression, anxiety, burnout, etc., so it is useful to be familiar with scales that help assess impostor feelings. The Harvey Impostor Phenomenon Scale (HPI; Harvey, 1981) was devised to measure 14 items, but was improved and surpassed by the subsequent "Clance Impostor Scale" consisting of 20 items focused on the perception of one's own effectiveness, as well as one's own defensive style, which includes the perceptions of others being aware of their failure, making its sufferers discount any positive comments that would reinforce a more competent self-image and validating those comments that could reveal their failure, which perpetuates the fraudulent self-image. Those with a score of 60 or higher are to be suffering from impostor syndrome.

To deal with this condition, it is essential to break the cycle of both social and internal feedback that holds us responsible for our failures and externalises our successes, deeming them to be a result of luck or chance (Chrisman, Pieper, Clance, Holland, & Glickauf-Hughes, 1995). One of the features that characterizes people affected by this syndrome is anxiety, which can become chronic if not treated, producing enduring personality changes that can become real disorders. This anxiety is their constant companion when facing challenges in the workplace, in their performance (fear when being evaluated), and in achieving results (even if they are successful, the feeling that they are not worthy will cause them anxiety). Another source of anxiety, which is no less important just because it is not often acknowledged, is the one provoked by violating classic gender roles. All this, sustained over time, can generate serious problems in connection with the perception of one's identity, which is the backbone of minimum emotional stability.

One of the relationships studied in patients affected by impostor syndrome is its correlation with burnout, as the two phenomena share a number of symptoms. Its status as a risk factor in terms of loss of professional ineffectiveness, its association with absenteeism and even an increase in medical errors are well-known (Villwock, Lindsay, Lindsey, & Tucker, 2016). The symptoms caused by both conditions are most likely to show up at the most critical moments of one's profession life, at times of change in which sufferers are most at risk of these conditions limiting their capacity to face challenges as successfully as may be expected.

SOLUTIONS AND RECOMMENDATIONS

When patients affected by this syndrome come in for treatment, it is usually for symptoms derived from this condition (or even a totally different condition). They seldom go explicitly because of impostor feelings, as what they have identified is anxiety or the physical symptoms associated with it. They do not usually focus their complaints on work-related matters or even mention their achievements, for example in the workplace. The therapist is the first one who usually detects these feelings and not the patient; this is another example of the difficulty they have at the cognitive level to identify their high levels of performance.

The simple action of detecting and recognizing that one suffers from this syndrome could be the first step in overcoming it. This can be the first step in breaking the vicious circle that perpetuates impostor syndrome. In addition, the patient's impostor syndrome cannot begin to be resolved if the therapy does not focus on it, and if it is not detected the patient's feeling that she is a fraud may even increase, as she will feel that, by hiding part of her self-image and the feelings that go along with that hidden part, she is giving her therapist an image that does not really correspond to her true self.

Therapists must first identify possible cases of impostor syndrome and then explore the patient's family roles and the dynamics in her birth family that may be favouring the cognitive processes that perpetuate the syndrome (Thompson, Davidson & Barder, 1995; Leung & Kwan,1998; Ferrari & Olivette, 2000). Oftentimes, several sessions of individual or group therapy are necessary to be able to begin to detect the presence of impostor syndrome, since initially the patient is so convinced that she is an impostor and that this is real that she believes there is no possibility of changing the situation. She also believes that expressing her feelings that she is a fraud would not make it any more understandable.

Once impostor syndrome is detected, it is necessary to bring it out into the open in order to make it "real". The therapist must explore both the emotions and the cognitive processes that perpetuate it. It is therapeutic in itself just to break the silence that surrounds it, for the patient to know that what is happening to her has a name and that she is not the only one with these feelings and thoughts. It is important to place special emphasis on the need to separate feelings from reality and underscore that the fact that someone feels a certain way does not mean she is that way (feeling like you are an impostor is not the same as being one).

Understanding mistakes or failures is an opportunity to gain more knowledge. Group therapy with other patients who experience this syndrome is usually highly recommended. When one patient reveals that she suffers from this condition, many others are inclined to share their experiences and it comes as a relief to them to break out of their feelings of loneliness (Yalom, 1998). It is also easier to recognize the mechanisms that perpetuate the symptoms of impostor syndrome in others than in oneself, and from this position, to recognize the need to modify them. The only way for patients to break out of the vicious circle is to become aware that they can aspire to more and that their performance at work is good - this is where the power of the group really comes into play. The person needs to become aware of the imaginary and unreal beliefs that perpetuate the syndrome.

Small tasks that bring about changes in their behaviour can also be introduced. For example, introducing a cognitive variable that implies doing things because "like this I'll do a good job" and not "because if I don't do it, I might fail" (a negative cognitive variable), without discounting the probabilities of success from the beginning.

Another task that allows patients to modify their perceptions would be to reduce their compulsive work habits, which perpetuate their feelings that their success is due to this extra work, although this needs to be done progressively in order to prevent these changes from becoming one more source of anxiety. Another type of therapy is role reversal, putting yourself in the other person's position and asking why she would think you are a fraud. Sometimes this reveals that, hidden deep down under the feelings of guilt and fraud, patients think they possess exceptional characteristics. The therapist can then work with the fears and guilt that sometimes accompany these feelings of being exceptional, allowing the patient to return to a more realistic self-image of her abilities, neither over nor underestimating them. It is important to work on the doom and gloom theories of what could happen if she recognizes her success and worth, which usually arise from childhood fears rooted in specific experiences.

The point is to stimulate the patient to be authentic and make her see that her image does not depend solely on the approval of others. The patient has to work on her resistance to these changes and allow herself to enjoy the successes she achieves. Many times this resistance is kept alive by social roles whose importance in maintaining social order will have to be questioned, no matter how much they have been kept alive over time. This helps defeat the idea that being a woman is incompatible with professional success, an idea that often brings about the feelings of impostor syndrome.

FUTURE RESEARCH DIRECTIONS

We must therefore formulate strategies that prevent the development of impostor syndrome and weaken its intensity, given that it occurs more frequently in women in important positions, including the medical profession, and neither disappears nor lessens with the achievements that come with greater work experience or a record that reinforce one's aptitudes. Sharing these feelings and not perpetuating the associated guilt could be a good start to avoiding the possible consequences, such as less competitive professionals who fear and reject new ideas due to the greater degree of exposure involved. These professionals miss out on the possibility of making new contributions to the scientific community, with the unquantifiable costs that this entails for scientific development.

CONCLUSION

We must be aware of the existence of this syndrome in the healthcare field, particularly among women, not forgetting the social construct of gender discrimination, especially when it is manifested unconsciously and perpetuates the symptoms of impostor syndrome. Impostor syndrome must become more visible in order for its sufferers to not feel alone, so that they are able to begin treatment and share their experiences with others as a way to break the barrier of silence that surrounds it.

The chapter only tries to make a first approach to this syndrome, of which currently do not exist in important statistic works that analyse its frequency and relationship with more recognized psychiatric pathologies.

It would be important to start doing these studies to gain a better understanding of the subject.

It would also be necessary to carry out a study on the different therapies used pasts patients, as well as the analysis of their results.

Possibly an important initial step is the one outlined in this chapter in terms of rethinking gender roles in an ever-evolving Society.

REFERENCES

Bonilla, G. (2010). Teoría feminista, ilustración y modernidad: Notas para un debate. *Cuadrenos de literatura del Caribe e Hispanoamericana.* Enero-junio 2010.

Chrisman, S. M., Pieper, W. A., Clance, P. R., Holland, C. L., & Glickauf-Hughes, C. (1995). Validation of the Clance Impostor Phenomenon Scale. *Journal of Personality Assessment*, *65*(3), 456–467. doi:10.120715327752jpa6503_6 PMID:16367709

Clance, P. & O`Toole, M. A. (1998). The impostor phenomenon: an internal barrier to empowerment and achievement. Special issue: Treating women's fear of failure. *Women & Therapy*, *6*, 51–64.

Clance, P. R., & Imes, S. (1978). The imposter phenomenon in high achicving womcn: Dynamics and therapeutic intervention. *Psychotherapy (Chicago, Ill.)*, *15*.

Clance, P. R. , & O'Toole, M. A. (1988). *The Imposter Phenomenon: An Internal Barrier To Empowerment and Achievement.* Philadelphia, PA: Haworth Press.

Dudău, D. P. (2014). The relation between perfectionism and impostor phenomenon. *Procedia: Social and Behavioral Sciences*, *127*, 129–133. doi:10.1016/j.sbspro.2014.03.226

Fernández, Evaristo, & Bermúdez, José. (2000). El pesimismo defensivo y el síndrome del impostor: análisis de sus componentes afectivos y cognitivos. *Revista de Psicopatología y Psicología Clínica*, *5*(2), 115–130.

Ferrari, J. R., & Olivette, M. J. (2000). Parental authority influences on the development females dysfunctional procrastination. *Journal of Research in Personality*, *7*, 495–502.

Harvey, J. C., & Katz, C. (1985). *If I'm So Successful, Why Do I Feel Like a Fake: The Impostor Phenomenon*. New York, NY: Random House.

Holmes, S. W., Kertay, L., Adamson, L. B., Holland, C. L., & Clance, P. R. (1993). Measuring the impostor phenomenon: A comparison of Clance's IPScale and Harvey's IPScale. *Journal of Personality Assessment*, *60*(1), 48–59. doi:10.120715327752jpa6001_3 PMID:8433268

Instituto de la Mujer y para la Igualdad de Oportunidades. (n.d.). Retrieved from http://www.inmujer.gob.es/MujerCifras/PoderDecisiones/RealesAcademias.htmhttp://www.ine.es/jaxi/Datos.htm?path=/t15/p416/serie/l0/&file=s01001.px

-Koligian, J. & Sternberg, R. J. (2000). Perceived fraudulence in young adults: Is there an imposter syndrome? *Journal of personality assessment, 56*(2), 308-326.

Leung, P. W. L., & Kwan, K. S. F. (1998). Parenting style, motivational orientation and self-perceived academic competence: A meditational model. *Merrill-Palmer Quarterly*, *44*, 1–19.

McIntosh, P. (1989). *Feeling like a fraud*. Wellesley, MA: Stone Center College.

Oriel, K., Plane, M. B., & Mindt, M. (2004, April). Family Medicine Residents and the impostor phenomenon. *Family Medicine*, *36*(4), 248–252. PMID:15057614

Pastor Gosálbez, M. I., Belzunegui Eraso, A. , & Pontón Merino, P. (2012). Mujeres en sanidad: Entre la igualdad y la desigualdad. *Cuadernos de Relaciones Laborales*, *30*(2), 497–518.

Reed, V., & Buddeberg-Fischer, B. (2001). Career obstacles for women in medicine: And overview. *Medical Education*, *35*(2), 139–147. doi:10.1046/j.1365-2923.2001.00837.x PMID:11169087

Servicio Madrileño de Salud, Dirección General de Recursos Humanos y Relaciones Laborales. (n.d.). Retrieved from http://www.comunidad.madrid/sites/default/files/doc/sanidad/rrhh/rrhh-portal_estadistico_mes_en_curso_02.pdf

Thompson, T. (2004). Failure-avoidance parenting, the achievement environment of the home and strategies for reduction. *Learning and Instruction*, *14*(1), 3–26. doi:10.1016/j.learninstruc.2003.10.005

Thompson, T., Davidson, J. A., & Barber, J. G. (1995). Self-worth protection in achievement motivation: Performance effects and attribution behavior. *Journal of Educational Psychology*, *87*(4), 598–610. doi:10.1037/0022-0663.87.4.598

<unknown>Ghorbanshirodi, S. (2012) The relationship between self-esteem and emotional intelligence with imposter syndrome among medical students of Guilan and Universidades Heratsi universities. Journal of Basic and Applied Scientific Research, 2(2), 1793–1802.</jrn>

Villwock, J. A., Sobin, L. B., Koester, L. A., & Harris, T. M. (2016). Impostor syndrome and burnout among American medical students: A pilot study. *International Journal of Medical Education*, *7*, 364–369. doi:10.5116/ijme.5801.eac4 PMID:27802178

Want, J., & Kleitman, S. (2006). Imposter phenomenon and self-handicapping: Links with parenting styles and self-confidence. *Personality and Individual Differences*, *40*(5), 961–971. doi:10.1016/j.paid.2005.10.005

Yalom, I. D. (1998). *The Yalom Reader. New York, NY:* Basic Books.

Chapter 11
The Imposter Phenomenon in the Medical Profession

Rebecca C. Grossman
Buckinghamshire Healthcare NHS Trust, UK

ABSTRACT

The imposter phenomenon, or imposter syndrome, is defined as an internal experience of feeling like an intellectual fraud, despite external evidence of an individual's accomplishments, and results in an inability to internalise a sense of success. It is common among high-achieving people, and appears to be more common in women and ethnic minorities. In this chapter, a systematic review of the literature will be presented on imposter syndrome in the medical profession. Topics covered include purported aetiology, implications (including the impact on mental health and career progression), limitations of research, potential coping strategies, and avenues for future research.

INTRODUCTION

The imposter phenomenon (IP), or imposter syndrome, was first described by Clance and Imes (1978). It is defined as an internal experience of feeling like an intellectual fraud, despite external evidence of an individual's accomplishments, and results in an inability to internalise a sense of success. This can manifest itself as a belief that the individual was mistakenly employed or admitted to a degree, and a fear of being discovered as an imposter. Individuals with IP tend to attribute any successes to external influences, such as luck, rather than their own abilities (Seritan & Mehta, 2016). IP is thought to be a contributing factor in the lack of women in senior leadership positions.

Imposter syndrome should not to be confused with Capgras syndrome (the delusion that a friend or family member has been replaced by an identical imposter); IP is not considered a psychiatric illness, and does not appear in the Diagnostic and Statistical Manual (DSM-5) criteria. IP is a psychological construct (Seritan & Mehta, 2016). It lies at the end of a spectrum of self-doubt: the "unconsciously competent" (LaDonna, Ginsburg, & Watling, 2018). At the opposite end of the spectrum are those who lack awareness of their deficits – the "unconsciously incompetent" – otherwise known as the Dunning-Kruger effect (Kruger & Dunning, 1999).

DOI: 10.4018/978-1-5225-9599-1.ch011

This chapter aims to review the literature on imposter syndrome in the medical profession, including in medical students, and to explore the aetiology (and reasons for its high prevalence in women), implications (including effects on career progression and mental health), and coping strategies for the condition.

BACKGROUND

IP was first noticed during psychotherapeutic sessions with high-achieving women (Clance & Imes, 1978). It has since been described extensively in adolescents (Sakulku & Alexander, 2011), teachers, accountants (Byrnes & Lester, 2016), business professionals (Fried-Buchalter, 1992), and nurses (Christensen et al., 2016), but it is less well researched among doctors. Many doctors and medical students have described the syndrome anecdotally (Koven, 2017; Russell, 2017; "Simon Gilbody: The importance of being active," 2017; Smith, 2003).

IP is increasingly being cited as a causative factor in the lack of women in senior leadership positions in the health services, to the extent that the Health and Care Women Leaders Network held a "tweetchat" (open online conversation on the social media platform Twitter) on the subject in March 2018 (Health & Care Women Leaders Network, 2018), with individuals sharing their experiences and advice on the topic using the hashtags (metadata tags) #ImposterSyndrome and #NHSwomen. Quotations from the tweetchat will be included in this chapter to illustrate how IP affects real people.

I have often felt that some success has been down to luck (right place/right time)... it's difficult to shake, however, luck only gets you so far – the rest is down to you. The gremlins push me to be better, learn & improve! (he_reeves, 2018)

THE STUDY OF THE IMPOSTER PHENOMENON

Most studies on the syndrome use the Clance Impostor Phenomenon Scale (CIS) (Clance, 1985; Chae, Piedmont, Estadt, & Wicks, 1995; Chrisman, Pieper, Clance, Holland, & Glickauf-Hughes, 1995) or Harvey's IP Scale (Harvey, 1981; Hellman & Caselman, 2004), with Clance's scale being slightly more sensitive and reliable (Holmes, Kertay, Adamson, Holland, & Clance, 1993). Both of these scales have been validated. The CIS is composed of 20 items that subjects rate on a 5-point Likert-type scale, and can be found at https://paulineroseclance.com/pdf/IPTestandscoring.pdf (Clance, n.d.). The Harvey scale consists of 14 items. Some researchers have used the shorter, unvalidated Young Imposter Quiz (Young, n.d.; Villwock, Sobin, Koester, & Harris, 2016). Normative data for these scales are limited, but estimated clinical cut-offs have been agreed, e.g. ≥ 62 for the CIS (Henning, Ey, & Shaw, 1998; Holmes et al., 1993).

REVIEWING IMPOSTER SYNDROME IN THE LITERATURE: METHODS

A systematic literature review was performed on imposter syndrome in the medical profession and in medical students. Pubmed and Google Scholar were searched using the keywords: "imposter syndrome" "impostor syndrome" "imposterism" "impostorism" "imposter phenomenon" and "impostor phenomenon". References were also examined for additional papers. Studies were not included if the participants consisted of students as a group (without being divided according to their subject), or of professionals as a group (without being divided according to their field). Qualitative studies, and quantitative studies of insufficient quality, were also excluded. A PRISMA flow diagram can be seen in Figure 1.

There were three papers on IP in doctors, and four papers on IP in medical students. Five papers used the CIS, and two used the Young Imposter Quiz. Four papers reported CIS as a continuous variable, and four studied the prevalence of IP, with a "diagnosis" of IP considered positive with a CIS score of ≥62, except for Egwurugwu et al. (2018), who quoted rates at scores of >60.

THE IMPOSTER PHENOMENON IN DOCTORS

There have been three key papers on IP in doctors. These were small studies, with a mean number of participants of 99 (range 48-185) doctors. The mean response rate of participants was 69% (range 55-87%). The percentage of female participants ranged between 30 and 53%.

The first study on IP in doctors was performed in Wisconsin family medicine residents, using postal surveys with incentives to respond (Oriel, Plane, & Mundt, 2004). The mean age of respondents was 33 years. This study revealed that there was no effect of year of training on IP rates, and that IP correlated with depressive symptoms, trait anxiety, state anxiety, and low self-esteem. Both mean CIS scores and prevalence of IP were found to be higher in female doctors than male doctors: 58.5 *versus* 54.3 ($p = 0.03$) and 41% *versus* 24% ($p = 0.02$) respectively. Interestingly, when results were controlled for trait anxiety, imposter feelings were no longer related to gender.

Figure 1. PRISMA flow diagram for the systematic review of imposter syndrome in the medical profession

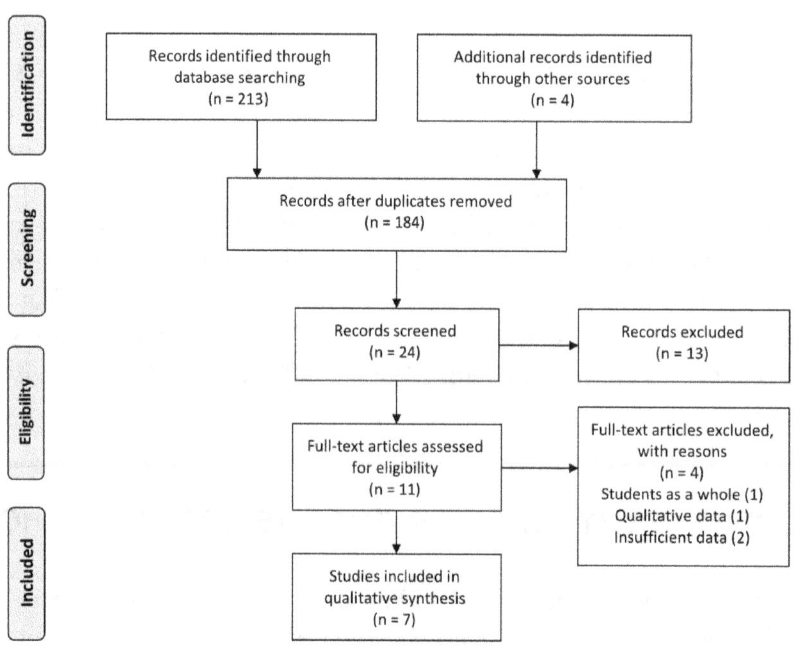

This was followed by a cross-sectional, single-institution study of internal medicine residents in Canada, using an anonymous postal survey (Legassie, Zibrowski, & Goldszmidt, 2008). The authors combined the use of the CIS and the Maslach Burnout Inventory-Human Services Survey (MBI-HSS) to assess wellbeing and burnout. More than a quarter of respondents in this study had graduated from medical school abroad, approximately two-thirds reported their marital status as single, and 83.3% of participants were below 30 years. This study confirmed that year of training had no effect on levels of IP, and that female residents had higher scores. Higher CIS scores were also found in foreign medical graduates. IP was found to be associated with burnout, and there was a negative correlation between IP and personal accomplishment.

The most recent study in doctors was performed in general surgeons and general surgery residents at two teaching hospitals in Minneapolis, USA, with a particular focus on burnout (Leach, Nygaard, Chipman, Brunsvold, & Marek, 2018). Over 90% of respondents to the email survey were Caucasian, 78% were married, and two-thirds had children. This study showed that trainees scored higher in the CIS than faculty (61 *versus* 51.1 respectively; $p = 0.017$). Interestingly, there was no association with gender, but clinical IP symptoms were again associated with burnout (Odds Ratio 3.95, $p = 0.017$).

The latter two studies reported mean CIS scores of 61.2 (Legassie et al., 2008) and 58.2 (Leach et al., 2018), giving an overall mean CIS of 60 in doctors.

THE IMPOSTER PHENOMENON IN MEDICAL STUDENTS

There have been four key papers on IP in medical students. These studies were slightly larger than the ones of doctors, with a mean number of participants of 192 (range 138-477) students. The mean response rate of participants was 66% (range 20-100%). The percentage of female participants ranged between 48 and 59%.

IP, and its relationship to perfectionism and psychological distress, were studied among medical, dental, nursing, and pharmacy students at a university in South Carolina (Henning et al., 1998). The authors used an anonymous questionnaire distributed during regularly scheduled classes, with a lottery incentive. In this study, 46% of participants were medical students. The majority of respondents were Caucasian (85%) and 63% reported never having married. The mean age of medical student respondents was 25.9 years. The authors found that CIS score was one of the strongest predictors of psychological distress among the students. Mean CIS scores were higher in women (57.83) than men (52.08) ($p < 0.001$). Prevalence of IP was higher in female students than male students (37.8% *versus* 22% respectively, $p < 0.001$).

Anonymous email surveys with the Young Imposter Quiz were used to assess the relationship between IP and burnout in a USA medical school (Villwock et al., 2016). Half of respondents were between 25-30 years old. The majority of respondents were Caucasian (84.67%) and there were 21.01-29.71% of respondents per year of training. The authors found that IP was more prevalent in the fourth (final) year of medical school, and was significantly associated with multiple burnout components. These included exhaustion, cynicism, emotional exhaustion, and depersonalisation. IP was more prevalent in women than men (49.4% *versus* 23.7% respectively, $p = 0.004$). IP was less prevalent in Asian and white participants (30%) compared with other races (72.7%) ($p = 0.057$). This study was limited by a low response rate (20%), and the fact that the Young Imposter Quiz is unvalidated.

One study examined IP in final year medical students only, in a cross-sectional, single institution study in Pakistan (Qureshi et al., 2017). The authors used anonymous self-administered printed versions of the Young Imposter Quiz. The mean age of participants was 24.08 years. Although it had a very high response rate, limited data were gleaned from this small study. The authors reported that, out of the 68 students considered "positive" for imposter syndrome, 45 were women and 23 were men.

Most recently, Egwurugwu et al. (2018) explored the relationship between self-esteem and IP in undergraduate medical students in Nigeria. Participants had a mean age of 21.35 years, and 12% were married. This study demonstrated no difference in CIS score between male and female medical students, but did show a negative correlation between self-esteem and IP, as well as a negative correlation between marital status and IP.

Mean CIS scores were reported in two studies: 54.7 (Henning et al., 1998) and 46.97 (Egwurugwu et al., 2018), giving an overall mean CIS of 51 – apparently lower than the scores in qualified doctors. There was, however, no difference in IP prevalence between doctors and students.

AETIOLOGY

An exploration of the deep-rooted psychological origins in childhood that may contribute to IP is beyond the scope of this chapter. In any case, the literature has not always been consistent (Kets de Vries, 2005). However, some clear associations with personality traits, and some overlap with psychiatric symptoms, have emerged from recent studies.

With respect to the Big Five personality traits as outlined by Digman (1990), IP appears to be related to high neuroticism (N. S. Bernard, Dollinger, & Ramaniah, 2002; Sakulku & Alexander, 2011; Vergauwe, Wille, Feys, De Fruyt, & Anseel, 2014). Neuroticism is a measure of one's tendency towards negative emotions, including anxiety and depression (Whitaker, 2018). The literature suggests that the relationship between IP and conscientiousness, which is a measure of self-discipline, organisation and a preference for planning, is more complicated, with most studies showing a negative correlation with conscientiousness (N. S. Bernard et al., 2002; Sakulku & Alexander, 2011; Vergauwe et al., 2014). Vergauwe et al. (2014) argued that the rather counter-intuitive negative association with conscientiousness (considering IP is more common among high achievers) could reflect individuals' lack of belief in their own competence and a lower self-discipline. How the Five Factor Model applies to the medical profession is contentious, as results on personality traits in doctors have often been contradictory between different studies (Grossman, 2018).

In addition to the Five Factor Model, studies have shown IP to be linked with excessive perfectionism (Thompson, Foreman, & Martin, 2000; Vergauwe et al., 2014). In particular, Vergauwe et al. (2014) demonstrated a positive association between IP and *maladaptive* perfectionism, and a negative association with *adaptive* perfectionism. Indeed, maladaptive perfectionism may be the catalyst, as those with IP set themselves excessively high, unrealistic goals, and then torture themselves when they cannot achieve their own expectations (Kets de Vries, 2005). Imposter tendencies are associated with perceptions of having less control, greater task anxiety, and a greater concern over mistakes than those without IP (Thompson et al., 2000).

Cokley et al. (2018) showed that the relationship between perfectionism and imposterism was partially mediated by self-esteem in university students. Self-esteem was negatively associated with IP in medical students (Egwurugwu et al., 2018) and doctors (Oriel et al., 2004). Sonnak and Towell (2001) have previously suggested that IP is an extension of poor self-esteem, rather than an independent state; this may account for discrepancies in findings in the relationship between IP and self-esteem. Vergauwe et al. (2014) studied Belgian employees from three different sectors, and did not find a significant association with self-esteem; they considered general self-esteem to be too broad a category to capture IP. They found individuals with IP to have low Core Self Evaluations (CSE), i.e. low self-appraisals and general negative affect. Those who suffer from IP frequently doubt their own knowledge and the validity of their achievements (LaDonna et al., 2018). Leary, Patton, Orlando, & Wagoner Funk (2000) showed that high imposterism scores correlate with more negative self-appraisals. However, there was no correlation with negative difference between self- and reflected appraisals, i.e. those with IP believed that others held the same negative opinions of them as they did. Outstanding performance offers no protection against IP, and those who do well are assumed to know they are doing well, and therefore receive less support (LaDonna et al., 2018).

As individuals with IP find themselves on the extreme end of the self-esteem spectrum, there will inevitably be some overlap with psychiatric illness. Indeed, those with imposter tendencies have impaired reality testing and a tendency to catastrophise (Kets de Vries, 2005), as well as associations with a more negative affect (Thompson et al., 2000). As will be discussed later, imposterism may play a causative role in anxiety and depression.

High Prevalence in Doctors and Medical Students

Medical students are by definition high achievers, as the competition for a place at medical school is fierce. Perfectionism is also a common trait among them. The relationship between perfectionism and IP in medical students is supported by the findings of Henning et al. (1998). Medical students have often come from being at the top of their class at school, to being just one in a large group of high achievers at medical school (Sakulku & Alexander, 2011). They are therefore already primed for imposter tendencies once they arrive. A foundation for imposter syndrome is then lain during medical school, as students with limited experience are treated by friends and family as qualified doctors, and are asked questions, when they know little more than the person asking the question (Cohen, Kay, Youakim, & Balaicuis, 2009). This is compounded by the anxiety-provoking routines of humiliation, grilling, and bullying in ward rounds (Cohen et al., 2009). The body of knowledge in medicine is, as a matter of course, enormous, never ending, and continuously evolving. As a student begins their final year of medical school, this fact begins to dawn on them, and IP becomes more prevalent (Villwock et al., 2016). Students then graduate and become doctors, and are let loose on the wards, armed with only a tiny proportion of that knowledge. The more experience the young doctor gains, the more they are aware of what they don't know, and the weight of responsibility sinks in. It is little wonder that CIS scores appear higher in doctors compared with medical students. The bullying and grilling also do not stop after graduation; trainees report feeling constantly "braced for critique" (LaDonna et al., 2018). High standards in healthcare leave little room for error (LaDonna et al., 2018). But to err is human, and with the focus on perfection, the inevitable errors can lead to guilt, anxiety, and self-doubt. These are not helped by the fact that errors are often kept to oneself, for fear of reprisals.

It [...] can be quite hard to share sometimes when you work in an environment that is fast-paced and it can feel like you need to just "get on with it" ... it helps to find a trusted peer or friend. (Pottinger, 2018)

Two papers demonstrated that year of training had no effect on levels of IP (Legassie et al., 2008; Oriel et al., 2004). There does, however, appear to be some relief once trainees are fully qualified, with Leach et al. (2018) finding lower CIS scores in surgical faculty than trainees. This is of course cross-sectional data, and should be interpreted with caution. LaDonna et al. (2018) proposed that triggers for IP may differ between trainees and fully qualified practitioners, with trainees worrying that their skills did not meet their own expectations, while consultants were concerned they didn't measure up to how *others* saw them.

High Prevalence in Women and Minorities

From a young age, women are more likely to be socialised to avoid appearing arrogant, and this can result in the common habit of minimising one's own success in response to praise (Goldhill, 2016). This is evidenced by common responses on social media to women who put their full title (Dr, Prof etc.) in their profiles (Riddell, 2018b). As a result, women make a habit not only of advertising their own shortcomings, but also of disparaging their own strengths (Koven, 2017). It is therefore unsurprising that IP has been shown to be more prevalent in women.[1] In particular, IP appears to be more common in women who achieve success in fields that conflict with the gender roles they grew up with, i.e. traditionally male-dominated industries (Kets de Vries, 2005; Sakulku & Alexander, 2011). IP is also exacerbated at key life junctures, such as marriage and having children, as women make career decisions that contrast with their own childhood experiences. As women are socialised to be demure, they are also socialised to work in traditionally feminine jobs, such as nursing and midwifery. It is no wonder that such women would subconsciously feel fraudulent in male-dominant fields (Kets de Vries, 2005).

My imposter syndrome was fuelled by a male boss who once told me that I needed to learn 'the power of silence' – that fuelled my self-doubt on the validity of my opinions. Speak up! (ChrissieMoz, 2018)

As well as being more prevalent among women, IP is also common among minorities. Both groups are often told explicitly or implicitly that they do not belong in certain careers. Both groups see a paucity of their peers represented in senior roles in these careers, and thus have a lack of identity fit (Peters, Ryan, Haslam, & Fernandes, 2012). Some are even told that they did not deserve their jobs, or that they didn't achieve the positions on merit, but rather through quotas, positive discrimination, or affirmative action (Kets de Vries, 2005). These biases eventually become internalised by the individual in question. Guilt may play a role here too, as those with IP feel they are "betraying" their origins with social mobility. This is supported by findings by Harvey (1981), that individuals with IP were more likely to report feeling "out of place" with respect to family status. However, this is contradicted by Sonnak and Towell's findings (2001) of a lack of correlation between IP scores and a discrepancy with one's family's educational background.

... it's about being a minority: gender, nationality, race, social class, sexuality all feed #ImposterSyndrome. Also environments where there's lots of critical peer review. (Garrett, 2018a)

IMPLICATIONS

The Imposter Cycle

The natural history of IP is that of a cycle (Clance, 1985; Clance, Dingman, Reviere, & Stober, 1995; Sakulku & Alexander, 2011). Imposter thoughts lead to anxiety and self-doubt; these result in over-preparation and/or procrastination. When the task is achieved, a momentary feeling of relief is followed promptly by a disregard of any positive feedback. The achievement is attributed to sheer effort or luck, the imposter thoughts return, and the cycle is complete. This cycle is exhausting, and peppered with anxious and depressive experiences.

As has been discussed above, IP does not seem to improve with progression through medical school and into clinical practice. Worryingly, IP can in fact worsen over time (Fitzpatrick & Curran, 2014), and trainees may not recover their perceived competence even when actual competence is achieved (LaDonna et al., 2018). However, trainees may find some solace in Leach et al.'s study (2018) that showed qualified consultants had lower scores than trainees.

I lost out on lots of early opportunities in life (e.g. work placements) due to #impostersyndrome because I had the mentality of 'I don't know enough yet (to do this)'. Thankfully, I have now developed a growth mindset. And I try and teach new grads about both ASAP! (integrativpsych, 2018)

Career Progression

IP is not just a lack of confidence, as people with IP can find their entire career path affected by their imposter feelings (Neureiter & Traut-Mattausch, 2016). As stated by Ross-Smith and Chesterman (2009), the quieter achievers get left behind. Those with IP may apply for fewer grants, and take fewer opportunities to advance their career, to avoid being "found out" (Woolston, 2016). If an individual portrays a lack of confidence, this can subconsciously influence others to lower their expectations of the individual's achievements, further slowing down career progression (Robinson-Walker, 2011).

As mentioned above, women had a higher prevalence of IP among doctors and medical students, with mean differences ranging from 13 to 26%. They also had higher mean CIS scores (mean difference 4-6). IP may therefore play a role in the lack of women in the most senior leadership positions in academia and medicine. With increasing women entering the medical profession, awareness of IP will become progressively more important for health service managers.

Individuals with strong IP tendencies report higher dissatisfaction in their jobs, and report lower Organizational Citizenship Behaviour (OCB), which measures how likely an employee is to contribute discretionary effort (Vergauwe et al., 2014). These associations are mitigated by strong social support. Interestingly, Vergauwe et al. (2014) also found that employees with higher IP scores are more likely to express an intention to stay in their organisation due to financial and psychological burdens associated with resigning. With respect to medicine, further research is required to determine how rates of attrition among medical students, trainees, and qualified practitioners vary according to imposter tendencies. Anecdotal data suggest that IP may be associated with higher attrition rates, with high achievers leaving prestigious positions due to low self-worth (Kets de Vries, 2005; Woolston, 2016). Vergauwe et al. (2014) argue that career transition is less likely among those with IP. This would suggest that current issues with recruitment to higher training (with greater numbers of foundation year doctors undertaking an optional

"Foundation Year 3" to delay specialist training, and taking time out to travel) may in part be related to imposter feelings. Note that anecdotal data from a 2014 internal report by Hewlett Packard revealed that men apply for a position when they meet 60% of the job specifications, whereas women only apply if they meet 100% (Clark, 2014). This is supported by anecdotal data from university Vice-Chancellors in Australia (Ross-Smith & Chesterman, 2009): many women were in their positions because they had been invited to apply, whereas many senior academic men had actively sought promotion. Women direct ambition towards careers in which they perceive they will succeed.

Although IP tends to be more common in women, men with imposter syndrome may have more severe reactions to performance stimuli than women, and experience higher state anxiety than women (Badawy, Gazdag, Bentley, & Brouer, 2018). This translates to decreased work effort and performance in men, whereas women may increase effort and performance in response to negative feedback.

Burnout and Poor Mental Health

Cowman and Ferrari (2002) found that university students with imposter tendencies were more likely to engage in behavioural self-handicapping, that is, attributing poor performance to obstacles. As outlined in the imposter cycle mentioned above, such behaviour includes procrastination until the last minute, potentially providing an "alibi" of lack of effort in the case of failure (Cozzarelli & Major, 1990). Performance anxiety may also lead people with IP to habitually over-prepare and over-work, leading to burnout (Robinson-Walker, 2011). This is logical if you consider that they are constantly fearful of being "found out" (Leary et al., 2000).

The effects of IP may also spill over onto colleagues. Individuals with the syndrome may enforce their unrealistic expectations of perfection not only on themselves, but also on their peers. Procrastination and an inability to finalise decisions may cause frustration. These situations can all lead to low morale (Seritan & Mehta, 2016).

A consistent finding in the systematic review covered earlier in this chapter was that imposter tendencies were associated with burnout in doctors (Leach et al., 2018; Legassie et al., 2008) and medical students (Villwock et al., 2016). This may be explained by the maladaptive behaviours mentioned above.

As discussed earlier, studies in other disciplines have shown that IP is positively correlated with anxiety, depression, and overall poor mental health (McGregor, Gee, & Posey, 2008; Sonnak & Towell, 2001). This was also demonstrated in doctors (Oriel et al., 2004) and medical students (Henning et al., 1998). Cowman and Ferrari (2002) also demonstrated a link between imposter tendencies in university students and being prone to shame and guilt. As mentioned above, these feelings are common in doctors and medical students, particularly in the context of medical errors; it is all too easy to forget that doctors are human and fallible. Those who suffer from IP may worry constantly that they are unworthy of their role or know less than their colleagues (Cohen et al., 2009). Students with IP are more anxious about exams, and expect to perform less well (Cozzarelli & Major, 1990). Unsurprisingly, they also cope less well with exam failure than those without IP. Coping mechanisms of individuals with IP vary depending on perceived levels of social support (Whitman & Shanine, 2012). Those with higher levels of support tend to employ "active" coping strategies (being aware of a stressor, and attempting to reduce the negative outcome), and those without support fall back on "avoidant" coping (ignoring the stressor, and attempting to stay in denial).

LIMITATIONS OF RESEARCH INTO IMPOSTER SYNDROME

The quality of studies on IP in the medical profession is variable. The way that IP was reported varies between studies, with some reporting absolute scores, and some reporting the prevalence of "positive" scores (above a certain cut-off, sometimes referred to as "clinical" IP). This makes it challenging to compare findings; this is particularly hindered by the lack of normative data for CIS among the population in general, in young professionals, and in different medical specialties (Henning et al., 1998). Furthermore, much of this research is based on self-reported, retrospective, or cross-sectional questionnaires, limited by selection bias. There is, however, an element of reassurance in the reproducibility of some of the data.

COPING WITH IMPOSTER PHENOMENON

I think the first step is to [acknowledge] imposter syndrome and realise it is more common than you think! (Oliver, 2018)

As IP is not a recognised clinical disorder, little research exists on effective management strategies. However, the literature does describe some techniques that individuals may find helpful in preventing the syndrome from affecting career progress (Dowd & Davidhizar, 1997).

The first step is recognising that it is an issue. By its very nature, this is not an easy feat; as with many types of neuroticism, a low level of imposterism and perfectionism contribute to high performance (Kets de Vries, 2005). Improving insight into the problem relies on raising awareness not only among those at risk, but also among colleagues and peers who may recognise the condition in others. Mentors, managers, and coaches should be trained in recognising signs of neuroticism in their charges. An individual may notice that progress in their career has stalled because they have been avoiding taking chances and making the most of opportunities. A quick way for the individual to explore whether they might be affected is to take the Clance IP Test online (Clance, n.d.). Mindfulness, defined as being aware of present-moment experiences with a mental stance of receptivity and non-judgment, can be a useful tool (Kabat-Zinn, 1994; Lindsay & Creswell, 2017). It allows an individual to pay attention to when one's mind goes to imposter thoughts in a balanced manner (Patzak, Kollmayer, & Schober, 2017). At the point that IP is recognised, the individual should seek support from others, including a mentor that they feel able to confide in.

Learning to accept praise can be one of the biggest challenges for individuals who suffer from IP, and this ties in with feeling guilty about one's success (Dowd & Davidhizar, 1997). To counter this, individuals need to become accustomed to responding positively to praise. This may involve coaching or Cognitive Behavioural Therapy exercises (Ilkhchi, Poursharifi, & Alilo, 2011). It is important to avoid minimising one's own achievements, and avoid responding to praise with words such as "just" and "only" when describing one's work (Woolston, 2016). If an individual can inspire confidence from other people, they may in turn absorb some of that confidence. It is perfectly acceptable to be proud of one's work and achievements.

As discussed above, discriminatory behaviour may contribute to IP. Dr Fern Riddell, an academic historian, suffered frequent micro-aggressions – subtle discriminatory actions and behaviours, both intentional and unintentional, that can accumulate over time, producing negative consequences (Gonzales et al., 2016; Sue et al., 2007) – in the form having her expertise questioned, and being referred to by her first name or by the wrong title. She posted the following on Twitter in response to those micro-aggressions:

My title is Dr Fern Riddell, not Ms or Miss Riddell. I have it because I am an expert, and my life and career consist of being that expert in as many different ways as possible. I worked hard to earn[...] my authority, and I will not give it up to anyone. (Riddell, 2018a)

The tweet received over 1,500 "retweets" (shares on Twitter) and 15,000 "likes" (favourites). It also received a number of comments, including a reply from a man calling Dr Riddell "immodest". This led to an online movement, with many women changing their profiles to include their hard-earned titles, and tweeting the hashtag #immodestwomen (Riddell, 2018b).

Individuals with imposter syndrome should be inspired by Dr Riddell, and should not be afraid to show confidence in their abilities: eventually this may change the culture of women being expected to downplay their achievements.

Of course, there are times when a trainee is not as competent as they need to be – but that does not make them any less worthy of their job. That is part of training: "With responsibility comes constructive criticism" (Kets de Vries, 2005). It is important for a trainee to recognise where their skills are lacking, and to focus their training on that area (Robinson-Walker, 2011). Realistic personal development plans, reflective practice, specific and accurate feedback, and regular appraisal meetings between a trainee and their educational supervisor all play important roles in identifying these areas. It is important for trainees, or any specialty and associate specialist grade doctors who work under consultant supervision, to know that they have the support of their clinical supervisor, and that they may approach them to discuss cases when they are in doubt. Part of training is to learn when "good enough" is a viable (and safe) alternative to perfection. Similarly, trying and failing is sometimes part of the job. These moments should be treated as learning opportunities (Fitzpatrick & Curran, 2014). If a surgeon never tries to operate independently, they won't fail, but they won't learn to be a surgeon either. Even at consultant level, nobody is perfect; no doctor can know everything.

I agree [that] organisations that allow staff to show doubt, make mistakes and be vulnerable are less likely to have staff who suffer from #ImposterSyndrome (Garrett, 2018b)

It is difficult to overcome the tendency to focus on negative feedback, as imposter feelings are fairly resistant to accolades (LaDonna et al., 2018). Spending a conscious effort to focus on the positive can go some way to compensating for this, with a view to eventually learning to internalise achievements. Reflective practice may be helpful here, as well as reviewing one's CV or portfolio, and making an accurate list of strengths and achievements (Weir, 2013). It may also help to look at previous feedback and reflective practice, and read the positive feedback several times over. Another method is to write a private journal entry about how one's achievements make the individual suitable for their current role, or one they aspire to attain. This written "interview" may help the individual realise they have achieved more than they remember. Comparing these achievements with those of average peers in their field may allow the individual to realise they did not get their job by luck, but because they deserved it. This is particularly true if they can remember to trust the system (Woolston, 2016). Application processes and examinations are fairly rigorous and robust, and it is unlikely for someone to be admitted into medical school by accident, and even less so for them to get through medical school without the requisite skills.

But for every moment when we feel inadequate, there is another moment when we realize a previous challenge is now mundane. (Russell, 2017)

Tutoring more junior colleagues and students is another way to help a person appreciate the gains they have made in their knowledge and the level of expertise they have now achieved (Weir, 2013). Supporting others through their self-doubt can also help with one's own confidence. "To really pick yourself up, bring someone else up with you" (Woolston, 2016).

It is also the responsibility of leaders and managers to create an atmosphere that fosters confidence in their employees. Ensuring that diverse role models are approachable can allow more junior staff to find an identity fit, particularly if these role models share their stories about how they achieved their positions (Peters et al., 2012). A flattened hierarchy in an organisation has been shown to enable all members of the team to feel valued. And of course, bullying and harassment must be eradicated.

It is also the responsibility of the doctor and medical student to remember self-care. This may be in the form of mindfulness or exercise, or by making a conscious effort to avoid comparing oneself to others.

The only person I now compare myself to is me. Am I better than I was a week, a month, a year ago? If there's growth, I am happy. (Garrett, 2018c)

FUTURE RESEARCH

The study of IP among doctors and medical students is in its relative infancy, and more research is needed to establish the significance of the phenomenon. Larger, high-quality studies are needed to elicit how IP relates to personality traits, risk of burnout, and mental health disorders in doctors and medical students. It would also be useful to compare levels of IP in different medical specialties.

Research in other fields suggest that there are different subdivisions within the IP umbrella: so called "true imposters" and "strategic imposters", who are less hampered by their self-doubt, and only say they are not as good as others believe (Leary et al., 2000; Leonhardt, Bechtoldt, & Rohrmann, 2017). "Strategic imposters" may employ interpersonal, self-presentational behaviours to lessen the consequences of low skill level. It is important that in future studies, the heterogeneity of the phenomenon is considered.

The imposter phenomenon appears to be more prevalent among foreign medical graduates (Legassie et al., 2008), and race has a significant effect on IP rates in medical students (Villwock et al., 2016). This is consistent with IP research in other disciplines; for example, D. L. Bernard, Hoggard, and Neblett (2018) showed that experience of racial discrimination is associated with increased rates of IP among American university students. These findings raise important questions about how best to support students and trainees from diverse backgrounds.

Finally, it is likely that IP would be made worse by a discrepancy in what others' lives appear to be like as depicted on social media, and the truth of others' experiences. Future research should include studying the effect of social media use on IP.

CONCLUSION

[Imposter syndrome] may not be talked about widely – but I've found it to be a common subject when I'm coaching others. Particularly with women leaders. (Bryan, 2018)

Many successful people have been affected by IP, and all great leaders doubted their abilities at some stage. Self-doubt was just another obstacle they overcame on their journey. As more people discuss the syndrome, it is likely that it will constrain the careers of fewer people, as insight appears to be extremely beneficial in tackling the affliction.

In an atmosphere where you are surrounded with pressure and often self-doubt, it is restorative to remember just how normal your abnormal life has become. (Russell, 2017)

REFERENCES

he_reeves. (2018, March 1). I have often felt that some success has been down to luck (right place/right time) it's difficult to shake, however, luck only gets you so far the rest is down to you. The gremlins push me to be better, learn [Tweet]. Retrieved from https://twitter.com/he_reeves/status/969245903956660226

integrativpsych. (2018, March 28). @hcwomenleaders I lost out on lots of early opportunities in life (e.g., work placements) due to #impostersyndrome because I had the mentality of "I don't know enough yet (to do this)". Thankfully, I have now developed a growth mindset. And [Tweet]. Retrieved from https://twitter.com/integrativpsych/status/979075774044045313

ChrissieMoz. (2018, March 28). My imposter syndrome was fuelled by a male boss who once told me that I needed to learn "the power of silence," that fuelled my self doubt on the validity of my opinions. Speak up! #NHSwomen [Tweet]. Retrieved from https://twitter.com/ChrissieMoz/status/979084803336232962

Badawy, R. L., Gazdag, B. A., Bentley, J. R., & Brouer, R. L. (2018). Are all impostors created equal? Exploring gender differences in the impostor phenomenon-performance link. *Personality and Individual Differences*, *131*, 156–163. doi:10.1016/j.paid.2018.04.044

Bernard, D. L., Hoggard, L. S., & Neblett, E. W. (2018). Racial discrimination, racial identity, and impostor phenomenon: A profile approach. *Cultural Diversity & Ethnic Minority Psychology*, *24*(1), 51–61. doi:10.1037/cdp0000161 PMID:28414495

Bernard, N. S., Dollinger, S. J., & Ramaniah, N. V. (2002). Applying the Big Five personality factors to the impostor phenomenon. *Journal of Personality Assessment*, *78*(2), 321–333. doi:10.1207/S15327752JPA7802_07 PMID:12067196

Bryan, P. [petrajbryan]. (2018, March 28). @MandipRandhawa7 @ChrisOliverNHS @hcwomenleaders Agree may not be talked about widely - but I've found it to be a common subject when I'm coaching others. Particularly with women leaders #NHSwomen [Tweet]. Retrieved from https://twitter.com/petrajbryan/status/979073494922211328

Byrnes, K. D., & Lester, D. (2016). The imposter phenomenon in teachers and accountants. *Psychological Reports*, *77*(1), 350–350. doi:10.2466/pr0.1995.77.1.350 PMID:7501775

Chae, J.-H., Piedmont, R. L., Estadt, B. K., & Wicks, R. J. (1995). Personological evaluation of Clance's Imposter Phenomenon Scale in a Korean sample. *Journal of Personality Assessment*, *65*(3), 468–485. doi:10.120715327752jpa6503_7 PMID:16367710

Chrisman, S. M., Pieper, W. A., Clance, P. R., Holland, C. L., & Glickauf-Hughes, C. (1995). Validation of the Clance Imposter Phenomenon Scale. *Journal of Personality Assessment*, *65*(3), 456–467. doi:10.120715327752jpa6503_6 PMID:16367709

Christensen, M., Aubeeluck, A., Fergusson, D., Craft, J., Knight, J., Wirihana, L., & Stupple, E. (2016). Do student nurses experience imposter phenomenon? An international comparison of final year undergraduate nursing students readiness for registration. *Journal of Advanced Nursing*, *72*(11), 2784–2793. doi:10.1111/jan.13034 PMID:27240171

Clance, P. R. (1985). *The Impostor Phenomenon: When Success Makes You Feel Like A Fake* (pp. 20–22). Toronto, Canada: Bantam Books.

Clance, P. R. (n.d.). Clance Impostor Phenomenon Test. Retrieved from https://paulineroseclance.com/pdf/IPTestandscoring.pdf

Clance, P. R., & Imes, S. A. (1978). The imposter phenomenon in high achieving women: Dynamics and therapeutic intervention. *Psychotherapy (Chicago, Ill.)*, *15*(3), 241–247. doi:10.1037/h0086006

Clark, N. F. (2014). Act now to shrink the confidence gap. *Forbes*.

Cohen, M. J. M., Kay, A., Youakim, J. M., & Balaicuis, J. M. (2009). Identity transformation in medical students. *American Journal of Psychoanalysis*, *69*(1), 43–52. doi:10.1057/ajp.2008.38 PMID:19295620

Cokley, K., Stone, S., Krueger, N., Bailey, M., Garba, R., & Hurst, A. (2018). Self-esteem as a mediator of the link between perfectionism and the impostor phenomenon. *Personality and Individual Differences*, *135*, 292–297. doi:10.1016/j.paid.2018.07.032

Cowman, S. E., & Ferrari, J. R. (2002). "Am I for real?" Predicting impostor tendencies from self-handicapping and affective components. *Social Behavior and Personality*, *30*(2), 119–125. doi:10.2224bp.2002.30.2.119

Cozzarelli, C., & Major, B. (1990). Exploring the validity of the impostor phenomenon. *Journal of Social and Clinical Psychology*, *9*(4), 401–417. doi:10.1521/jscp.1990.9.4.401

Digman, J. M. (1990). Personality structure: Emergence of the Five-Factor Model. *Annual Review of Psychology*, *41*(1), 417–440. doi:10.1146/annurev.ps.41.020190.002221

Dowd, S. B., & Davidhizar, R. (1997). Do you feel like an impostor? *The Health Care Supervisor*, *15*(3), 51–56. PMID:10165429

Egwurugwu, J., Ugwuezumba, P., Ohamaeme, M., Dike, E., Eberendu, I., & Egwurugwu, E. (2018). Relationship between self-esteem and impostor syndrome among undergraduate medical students in a Nigerian university. *International Journal of Brain and Cognitive Sciences*, *7*(1), 9–16. doi:10.5923/j.ijbcs.20180701.02

Fitzpatrick, T. A., & Curran, C. R. (2014). Waiting for your coronation: A career-limiting trap. *Nursing Economics*, *32*(3), 162–165. PMID:25137816

Fried-Buchalter, S. (1992). Fear of success, fear of failure, and the imposter phenomenon: A factor analytic approach to convergent and discriminant validity. *Journal of Personality Assessment, 58*(2), 368–379. doi:10.120715327752jpa5802_13 PMID:16370869

Garrett, J. [JenniferGarrett]. (2018a, March 28). Good point Chris, it's about being a minority: gender, nationality, race, social class, sexuality all feed #ImposterSyndrome Also environments where there's lots of critical peer review #nhswomen https://t.co/1POhv8ETEQ [Tweet]. Retrieved from https://twitter.com/JenniferGarrett/status/979074080010899457

Garrett, J. [JenniferGarrett]. (2018b, March 28). I agree @ana_brankovic organisations that allow staff to show doubt, make mistakes and be vulnerable are less likely to have staff who suffer from #ImposterSyndrome #NHSwomen https://t.co/WHScauj0jV [Tweet]. Retrieved from https://twitter.com/JenniferGarrett/status/979074514788212736

Garrett, J. [JenniferGarrett]. (2018c, March 28). This is an important point, the only person I now compare myself to is me. Am I better than I was a week, a month, a year ago? If there's growth, I am happy #impostersyndrome #nhswomen #ditchcomparison https://t.co/zS0kxKrbGH [Tweet]. Retrieved from https://twitter.com/JenniferGarrett/status/979078285199015936

Goldhill, O. (2016, Feb. 1). Is imposter syndrome a sign of greatness? *Quartz.*

Gonzales, K. L., Noonan, C., Goins, R. T., Henderson, W. G., Beals, J., Manson, S. M., ... Roubideaux, Y. (2016). Assessing the everyday discrimination scale among American Indians and Alaska Natives. *Psychological Assessment, 28*(1), 51–58. doi:10.1037/a0039337 PMID:26146948

Grossman, R. (2018). The surgical personality: Does it matter? *The Bulletin of the Royal College of Surgeons of England, 100*(3), 130–132. doi:10.1308/rcsbull.2018.130

Harvey, J. C. (1981). The impostor phenomenon and achievements: A failure to internalize success (Doctoral thesis: Temple University, 1981). *Dissertation Abstracts International, 42*, 4969B.

Health & Care Women Leaders Network [hcwomenleaders]. (2018, March 27). Some have never heard of it. Some know it only too well. That confidence-sapping feeling that it's luck rather than ability that lies behind your success. Share your thoughts, experiences and coping strategies in our tweet chat, tomorrow from 8pm [Tweet]. Retrieved from https://twitter.com/hcwomenleaders/status/978646347082616839

Hellman, C. M., & Caselman, T. D. (2004). A psychometric evaluation of the Harvey Imposter Phenomenon Scale. *Journal of Personality Assessment, 83*(2), 161–166. doi:10.120715327752jpa8302_10 PMID:15456652

Henning, K., Ey, S., & Shaw, D. (1998). Perfectionism, the impostor phenomenon and psychological adjustment in medical, dental, nursing and pharmacy students. *Medical Education, 32*(5), 456–464. doi:10.1046/j.1365-2923.1998.00234.x PMID:10211285

Holmes, S. W., Kertay, L., Adamson, L. B., Holland, C. L., & Clance, P. R. (1993). Measuring the impostor phenomenon: A comparison of Clance's IP Scale and Harvey's I-P Scale. *Journal of Personality Assessment, 60*(1), 48–59. doi:10.120715327752jpa6001_3 PMID:8433268

Ilkhchi, S. V., Poursharifi, H., & Alilo, M. M. (2011). The effectiveness of Cognitive-Behavioral Group Therapy on self-efficacy and assertiveness among anxious female students of high schools. *Procedia: Social and Behavioral Sciences*, *30*, 2586–2591. doi:10.1016/j.sbspro.2011.10.506

Kabat-Zinn, J. (1994). *Wherever you go, there you are*. New York, NY: Hyperion.

Kets de Vries, M. F. R. (2005). The dangers of feeling like a fake. *Harvard Business Review, 83*(9), 108–16–159.

Koven, S. (2017). Letter to a young female physician. *The New England Journal of Medicine*, *376*(20), 1907–1909. doi:10.1056/NEJMp1702010 PMID:28514609

Kruger, J., & Dunning, D. (1999). Unskilled and unaware of it: How difficulties in recognizing one's own incompetence lead to inflated self-assessments. *Journal of Personality and Social Psychology*, *77*(6), 1121–1134. doi:10.1037/0022-3514.77.6.1121 PMID:10626367

LaDonna, K. A., Ginsburg, S., & Watling, C. (2018). Rising to the level of your incompetence. *Academic Medicine*, *93*(5), 763–768. doi:10.1097/ACM.0000000000002046 PMID:29116983

Leach, P. K., Nygaard, R. M., Chipman, J. G., Brunsvold, M. E., & Marek, A. P. (2018). Impostor phenomenon and burnout in general surgeons and general surgery residents. *Journal of Surgical Education*, 1–8. doi:10.1016/j.jsurg.2018.06.025 PMID:30122638

Leary, M. R., Patton, K. M., Orlando, A. E., & Wagoner Funk, W. (2000). The impostor phenomenon: Self-perceptions, reflected appraisals, and interpersonal strategies. *Journal of Personality*, *68*(4), 725–756. doi:10.1111/1467-6494.00114 PMID:10934688

Legassie, J., Zibrowski, E. M., & Goldszmidt, M. A. (2008). Measuring resident well-being: Impostorism and burnout syndrome in residency. *Journal of General Internal Medicine*, *23*(7), 1090–1094. doi:10.100711606-008-0536-x PMID:18612750

Leonhardt, M., Bechtoldt, M. N., & Rohrmann, S. (2017). All impostors aren't alike – differentiating the impostor phenomenon. *Frontiers in Psychology*, *8*, 424. doi:10.3389/fpsyg.2017.01505 PMID:28936188

Lindsay, E. K., & Creswell, J. D. (2017). Mechanisms of mindfulness training: Monitor and Acceptance Theory (MAT). *Clinical Psychology Review*, *51*, 48–59. doi:10.1016/j.cpr.2016.10.011 PMID:27835764

McGregor, L. N., Gee, D. E., & Posey, K. E. (2008). I feel like a fraud and it depresses me: The relation between the imposter phenomenon and depression. *Social Behavior and Personality*, *36*(1), 43–48. doi:10.2224bp.2008.36.1.43

Neureiter, M., & Traut-Mattausch, E. (2016). An inner barrier to career development: Preconditions of the impostor phenomenon and consequences for career development. *Frontiers in Psychology*, *7*, 53. doi:10.3389/fpsyg.2016.00048 PMID:26869957

Oliver, C. [ChrisOliverNHS]. (2018, March 28). @NHSE_Paul @hcwomenleaders I think the first step is to aknowlege imposter syndrome and realise it is more common than you think! #nhswomen [Tweet]. Retrieved from https://twitter.com/ChrisOliverNHS/status/979074441429872641

Oriel, K., Plane, M. B., & Mundt, M. (2004). Family medicine residents and the impostor phenomenon. *Family Medicine*, *36*(4), 248–252. PMID:15057614

Patzak, A., Kollmayer, M., & Schober, B. (2017). Buffering impostor feelings with kindness: The mediating role of self-compassion between gender-role orientation and the impostor phenomenon. *Frontiers in Psychology*, *8*, 1289. doi:10.3389/fpsyg.2017.01289 PMID:28798714

Peters, K., Ryan, M., Haslam, S. A., & Fernandes, H. (2012). To belong or not to belong. *Journal of Personnel Psychology*, *11*(3), 148–158. doi:10.1027/1866-5888/a000067

Pottinger, H. [HPottinger]. (2018, March 28). @hcwomenleaders It is can be quite hard to share sometimes when you work in an environment that is fast paced and it can feel like you need to just "get on with it" … it helps to find a trusted [Tweet]. Retrieved from https://twitter.com/HPottinger/status/979078359228604416

Qureshi, M. A., Taj, J., Latif, M. Z., Rafique, S., Ahmed, R., & Chaudhry, M. A. (2017). Imposter syndrome among Pakistani medical students. *Annals of King Edward Medical University*, *23*(2), 1–6. doi:10.21649/akemu.v23i2.1647

Riddell, F. [FernRiddell]. (2018a, June 13). My title is Dr Fern Riddell, not Ms or Miss Riddell. I have it because I am an expert, and my life and career consist of being that expert in as many different ways as possible. I worked hard to [Tweet]. Retrieved from https://twitter.com/FernRiddell/status/1006870044331200512

Riddell, F. [FernRiddell]. (2018b, June 16). We need #ImmodestWomen when so many men are unable to accept female expertise. *New Statesman*. Retrieved from https://www.newstatesman.com/politics/feminism/2018/06/we-need-immodestwomen-when-so-many-men-are-unable-accept-female-expertise

Robinson-Walker, C. (2011). The imposter syndrome. *Nurse Leader*, *9*(4), 12–13. doi:10.1016/j.mnl.2011.05.003

Ross-Smith, A., & Chesterman, C. (2009). "Girl disease": Women managers' reticence and ambivalence towards organizational advancement. *Journal of Management & Organization*, *15*(5), 582–595. doi:10.1017/S1833367200002431

Russell, R. (2017). On overcoming imposter syndrome. *Academic Medicine*, *92*(8), 1070. doi:10.1097/ACM.0000000000001801 PMID:28742562

Sakulku, J., & Alexander, J. (2011). The impostor phenomenon. *International Journal of Behavioral Science*, *6*(1), 73–92.

Seritan, A. L., & Mehta, M. M. (2016). Thorny laurels: The impostor phenomenon in academic psychiatry. *Academic Psychiatry*, *40*(3), 418–421. doi:10.100740596-015-0392-z PMID:26152516

Simon Gilbody: The importance of being active. (2017). Simon Gilbody: The importance of being active. *BMJ (Clinical Research Ed.)*, *359*, j5371. doi:10.1136/bmj.j5371 PMID:29187359

Smith, R. (2003). Thoughts for new medical students at a new medical school. *BMJ (Clinical Research Ed.)*, *327*(7429), 1430–1433. doi:10.1136/bmj.327.7429.1430 PMID:14684637

Sonnak, C., & Towell, T. (2001). The impostor phenomenon in British university students: Relationships between self-esteem, mental health, parental rearing style and socioeconomic status. *Personality and Individual Differences*, *31*(6), 863–874. doi:10.1016/S0191-8869(00)00184-7

Sue, D. W., Capodilupo, C. M., Torino, G. C., Bucceri, J. M., Holder, A. M. B., Nadal, K. L., & Esquilin, M. (2007). Racial microaggressions in everyday life: Implications for clinical practice. *The American Psychologist*, *62*(4), 271–286. doi:10.1037/0003-066X.62.4.271 PMID:17516773

Thompson, T., Foreman, P., & Martin, F. (2000). Impostor fears and perfectionistic concern over mistakes. *Personality and Individual Differences*, *29*(4), 629–647. doi:10.1016/S0191-8869(99)00218-4

Vergauwe, J., Wille, B., Feys, M., De Fruyt, F., & Anseel, F. (2014). Fear of being exposed: The trait-relatedness of the impostor phenomenon and its relevance in the work context. *Journal of Business and Psychology*, *30*(3), 565–581. doi:10.100710869-014-9382-5

Villwock, J. A., Sobin, L. B., Koester, L. A., & Harris, T. M. (2016). Impostor syndrome and burnout among American medical students: A pilot study. *International Journal of Medical Education*, *7*, 364–369. doi:10.5116/ijme.5801.eac4 PMID:27802178

Weir, K. (2013, November). Feel like a fraud? *gradPSYCH Magazine*. doi:10.1002/j.2161-1912.2013.00029.x/abstract

Whitaker, M. (2018). The surgical personality: Does it exist? *Annals of the Royal College of Surgeons of England*, *100*(1), 72–77. doi:10.1308/rcsann.2017.0200 PMID:29260896

Whitman, M. V., & Shanine, K. K. (2012). Research in Occupational Stress and Well-Being: Vol. 10. *Revisiting the impostor phenomenon: how individuals cope with feelings of being in over their heads* (pp. 177–212). doi:10.11081479-3555(2012)0000010009

Woolston, C. (2016). Psychology: Faking it. *Nature*, *529*(7587), 555–557. doi:10.1038/nj7587-555a PMID:26824109

Young, V. (n.d.). Impostor Syndrome Quiz. Retrieved from https://impostorsyndrome.com/quiz/

ADDITIONAL READING

Cohen, M. J. M., Kay, A., Youakim, J. M., & Balaicuis, J. M. (2009). Identity transformation in medical students. *American Journal of Psychoanalysis*, *69*(1), 43–52. doi:10.1057/ajp.2008.38 PMID:19295620

Goldhill, O. (2016, February 1). Is imposter syndrome a sign of greatness? *Quartz*.

Kets de Vries, M. F. R. (2005). The dangers of feeling like a fake. *Harvard Business Review*, *83*(9), 108–16– 159.

LaDonna, K. A., Ginsburg, S., & Watling, C. (2018). Rising to the level of your incompetence. *Academic Medicine*, *93*(5), 763–768. doi:10.1097/ACM.0000000000002046 PMID:29116983

Leary, M. R., Patton, K. M., Orlando, A. E., & Wagoner Funk, W. (2000). The impostor phenomenon: Self-perceptions, reflected appraisals, and interpersonal strategies. *Journal of Personality*, *68*(4), 725–756. doi:10.1111/1467-6494.00114 PMID:10934688

Riddell, F. [FernRiddell]. (2018b, June 16). We need #ImmodestWomen when so many men are unable to accept female expertise. *New Statesman*. Retrieved January 19, 2019, from https://www.newstatesman.com/politics/feminism/2018/06/we-need-immodestwomen-when-so-many-men-are-unable-accept-female-expertise

Russell, R. (2017). On overcoming imposter syndrome. *Academic Medicine*, *92*(8), 1070. doi:10.1097/ACM.0000000000001801 PMID:28742562

Vergauwe, J., Wille, B., Feys, M., De Fruyt, F., & Anseel, F. (2014). Fear of being exposed: The trait-relatedness of the impostor phenomenon and its relevance in the work context. *Journal of Business and Psychology*, *30*(3), 565–581. doi:10.100710869-014-9382-5

KEY TERMS AND DEFINITIONS

Active coping: Being aware of a stressor, and attempting to reduce the negative outcome.

Avoidant coping: Ignoring the stressor, and attempting to stay in denial.

Big Five personality traits: Otherwise known as the five-factor model. A classification system for personality traits based on factor analysis, which recognises five broad dimensions most often used to describe the human personality: neuroticism, conscientiousness, openness to experience, extraversion, and agreeableness.

Conscientiousness: A measure of self-discipline, organisation, and a preference for planning.

Hashtag: Metadata tag on social media to link discussions according to topic.

Imposter syndrome: An internal experience of feeling like an intellectual fraud, despite external evidence of an individual's accomplishments, and an inability to internalise a sense of success.

Micro-aggression: Subtle discriminatory actions and behaviours, both intentional and unintentional, that can accumulate over time, producing negative consequences.

Mindfulness: Being aware of present-moment experiences with a mental stance of receptivity and non-judgment.

Neuroticism: A measure of one's tendency towards negative emotions, including anxiety and depression.

Tweetchat: An open online conversation on the social media platform Twitter.

ENDNOTES

1 Interestingly, at the other end of the spectrum, Kruger and Dunning (1999) found no effect of gender on the inability to recognise one's own incompetence.

Chapter 12
Who Will Take Care of Me? The Future of Human Resources in Anaesthesiology, Critical Care, and Emergency Medicine in Europe.

Cristina Honorato-Cia
School of Medicine, University of Navarra, Spain

Stefan De Hert
Ghent University, Belgium

Edoardo De Robertis
Department of Surgical and Biomedical Sciences, University of Perugia, Perugia, Italy

Ioana Grigoras
University of Medicine and Pharmacy "Grigore T. Popa" Iasi, Romania

ABSTRACT

Foreseeing the needs and availability of anaesthesiologists across Europe is a challenging task. This is influenced by different factors that include the composition of the workforce and the organization and structure of health services in every country. Some trends call for attention, such as changes in work patterns brought about by an ageing specialist population, the increasing numbers of women in anaesthesia, or cultural and societal shifts towards work-life balance. Anaesthesiology is a challenging specialty with an expanding scope of practice, requiring highly motivated professionals, frequent long work hours, and addressing stressful situations often. To ensure quality anaesthesia provision, the wellbeing of this diverse population of anaesthesiologists should be addressed. Achieving rational and flexible work hours, adequate compensation, and promotion of a workplace culture that fosters safety, motivation to learn, and equal opportunities for leadership or academia positions are challenges to be addressed to make sure that excellence in patient care is maintained.

DOI: 10.4018/978-1-5225-9599-1.ch012

INTRODUCTION

Foreseeing in advance the needs and availability of anaesthesiologists across Europe is a challenging task. It is a very complex issue influenced by different factors including the composition of the workforce and the different organizations and structures of health services in every country. Some trends call for attention, such as changes in work patterns brought about by an ageing specialist population, the increasing numbers of women working in anaesthesia, or cultural and societal shifts towards work-life balance.

Anaesthesiology is a challenging specialty with an expanding scope of practice, requiring highly motivated professionals, frequent long working hours including nights, and very often addressing sudden stressful situations. To ensure high quality anaesthesia care, the wellbeing of this diverse population of anaesthesiologists should also be addressed. Achieving rational and flexible work hours, adequate compensation, and promotion of a workplace culture that fosters safety, motivation to learn and equal opportunities for (also flexible) leadership or academic positions are key challenges that should be tackled if we want to make sure that excellence in patient care is maintained (De Hert, 2018).

Current Situation in Anaesthesia, Critical Care, and Emergency Medicine

Anaesthesia departments across Europe are facing a higher workload due to their involvement in many hospital areas, which are growing or expanding their scope of practice. Anaesthesiologists are asked to provide round the clock services ensuring quality and safety in critical care, operating theatres, pain clinics, emergency patient care (both in and out of hospital) and palliative care.

The question is, as the population in Europe gets older, demand for specialized healthcare services is expected to keep growing. The burden of disease grows at an estimated 10% per year (Benziger, Roth, & Moran, 2016). Noncommunicable - or chronic - diseases are responsible for more than 60% of deaths on the continent. As average life expectancy in Europe is growing (76.7 years in 2010 to 77.9 years in 2015) (World Health Organization, 2018) so are the health problems associated with age and sedentary lifestyles. Although the obesity rate in Europe is still far from the numbers reported in North America, an increasing number of Europeans are joining the ranks (*Health at a Glance: Europe 2018*, 2018).

One reason for concern is the fact that resources are not growing at the same rate. Socialized health care systems as available in most European countries are closely monitored to optimize spending and efficiency. An estimated 10% of GDP in the EU is directed to healthcare, with countries like Germany, Sweden or France allocating even more than that. Yet, the annual average growth rate in healthcare spending in Europe went from 3.1% in 2005-2009, before the 2008 economic crisis, to 0.7% in the 2010-2015 period (*Health at a Glance: Europe 2018*, 2018). This affects both the material setup and management of the hospital as well as the possibilities to recruit and compensate available workers.

The Demographics of Anaesthesia and Critical Care

Age

A recent review by Giacalone et al (Giacalone, Zaouter, Mion, & Hemmerling, 2016) highlighted the fact that European anaesthesiologists are aging, too. In France, about 50% of the anaesthesiologists working in 2005 will be retired before 2020, and there is no sufficient replacement. The government has suggested an increase in retirement age to 72 years of age to compensate. In the UK it is estimated that up to 70% of the actual medical workforce will not retire before they are 68 years old. A similar pattern is observed in Canada and the US, where in 2013 close to 30% of anaesthesiologists were older than 55 years of age, and 8-10% (depending on source of information) were older than 65 years old. Replacement, again, is not guaranteed, let alone covering the growing demands for anaesthesia services (A. D. Baxter, Boet, Reid, & Skidmore, 2014).

Older anaesthesiologists provide great care and bring their extensive experience into the workplace. But they have their needs and concerns, too. Older physicians have a higher rate of burnout, anxiety, and depression. Their job satisfaction in lower than that of younger colleagues (Katz, 2016). On top of that, age related physiologic changes may reduce their physical tolerance to on-call duties, their ability to concentrate or listen in noisy environments, and the speed at which decisions are made (A. D. Baxter et al., 2014; Giacalone et al., 2016). All these skills apply in the daily work of an anaesthesiologist, and all the more so during nights on call. Of course, the aging process can be very different among individuals, and some older doctors may be performing at the same level as younger ones, but a systematic review from the US showed that quality of care tends to diminish with age, as elderly physicians are less likely to follow guidelines or be up to date in medical knowledge (Choudhry, Fletcher, & Soumerai, 2005). Although this had no effect on outcomes (experience probably acted as a counterbalance), it is certainly something to take into account.

As such, this population can therefore have widely variable needs and expectations. Some doctors may keep working because they love their job and feel fit to practice it; others may lack the financial stability to retire. Some may be happy limiting their clinical time in favour of administrative, teaching or research duties. Others may prefer to work less than full time (LTFT) but take only clinical work, or skip being on call entirely. Their continuing education needs may also be different, and it has been suggested that they may benefit especially from crisis management simulation to keep peak performance in the operating theatre and other acute care scenarios (A. D. Baxter et al., 2014; A. Baxter, Thompson, & McCartney, 2016).

All this adds complexity to an already complex situation; namely, managing an anaesthesia department. But in order to provide the best possible care and not waste the best that every physician has to offer, an individualized and flexible approach sounds like the most sensible option. Some departments already have "winding down" plans, including considering stopping "overnight on-call" at 60 years old, no further high acuity cases at 65, or retirement from main operating theatre practice at 70 (A. Baxter et al., 2016).

Women

As in many other areas in medicine, there is a higher number of female than male physicians in Anaesthesia. This was first highlighted by a 2007 study of the Anaesthesia workforce in Europe, which looked at the future considering the increasing presence of women in the field, and the impact of future medical immigration within Europe (Egger Halbeis et al., 2007). In that study, approximately 47% of anaesthesiologists in Europe were women; in trainees, the number ascended to 53%. In 2018, the European Society of Anaesthesia sent a survey to active and affiliate members, showing percentages of 49.5% for male and 50.5% for female anesthesiologists (De Hert & Honorato-Cia, 2018). Not surprisingly, the biggest net increase per age group happened in the younger cohort (Baird, Daugherty, Kumar, & Arifkhanova, 2015). This is interesting considering the future of the specialty. The trend is likely to keep on growing, as female medical students now account for 50-55% in most medical schools (Leslie, Hopf, Houston, & O'Sullivan, 2017). The general situation in the developing world is very similar to Europe (Baird et al., 2015; Leslie et al., 2017)

When studying gender differences in anaesthesia and critical care, the focus has been directed at the higher number of women working part-time, and, consequentially, the difference in compensation (Baird et al., 2015; Egger Halbeis et al., 2007; Haller, Delhumeau, Mamie, Zoccatelli, & Clergue, 2016; Miller & Katz, 2018). The 2018 ESA survey showed that, in Europe, substantially more women than men work part-time (29% women vs 12% men). More men than women are thus in the higher income range (5,000–10,000 € and > 10,000 €). It is difficult to ascertain if this can be solely related to the different work pattern. A recent study from Switzerland (Haller et al., 2016) showed that more women were paid with a fixed salary (59.2% vs 46.6%) as compared to men, and that services carrying an extra compensation were more often taken by men (36.9% vs 22.9%) than by women. This reflects the situation in other European countries.

The general assumption is that most women will be the primary caregivers for children, parents or other older relatives. The demands imposed of them by this effort make them more likely to prefer LTFT work, or at least to be able to have a relatively flexible schedule. But women also seem to be more frequently involved in some work areas more than others, dealing with ambulatory or paediatric anaesthesia, or being more active in pain management. There seems to be an implicit understanding that a woman will fare better in less aggressive and physically demanding areas of the specialty, which is notoriously one that deals with emergencies and complex or critical cases requiring many talents and strengths, and that frequently involves long shifts or night work. It is difficult to ascertain whether these preferences are anecdotal or real, and, in that case, if the proportion is really significant. Also, there is a lack of data on what may cause women to gravitate towards those areas: schedule, flexibility, type of patient, type of work environment?

The Swiss study mentioned earlier (Haller et al., 2016) also highlighted another issue that is widely recognized and that has generated a large amount of interest in the past two or three years: the fact that women are majorly underrepresented in academia, leadership and management positions. A 2017 study comparing Australia, New Zealand, Ireland, Canada, the UK and the US, found that female trainees accounted for 40-50% depending on country, but that chairs of department, academic leaders or board members barely reached 20% in average (Leslie et al., 2017). Another 2017, worldwide analysis in Critical Care diversity showed that the representation of women in conferences, guideline recommendation or clinical practice guidelines was also very low (around 13% of 413 guidelines published between 2012 and 2016) (Mehta et al., 2017). In the 2018 ESA survey the disparity was also very apparent, with twice as many men than women in a position of professor and hospital medical director and even 3 times more men in the position of head of the department (De Hert & Honorato-Cia, 2018).

The reasons behind this situation are varied and complex, and may vary slightly within different areas or countries in Europe. They may not be intentional, but they are not random, either. This situation is not exclusive of the medical field, and as a matter of fact has been extensively documented and researched, especially in the business world. There is no doubt as to the capability, competence or expertise of women in their respective fields of knowledge, so there must be other reasons holding them back. Personal preferences aside (any woman -or man- may choose to prioritize family, health, social work or other aspects of their life, or just not be interested in academia or leadership), many reasons have been researched that may explain the disparity. One is cultural bias, when people implicitly assign gender-specific roles such as caring for children in women or expecting a focus in career success for men (Ibarra, Ely, & Kolb, 2013). This is frequently unconscious and includes gender but also race, country of origin, or age. Women´s competence appears to be evaluated using different standards than men and takes personality more into account (assertive women as seen as "bossy" while the same attitude in a man would be acceptable and even expected). These biases affect both men and women, with many successful women falling into what is called a "second-generation bias" in which they tend to minimize the effort and hurdles they had to overcome. This happens partly because women tend to expect their efforts to be recognized while men are apparently more forward and make sure that their hard work is visible (Gravett, 2013; Ibarra et al., 2013).

In the past five years, a considerable effort has been made to educate everyone on those biases and to promote and facilitate the access of women to higher positions (De Hert & Honorato-Cia, 2018; Leslie et al., 2017; Mehta et al., 2017; Toledo et al., 2017). Both the ASA (Leslie et al., 2017) and the ESA (De Hert & Honorato-Cia, 2018) have made it public that they are committed to advocate for changes and have taken steps to ensure data transparency, equality in boards and conferences and to promote workplace change through education. These measures will be discussed later, as they affect some of the other issues in this chapter.

Diversity in the Workplace

Diversity is a very broad term. Currently, and in Medicine, who does it refer to? What is the norm that is not being met? A possible approach would be to consider that most European health care systems were originally designed with one type of physician in mind – the most common one at the time. That would be a Caucasian male, head of a family, culturally close to the community he was serving, and available to put in as many hours as needed as family support was guaranteed. From that perspective, aging physicians and women are probably the biggest "diverse" groups we are dealing with right now.

Over the past forty years, European society has changed beyond recognition, and it is safe to say that that kind of physician is not anymore the norm. There is a different approach to work-life balance, women are currently half or more of the medical workforce, and economic pressures are much higher. The way we work in hospitals has also changed, and anesthesiologists are currently seeing how their scope of practice is growing to perioperative medicine, emergency care, pain management and so on. Training and continuing education are more challenging as new technologies emerge and are incorporated into daily work.

While this is challenging enough for just about anyone, doctors from different cultural or religious backgrounds or that trained abroad and returned may face additional pressure. Medical migration in Europe was first addressed in the 2007 survey mentioned before, and at the time it showed that most of the movement was happening from Eastern to Western Europe, with a small number of anesthesiologists coming from the Middle East or Asia. Some countries such as Estonia or the Slovak Republic lost up to 15% and 20% of their anaesthesiologists (Egger Halbeis et al., 2007). Although this trend seems to have slowed down in recent years, there is still a considerable number of physicians working outside their home countries for a variety of reasons. The needs and concerns of these groups might be hard to reach as they may take some time to become fully integrated in medical professional associations.

IN SUMMARY

Providing the best possible care to our patients requires well trained, highly motivated anaesthesiologists. To ensure this, it is important to look at the composition of the workforce, both now and in the years to come. Their needs have to be addressed to make sure that they can develop their careers in a balanced, integrated way, and that they stay motivated to deliver good care, do research and teach future anaesthesiologists. A good way to make sure of this is to ensure adequate representation and access to leadership positions; it is well known that diversity is associated with better results in the business world, and there is no reason that suggests otherwise in medicine. This seems to be related to the fact that other points of view are taken into account when making managing decisions, and also to the possibility of finding different ways to solve problems.

Most of the work already done has been in the field of gender equality, but the possibilities and mechanisms affect all groups. Before looking at what has already worked and what else can be done, we are going to analyse the impact of other key influences: how technology (and especially communications technology) affects us and how we work; and the increasing problem of burnout and ensuring physician wellbeing.

LIFE ITSELF

If there is a generalization that a vast majority of us will accept, it is this one: the happier you are, the better professional you will be. This should specially ring true for doctors, whose empathy and compassion towards patients will directly affect the quality of their work. But will also affect their motivation for career development, research, learning, and teaching. And ultimately, their decision to stay in medicine or quit, or to retire early. Satisfaction at work is affected by many variables, and is highly personal. It is affected by cultural background and gender, but also by whether you are a baby boomer, a millennial or belong to generation X. A detailed analysis is beyond the scope of this work, but one issue remains critical: whatever can be done to increase wellbeing will ultimately affect the quality of care.

Technology and Connectivity in the Workplace

Connectivity is changing how we work and relate to others and has had a major impact on how doctors deal with their patients, the hospital workflow, and how and what they need to learn in order to stay current and motivated. Surgeries of about 2h can experience an average of 9 interruptions per hour (one every 7 minutes!) of varying importance (Antoniadis, Passauer-Baierl, Baschnegger, & Weigl, 2014). Some are related to time dedicated to enter data into anesthesia information management systems, and a good number of others to the use of the phone, by talking or by texting. This use is not always work related and it is debatable whether work-only use can possibly be demanded. In a 2012 analysis, the ASA Closed Claims database reported 13 adverse outcomes in 5822 claims related to distractions such as reading, phone use, or loud music. There was no report involving social networks or other Internet uses. These events were labelled substandard care and were associated with payments in 80% of the cases. The median payment was $725,937 (Domino & Sessler, 2012). Clearly, patients consider that doctor´s focus is important.

It´s not a mere question of whether this affects outcomes, although that is a serious concern. It affects the whole way we communicate and the pressures that we experience. It certainly affects psychological energy and focus. And it requires a high standard of professionalism, requiring an effort to minimize anything that distracts from good care, to facilitate the avoidance of alert fatigue, and of course the inappropriate use of social networks (Cammarata & Thomas, 2014). That is today´s world, after all. If you are in Belgium, you look at your phone an average of 34 times/day. In the US, it would be 52. In Norway and Sweden, 61% of people use their phone at work for personal purposes. In France, this number goes up to 92% ("2018 Global mobile consumer trends. Deloitte.," 2018).

How many times each of us, or someone close, has stated that they use their phones too much but don´t actually know how to change that behaviour? Internet addiction was defined more than 20 years ago (in 1996, to be precise). Technology has many benefits and has changed our lives for the better in countless ways, but we have to own it, not the other way around. More than never, each anaesthesia provider now holds the responsibility for how they provide care, and of what they publish in social media. It´s not just about respecting the privacy of patients – there are some cases of doctors who were fired because of racist or highly inappropriate comments about their (anonymous) patients.

To add another layer of pressure to an environment already loaded with them, in many hospitals in Europe texting through chat apps such as WhatsApp™ has become the preferred way of delivering department alerts or requests. This means that a medical professional may receive his/her week schedule, case list, and any changes in them without actually talking to anyone, be it the operating theatre manager, the department chief or whoever is in charge of organizing and distributing work. It´s practical and easy, but many of the nuances of communication are completely lost. Is that anaesthesiologist all right with a sudden change? How did the last case affect this professional emotionally? Face to face communication may not always be the most practical approach, but it should not be cornered that easily. Healthcare professionals, after all, are notorious for minimizing their own pains and aches in favour of patient care.

How Technology is Shaping the Work Environment

Being constantly connected is not the only way in which technology affects the way an anesthesia professional (or any other medical doctor) works. The development of artificial intelligence (AI) and self-learning algorithms is aimed primarily at the automation of tasks that formerly required a human being, like EKG reading or radiologic and ultrasound interpretation. Mobile apps are being developed for diagnosing diabetic retinopathy or melanoma, and are becoming increasingly accurate. All this technology might not be ready yet, but for sure is not going to take long (Chuchu et al., 2018). Some of them are already available for the general public to download and use. Virtually anyone will be able to diagnose skin cancer or atrial fibrillation. Will be eventually stop needing doctors altogether?

In anesthesia, automated closed-loop systems have been under development for quite a while, guiding drug dosage through processed electroencephalograms, with positive results: lower use of drugs, stable anesthesia depth, shorter recovery times (Pasin et al., 2017). Other physiologic variables such as variability in heart rate or stroke volume have also been used to guide fluid therapy or analgesia delivery (De Jonckheere, Jeanne, Keribedj, Delecroix, & Logier., 2018; Joosten et al., 2016). All this does not yet replace a human anaesthesia provider (for the time being, we are still better than machines at rapid danger recognition and at integrating information). The question here is *when?* (probably sooner than we may think) and also *how?* - and here the answer is: *we don´t know yet*. The way we work is going to change, and sooner rather than later. The way anesthesiologists will work in, let´s say, ten or twenty years from now, may be very different from what we do now. We will still need human providers but they may have a somewhat different set of skills and knowledge. With robots and AI guiding the more technical aspects of anesthesia delivery and physiologic homeostasis, the role of the anaesthesiologist might very well lean towards team coordination, preanesthesia counselling, and a humane, compassionate approach to surgical and critical care patients and their families.

Does this mean we won´t need as many doctors in a few years? It´s difficult to foresee, but it certainly looks possible. What is clear is that there is something no robot can deliver: the human touch. The understanding, the comforting, the compassion – who wouldn´t want a knowledgeable physician providing this, and coordinating our care, in those moments of critical illness or surgery?

Burned-Out Anaesthesiologists

The problem with human touch is that it implies that the anaesthesiologist is capable of this empathy and compassion. There has been for long now a discussion on why doctors seem to stop less by the bedside nowadays. A 2017 review showed that, in UK anesthesia departments, two thirds of patients' complaints were related to the ethics and professionalism of healthcare workers, and only one third to medical or technical issues (Pieri et al., 2016). What´s going on here? There is not one single reason. Anaesthesia is one of the medical fields at high risk of psychological stress. Anaesthesiologists are exposed daily to heavy workloads, stressful situations with patients and colleagues and many responsibilities. They work nights, weekends and holidays. They miss on social life, and may feel isolated. They don´t always have a solid social or institutional support. On top of this, and as a recent article in *The Lancet* stated, physicians become "disillusioned by the productivity orientation of administrators and absence of affirmation for the values of relationships that sustain their sense of purpose" (Epstein & Privitera, 2016). This affects morale, and, when it all together becomes too much, or the individual doesn´t find a mechanism to deal with it, burnout may ensue.

This syndrome seems to have reached epidemic levels in the medical field with a reported prevalence around 50% in all specialties, and well over it in fields related to emergency or critical care (Sanfilippo et al., 2017). Burnout in anesthesia is known to appear in response to chronic stressors, such as poor temporal structuring of work, conflicting interpersonal relations, or lack of control over the activity itself (De Oliveira, 2017). Burnout syndrome is broadly accepted to have three main components: depersonalization (physicians become cynical and detached), emotional exhaustion (loss of motivation and hope) and low personal accomplishment (they feel ineffective and helpless) (Epstein & Privitera, 2016). Who doesn´t know of someone experiencing this to some extent?

The consequences impact the workplace heavily (impaired job performance, poor display of empathy towards patients, a trend to leave the practice); but especially the person, with reports of poorer health (higher incidence of hypertension, sleep problems or gastric disorders), increased interpersonal and marital conflicts, depression and other mental problems, some leading to substance abuse. It may even lead to suicidal ideation or even attempts to take one´s life (Rama-Maceiras, Jokinen, & Kranke, 2015).

To top this, women consistently report higher levels of burnout. This begins early in their careers, and with early we mean *very* early: six months into residency, female residents have higher levels of stress and burnout than their male counterparts (Guille et al., 2017). We have cited before the many cultural reasons and biological factors that have been advocated to account for this difference. Age, on the contrary, seems to have the opposite effect: older anesthesiologists report lower levels of burnout, as they have probably developed adequate coping mechanisms over time (Wong & Olusanya, 2017).

A considerable effort has been devoted to identifying both risk and protective factors. Developing resilience and coping mechanisms is useful, as are stress management strategies. Individuals are encouraged to give self-care its due importance, establishing the best possible work life balance achievable, identifying specific stressors and trying to change either the setting or the emotion associated with them (Rama-Maceiras et al., 2015).

However, physician-oriented strategies are overall less effective than organization-oriented interventions like reducing workload, rescheduling shifts or organizing multidisciplinary meetings to enhance teamwork (Panagioti et al., 2018). Promoting a positive climate, group cohesion, communication, and participation are also approaches that institutions can take. Engagement can be promoted, and especially in anesthesia, by giving certain extent of control over work schedules, by promoting flexibility and part time schedules that don´t curtail the physician capability to pursue research or teaching. Other way to increase control is to promote clinical pathways designed by multidisciplinary teams.

All this is going to require quite a cultural change. Big academic hospitals with a never-ending workload – how will they avoid rewarding a faster (but chaotic) pace and promote quality? Smaller institutions – will they have the capability to actively measure climate in the workplace and provide counsellor help when needed? Will they have the resources to provide flexibility in work schedule? And all of them, how to deal with the stigma associated with psychological distress? Not to say when things go even further and substance abuse becomes the coping mechanism selected. Anesthesia is notorious for having a risk of addiction 2.7 times higher than other specialties. Opioids addictions (mostly fentanyl) account for 55%, alcohol for 28%, and stimulants for 8% of the substances used by anesthesiologists as a "coping strategy" (Lefebvre & Kaufmann, 2017).

Emotional and medical education since early in medical school, and promoting engagement and a good social support are good strategies to help prevent and deal with psychological distress, burnout or, if it comes to that, substance abuse or any other kind of addiction.

IN SUMMARY

The work environment of anesthesiologists has seen a degree of change in the past 15 years. Technology has provided new ways of working, automating processes and highlighting the human interaction provided by the anesthesia team, and their role in leadership and coordination of care. Connectivity has also made communication easier and faster, although it might also become a distraction sometimes. Anesthesiologists need to be aware and in control of how they use these tools so that they don´t compromise quality of care. This faster pace, along with the characteristics of the anaesthesiologist work, has made apparent the psychological distress that doctors may suffer when hospitals are managed based solely on economic factors. Burnout syndrome and substance abuse to a much lesser extent, are real problems that require action from both the individual and the institution in order to avoid harm for both the medical provider and the patient.

MAKING SURE THE FUTURE LOOKS BRIGHT

There is a general acknowledgement that we need a vast cultural change, both for men and for women, individuals and institutions. This is the workforce that we have, when we look into the future:

- A significant portion of aging physicians that can offer magnificent expertise and very valuable experience, but that need winding down from the physically challenging aspects of anesthesia;
- An increasingly higher proportion of women whose talent and contribution are currently underutilized due to cultural constricts and a rigid, outdated work organization;
- A more diverse workforce that values work-life balance.

The way they develop their work needs to change, or we will see a good number of them leaving the specialty or providing low quality care due to burnout. We need to find a way to create better structures that could allow for a more psychologically safe work environment. We need to see how we can develop a work culture that keeps medical professionals highly motivated in staying up to date and developing research; providing safe, high quality medical care, putting the patient at the centre of their practice; and making sure that they can balance their personal and professional lives.

What do we Know that we can Apply?

Of all the issues we have talked about in this chapter, the most extensively researched are gender equity and burnout. There are no strong evidences to support any specific intervention, because there are many factors involved and their complexity is considerable. Not only every country is different, there are also big differences in workplace culture in neighbouring institutions.

Individual Based Strategies

Women physicians, as we have seen, face many barriers is career development. Throughout the past several decades, there has been an increase of initiatives to teach women how to navigate the male-centered work environment, how to negotiate, or how to develop a better work-life balance. This has been best achieved through peer-to-peer networking, mentoring programs (where the mentor can be either male or female), aiming at a better sharing of household responsibilities with partners, and seminars promoted by different organizations. Social support is seen as crucial. Awareness programs aimed at noticing and managing conscious and unconscious bias, and low intensity, often non malicious sexual harassment (such as sexist remarks or behaviours), have also proven very helpful (Mehta et al., 2017; Pfleiderer, Bortul, Palmisano, Rodde, & Hasebrook, 2018; Wong & Olusanya, 2017).

In dealing with burnout, physician directed interventions usually comprise cognitive behavioural techniques, courses on mindfulness, communication skills and coping strategies, like enhancing peer-to-peer networking, or enriching social life outside of work. Physical exercise or hobbies are also encouraged. Again, social support is seen as crucial (Rama-Maceiras et al., 2015).

Institution Based Strategies

Not surprisingly, the biggest challenge lies in changing the workplace environment and burnout than physician-oriented interventions (Wong & Olusanya, 2017). In gender equity, there is simply no other way to promote change.

Many academic hospitals, to provide an example, directly do not have work conditions suitable for a woman of any age, but especially young, trying to juggle family, clinical time, research and teaching. Female physicians tend to choose working environments that are more flexible, work less than full time and in average earn less than their male counterparts for doing the same job (Baird et al., 2015; Pfleiderer et al., 2018). Hospital managers need to be aware of this and address the issue accordingly. Human resources management has to be aligned with economic, academic and clinical management. This can only be achieved if the institution takes the problem seriously and commits to find solutions to remove barriers in work scheduling and career progression. Quotas have been long looked at suspiciously, but the fact is that, if you promote gender equality in boards, then women's problems and needs will be recognized and addressed much earlier, and the solutions will be better fitted for them.

Gender equality in leadership positions is also beneficial as it creates more role models, a more open and welcoming environment, and an increase in visibility. In the short term, specific grants and scholarships can also help younger women establish a research career. In the long term, institutions have to find a way to accommodate the needs and dynamics of female doctors. The magic word here is flexibility.

This is a similar approach to addressing burnout from an organizational point of view. Changes in shift models that allow for reasonable rest time, comfortable on call rooms, varied job plans and planned sabbaticals are useful in improving the work environment and climate. Transparency from management, participation in decisions, team building exercises improve sense of value for the physician. And very importantly, the sense of fairness in work distribution and rewards is an important part of this work climate.

If we look at what these approaches have in common, two things stand out: there needs to be a commitment from top to down to change things; and flexible work plans within the possibilities of every institution should be implemented and actively supported.

CONCLUSION

It is virtually impossible to foresee in advance the needs and availability of anaesthesiologists across Europe. There are many different factors and every country has its own idiosyncrasy in what comes to culture, organization and structure of health services. We have reviewed the impact of some trends, such as the ageing specialist population, the increasing numbers of women working in anaesthesia, or cultural and societal changes in perception towards work-life balance.

Anaesthesiology is a challenging specialty and requires a high degree of engagement and motivation to endure long work hours, stressful situations and often tense work environments. To ensure quality and sustainable anaesthesia provision, wellbeing of this diverse population of anaesthesiologists needs be addressed. There are some individual interventions that are useful, but the biggest impact come from organizational, top to down changes. Achieving rational and flexible work hours, adequate compensation, and promotion of a workplace culture that fosters safety, would be key points to ensure the culture of safety, quality and motivation that will provide, in years to come, the doctor that will care of us.

REFERENCES

Antoniadis, S., Passauer-Baierl, S., Baschnegger, H., & Weigl, M. (2014). Identification and interference of intraoperative distractions and interruptions in operating rooms. *The Journal of Surgical Research*, *188*(1), 21–29. doi:10.1016/j.jss.2013.12.002 PMID:24405613

Baird, M., Daugherty, L., Kumar, K. B., & Arifkhanova, A. (2015). Regional and gender differences and trends in the anesthesiologist workforce. *Anesthesiology, 123*(5), 997–1012. doi:10.1097/ALN.0000000000000834 PMID:26291778

Baxter, A., Thompson, C., & McCartney, C. (2016, October). "Winding down" guidelines for anesthesiologists: The Ottawa Hospital plan. *Canadian Journal of Anaesthesia = Journal Canadien d'anesthesie*. United States. doi:10.100712630-016-0692-0

Baxter, A. D., Boet, S., Reid, D., & Skidmore, G. (2014). The aging anesthesiologist: a narrative review and suggested strategies. *Canadian Journal of Anaesthesia = Journal Canadien d'anesthesie, 61*(9), 865–875. doi:10.100712630-014-0194-x

Benziger, C. P., Roth, G. A., & Moran, A. E. (2016). The Global Burden of Disease Study and the Preventable Burden of NCD. *Global Heart, 11*(4), 393–397. doi:10.1016/j.gheart.2016.10.024 PMID:27938824

Cammarata, B. & Thomas, B. (2014). Technology's Escalating Impact on Perioperative Care: Clinical, Compliance, and Medicolegal Considerations - Anesthesia Patient Safety Foundation. *APFS Newsletter, 29*(1). Retrieved from https://www.apsf.org/article/technologys-escalating-impact-on-perioperative-care-clinical-compliance-and-medicolegal-considerations/

Choudhry, N. K., Fletcher, R. H., & Soumerai, S. B. (2005). Systematic Review: The Relationship between Clinical Experience and Quality of Health Care. *Annals of Internal Medicine, 142*(4), 260. doi:10.7326/0003-4819-142-4-200502150-00008 PMID:15710959

Chuchu, N., Takwoingi, Y., Dinnes, J., Matin, R. N., Bassett, O., & Moreau, J. F., … Group, C. S. C. D. T. A. (2018). Smartphone applications for triaging adults with skin lesions that are suspicious for melanoma. *Cochrane Database of Systematic Reviews*, (12). doi:10.1002/14651858.CD013192 PMID:30521685

De Hert, S. (2018). Burnout Among Anesthesiologists: It's Time for Action! *Journal of Cardiothoracic and Vascular Anesthesia, 32*(6), 2467–2468. doi:10.1053/j.jvca.2018.06.010 PMID:30093191

De Hert, S. & Honorato-Cia, C. (2018). Gender and leadership positions in Anaesthesiology: take on the challenge. *ESA Newsletter*, Issue 75. Retrieved from http://newsletter.esahq.org/gender-leadership-positions-anaesthesiology-take-challenge/

De Jonckheere, J., Jeanne, M., Keribedj, A., Delecroix, M., & Logier., R. (2018). Closed-loop administration of analgesic drugs based on heart rate variability analysis*. In *2018 40th Annual International Conference of the IEEE Engineering in Medicine and Biology Society (EMBC)* (Vol. 2018, pp. 506–509). IEEE. doi:10.1109/EMBC.2018.8512330

De Oliveira, G. S. J. (2017, September). Biological evidence of the impact of burnout on the health of anesthesiologists. *Journal of Clinical Anesthesia*. United States. doi:10.1016/j.jclinane.2017.06.011

Domino, K. B., & Sessler, D. I. (2012). Internet Use during Anesthesia Care. *Anesthesiology, 117*(6), 1156–1158. doi:10.1097/ALN.0b013e31827515fb PMID:23099739

Egger Halbeis, C. B., Cvachovec, K., Scherpereel, P., Mellin-Olsen, J., Drobnik, L., & Sondore, A. (2007). Anaesthesia workforce in Europe. *European Journal of Anaesthesiology, 24*(12), 991–1007. doi:10.1017/S0265021507000762 PMID:17608964

Epstein, R. M. & Privitera, M. R. (2016). *Doing something about physician burnout, 388*(10057), 2216–2217. doi:10.1016/S0140-6736(16)31332-0

Giacalone, M., Zaouter, C., Mion, S., & Hemmerling, T. M. (2016). Impact of age on anaesthesiologists' competence: A narrative review. *European Journal of Anaesthesiology, 33*(11), 787–793. doi:10.1097/EJA.0000000000000534 PMID:27635955

2018 . Global mobile consumer trends. Deloitte. (2018). Retrieved from https://www2.deloitte.com/global/en/pages/technology-media-and-telecommunications/articles/gx-global-mobile-consumer-trends.html

Gravett, G. (2013). Tell Me Something I Don't Know About Women in the Workplace. *Harvard Business Review*, (August). Retrieved from https://hbr.org/2013/08/tell-me-something-i-dont-know

Guille, C., Frank, E., Zhao, Z., Kalmbach, D. A., Nietert, P. J., Mata, D. A., & Sen, S. (2017). Work-Family Conflict and the Sex Difference in Depression Among Training Physicians. *JAMA Internal Medicine, 177*(12), 1766. doi:10.1001/jamainternmed.2017.5138 PMID:29084311

Haller, G., Delhumeau, C., Mamie, C., Zoccatelli, D., & Clergue, F. (2016, August). Gender difference in career advancement and job satisfaction in anaesthesia: A cross-sectional study. *European Journal of Anaesthesiology*. England. doi:10.1097/EJA.0000000000000471

Health at a Glance: Europe 2018. (2018). OECD. doi:10.1787/health_glance_eur-2018-en

Ibarra, H., Ely, R., & Kolb, D. (2013). Women rising: the unseen barriers. *Harvard Business Review*, (September). Retrieved from https://hbr.org/2013/09/women-rising-the-unseen-barriers

Joosten, A., Delaporte, A., Cannesson, M., Rinehart, J., Dewilde, J. P., Van Obbergh, L., & Barvais, L. (2016). Fully Automated Anesthesia and Fluid Management Using Multiple Physiologic Closed-Loop Systems in a Patient Undergoing High-Risk Surgery. *A & A Case Reports, 7*(12), 260–265. doi:10.1213/XAA.0000000000000405 PMID:27669030

Katz, J. D. (2016). The aging anesthesiologist. *Current Opinion in Anaesthesiology, 29*(2), 206–211. doi:10.1097/ACO.0000000000000299 PMID:26705128

Lefebvre, L. G. & Kaufmann, I. M. (2017). The identification and management of substance use disorders in anesthesiologists. *Canadian Journal of Anaesthesia = Journal Canadien d'anesthesie, 64*(2), 211–218. doi:10.100712630-016-0775-y

Leslie, K., Hopf, H. W., Houston, P., & O'Sullivan, E. (2017). Women, minorities, and leadership in anesthesiology: Take the pledge. *Anesthesia and Analgesia, 124*(5), 1394–1396. doi:10.1213/ANE.0000000000001967 PMID:28426582

Mehta, S., Burns, K. E. A. A., Machado, F. R., Fox-Robichaud, A. E., Cook, D. J., Calfee, C. S., ... Herridge, M. S. (2017). Gender parity in critical care medicine. *American Journal of Respiratory and Critical Care Medicine, 196*(4), 425–429. doi:10.1164/rccm.201701-0076CP PMID:28240961

Miller, J., & Katz, D. (2018). Gender Differences in Perception of Workplace Experience Among Anesthesiology Residents. *The Journal of Education in Perioperative Medicine: JEPM, 20*(1), E618. Retrieved from http://www.ncbi.nlm.nih.gov/pubmed/29928665 PMID:29928665

Panagioti, M., Geraghty, K., Johnson, J., Zhou, A., Panagopoulou, E., Chew-Graham, C., ... Esmail, A. (2018). Association Between Physician Burnout and Patient Safety, Professionalism, and Patient Satisfaction. *JAMA Internal Medicine, 178*(10), 1317. doi:10.1001/jamainternmed.2018.3713 PMID:30193239

Pasin, L., Nardelli, P., Pintaudi, M., Greco, M., Zambon, M., Cabrini, L., & Zangrillo, A. (2017). Closed-loop Delivery Systems Versus Manually Controlled Administration of Total Iv Anesthesia: A Meta-analysis of Randomized Clinical Trials. *Anesthesia &amp, 124*(2), 456–464. doi:10.1213/ane.0000000000001394

Pfleiderer, B., Bortul, M., Palmisano, S., Rodde, S., & Hasebrook, J. (2018). Improving female physician's careers in academic medicine: Chances and challenges. *Best Practice & Research. Clinical Anaesthesiology, 32*(1), 15–23. doi:10.1016/j.bpa.2018.04.006 PMID:30049335

Pieri, M., Bonizzoni, M. A., Lembo, R., Dalessandro, V., Alba, A. C., Zangrillo, A., & Landoni, G. (2016, October). Intensive Care and Anesthesia Specialists Would Do More Research If They Could. *Journal of Cardiothoracic and Vascular Anesthesia*. United States. doi:10.1053/j.jvca.2016.04.024

Rama-Maceiras, P., Jokinen, J., & Kranke, P. (2015). Stress and burnout in anaesthesia: A real world problem? *Current Opinion in Anaesthesiology, 28*(2), 151–158. doi:10.1097/ACO.0000000000000169 PMID:25695803

Sanfilippo, F., Noto, A., Foresta, G., Santonocito, C., Palumbo, G. J., & Arcadipane, A., … Maybauer, M. O. (2017). Incidence and Factors Associated with Burnout in Anesthesiology: A Systematic Review. *BioMed Research International*. doi:10.1155/2017/8648925

Toledo, P., Duce, L., Adams, J., Ross, V. H., Thompson, K. M., & Wong, C. A. (2017). Diversity in the American Society of Anesthesiologists Leadership. *Anesthesia and Analgesia, 124*(5), 1611–1616. doi:10.1213/ANE.0000000000001837 PMID:28277321

Wong, A. V.-K., & Olusanya, O. (2017). Burnout and resilience in anaesthesia and intensive care medicine. *BJA Education, 17*(10), 334–340. doi:10.1093/bjaed/mkx020

World Health Organization. (2018). European Health Report. Retrieved from http://www.euro.who.int/en/data-and-evidence/european-health-report/european-health-report-2018

KEY TERMS AND DEFINITIONS

Burnout: Syndrome comprised of three main components: depersonalization (cynicism and detachment), emotional exhaustion (loss of motivation and hope) and low personal accomplishment (feelings of ineffectiveness and helplessness).

Coping Mechanisms: Set of psychological skills an individual uses consciously to deal with personal, interpersonal or environmental problems in order to minimize and manage stress and conflict.

Diversity: Understanding and acceptance of each individual uniqueness and value; it implies acceptance, respect and recognition that every individual can provide value to a community or organization.

Equality: Assumption that rights, responsibilities and opportunities will not depend on a specific trait such as being male or female, or belonging to a specific race or social group.

Equity: Assumption that there will be fairness of treatment for everyone according to their respective needs.

Resilience: Mental processes and behaviours an individual uses to bounce back from a crisis or manage difficulty.

Second Generation Gender Bias: Practices that may appear neutral or non-sexist because they are applied to everyone, but which end up discriminating against women because they reflect the values of the men who created or developed the setting, usually a workplace. First-generation bias refers by contrast to a deliberate and intentional exclusion.

Winding Down Strategies: Set of strategies developed with the intention of gradually replacing more demanding or physical work by other type of work or work schedule, usually oriented to ageing professionals.

Workplace Connectivity: Work environment in which information and professionals are available constantly and with very little time delay through digital and mobile devices.

Chapter 13
Gender Equity Evaluated by Five Successful Women in the Medical Profession

Ana Jorge
Hospital Garcia de Orta, Portugal

Helena Alves
Instituto Nacional de Saúde Dr. Ricardo Jorge, Portugal

Fátima Carvalho
Centro Hospitalar do Porto, Portugal

Maria Amélia Ferreira
Faculty Medicine, University of Porto, Portugal

Maria-Ceu Machado
Faculty of Medicine, Lisbon University, Portugal

ABSTRACT

The authors (five women with successful experiences in different medical specialties, researchers, academics, Hospital Service Director, Presidents of Board of Health Institutions and National Agency, Minister of Health and Director of the Medical Faculty), make a reflection about gender equity in Portugal and the impact of 45 years of democracy. The medical profession in Portugal has a high rate of women, but this is not the same in leadership positions. The role of women in the medical profession needs to be re-evaluated, especially in top positions. This chapter is divided into four sub-chapters: "The role of organizations and professional associations to improve gender equality", "Gender equity in Academia: past, present and future", "Gender Equity in the Medical Profession as a Management Strategy", and "The role of gender to the networks in research and medical education", by Fátima Carvalho and Helena Alves, Maria do Céu Machado, Ana Jorge and Maria Amélia Ferreira.

DOI: 10.4018/978-1-5225-9599-1.ch013

THE ROLE OF ORGANIZATIONS AND PROFESSIONAL ASSOCIATIONS TO IMPROVE GENDER EQUALITY

The History of the involvement of medical women in political and associative movements tending to the installation of democracy in Portugal and the greater participation of women in public life, dates to the late 19th and early 20th centuries. In the end of the 19th century the progressive Portuguese periodicals *A Voz Feminina* and *O Progresso (The Feminine Voice* and *The Progress)* marked the beginning of the debate about the cause of women's rights in Portugal.

Female Doctors were leaders in the feminist movement organized in Portuguese associations since the beginning of the 20th century.

Portuguese feminism emerged in the struggle against the monarchy.

The end of the monarchy and the installation of the Portuguese Republic took place in 1905. A few years later emerged the Republican League of Portuguese Women (1909-1918), the Feminist Propaganda Association (1911-1918) and in 1914 was founded the National Council of Portuguese Women, founded by the physician Adelaide Cabete (1867-1935), that was the third Portuguese woman to be trained in Portugal (1909-1918). (Gomes A. (2004)).

Adelaide Cabete started her basic studies at age 22, after being married. She graduated at the Medical School in 1900 defending the thesis: *"Protection of poor pregnant women as a means of promoting the Physical Development [of new] generations"*.

Adelaide Cabete was not just a famous physician, but also a social activist, being in the origin of the foundation of the National Council of Women Portuguese (Conselho Nacional das Mulheres Portuguesas - CNMP) where she was reelected successively President up to the 30s (Lousada I, 2010).

Adelaide Cabete and Carolina Beatriz Ângelo (1878-1911) other female physician known to be the first woman to vote in Portugal and the first woman to practice surgery in Portugal, founded the Feminist Propaganda Association in Medicine (Associação Portuguesa de Propaganda Feminista) (1911-1918), (Janz &Schonpflug, 2014, Lousada I, 2010) less connected with political power, but very close to Freemasonry. All the leaders were Freemasons, in the independent feminine shop Humanity, with the exception of Maria O'Neill.

After the fight against monarchy, women faced the disappointment of the diminution of rights that the Republic recognized to women. Regrettably, the right to vote that was denied to them.

Carolina Beatriz Ângelo passed away young, at the age of 33 years. After a very active political and social intervention, her death was an important loss for the feminist cause.

In 1924 there were only one feminist association, the National Council of Portuguese Women, headed by Adelaide Cabete.

The Council of Portuguese Women was part of the International Council of Women, an international federation of the various national women's councils from many European countries and America. There was a common program at the basis of the different national Councils, mainly: improving the legal status of women in the family and in the State; women's right to vote; improvement of public health; creation of a consultation bureau for professions, education and protection of migrants, especially women and children.

In 1924, the Council included several feminists, from different social backgrounds, educational and welfare associations, such as a group of the Seamstresses "Tuna das Costureiras de Lisboa", the Boxes of Aid to Poor Female Students "Caixas de Auxílio aos Estudantes Pobres do Sexo Feminino", the Portuguese Feminist Group, the Association of Teachers of Free Teaching the Portuguese League of Educators. Health, Education and equal opportunities were central subjects.

In May 1924 was held the first National Women's Congress in Lisbon, at a time when similar events took place in Europe and the United States. Feminism was affirming itself as what it would today be called as the globalization movement in the Western world. The event was socially important, and it was solemnly inaugurated by Teixeira Gomes, the President of the Portuguese Republic.

At that Congress, Adelaide Cabete presented 2 conferences: "Protection of pregnant women and children" and "The role of the study of childcare, first-aid teaching, maternal pedagogy in domestic education".

Adelaide Cabete presented also one very advanced proposal for the time, claiming that working women should be entitled to one month of rest before the expected day to give birth (now obligatory in the holiday legislation in the Nordic countries) (Gomes A. (2004)).

Several other claims were made, as equal pay for equal work, legal equality in the couple and women's suffrage, that were integrated only in the legislation 50 years later, after the 25th April 1974.

As a historical moment in the paths of women, the Feminist and Education Congress, promoted by a female doctor, after 95 years of radical social change, is still a project to be concluded, even after 45 years of democracy.

The political revolution that occurred in Portugal on the 25th April 1974, gave rise to the new establishment of the Constitution of the Portuguese Republic in which equality of gender became a social right and it is stated in articles 12 and 14.

In the meantime, much has been spoken about gender equality with respect to its rights. Since men and women are biologically different and considering current scientific knowledge with insurmountable differences, probably this debate should be centered on equality of opportunities.

With the democratic regime installed in Portugal, discrimination in access to education was minimized; a touchstone of social evolution. Until then, women were many times deprived of continuing their education and participating in the so-called intellectual community.

Many of the active women doctors grew up in a time when gender identification did not limit access to education or professions and general progress in a professional career was based on individual capacity. Some women naturally occupied intermediate/top positions and they revealed that they were up to this challenge.

However, in professions in which the degree of schooling is less, the differences in opportunities and social status between men and women is still excessively dissimilar and this translates into different salaries for same functions.

Even in Portugal where many steps were taken towards the right direction in gender equality, mitigating discrepancy, the truth is that this is still a reality. It is perhaps in these groups that professional associations and unions have room to fight for this equality of rights and opportunities.

Portugal has seen a rapid increase in the number of women in the medical profession.

In truth, currently, the majority of medical students are women, and this difference has grown from year to year.

There is still a differential in academia and in the number of doctorates in favour of men but it is becoming attenuated in the last years.

In healthcare institutions, at both hospital and primary care level, women are starting to enter in a higher number. Consequently, this reality has reflected in accepting intermediate management positions (department heads) and sometimes top positions (clinical directors and chairperson of board of directors). In healthcare, salaries depend solely on professional category and management positions.

Since 1975, that is, during the democratic regime, Portugal has had 14 male and 5 female Health Ministers, but just one, Ana Jorge, was a female doctor.

Also, in the post of President of the Portuguese Medical Association, no woman was ever appointed.

This asymmetry may be due to various factors that depend on the past and the historical tradition of these political positions being mainly occupied by men, but also by the smaller number of women that dedicate themselves to politics, even nowadays, because of familiar duties.

The mandatory dues of the political parties have brought more women to the limelight.

Participation in politics must be achieved by free will and personal effort from individuals of either gender.

The Medical Association as a public professional association has increased responsibilities in this matter. Making its members aware of the importance of political participation is a way to motivate and alert them to the importance of being a socially active voice. In the same manner it has taken on the role of battling social differences in access to healthcare, it has also the duty to safeguard equality of opportunities in both the internal structure of the Medical Association and promoting the same equality in medical society.

There is still a way to go. A path that includes more and better information. The democratization of knowledge is essential for equality of opportunities.

Medical associations can contribute:

- Organizing and participating in internal debates at a regional and national level that approach the multiple dimensions involving gender equality and proposing internal and external recommendations in the defense of the justice of opportunities. To have a policy placing equal opportunities in all areas of the Medical Association from education to training passing through humanization and communication integrating and highlighting human rights.
- In the same manner, promoting the importance of equality of opportunities for the evolution of medicine and civil society, will be essential as a trademark of the Medical Association.
- To think out and develop a national campaign under the tutelage of the Medical Association that emphasizes the virtues of equality of opportunities may be one way, together with the community, that may give rise to a fairer, more plural and fearless society.

GENDER EQUITY IN ACADEMIA: PAST, PRESENT AND FUTURE

My grandfather was a medical doctor, graduated in 1916, in Coimbra Medical School. Every year he and his colleagues (20 male doctors and one female doctor) met for lunch and he used to comment: "she didn't get married. Nobody wants to marry a lady who is a doctor" (Author's note).

In 1960, Portugal was an undeveloped country with a weak economy and half of the population was illiterate. Considering all fields of study, less than 1% of students were attending the university and scarcely 0,4% were female. (Mariana G. Alves et al.)

During the 70' and 80' decades, better social and economic conditions were decisive for European development and for the education of the Portuguese population. Mandatory schooling directed much more young people to the universities. In 2011, college students increased to 14,9% and up until 16,9% of them were female student, in all universities.

And what is the current scenario in medical schools? There is a phenomenon of student's feminization all around the world. And in Portugal during the last decades? And did this feminization result on more women entering on PhD programs and with more leadership positions in academia as university professors?

Believe it or not, women did play a significant role in medicine in Europe from the 13th to the 17th centuries. They were allowed in medicine, but often as singular anomalies or aberrations of nature (Miller CA.):

[...] allowed membership of guilds of surgeons, to practice blood-letting or amputations as widows if this had been their husband's craft [...] [France, 13th to 17th centuries].

[...] the Apothecary Guild regulation did not explicitly exclude women [...] but rules were immediately changed after the first female application [England, 18th century].

[...] later, approved the application to a medical school but not to residency or training; allowance to provide care on other women, children or poor people [England, 19th century].

[...] the first woman physician was Elizabeth Blackwell, a British with American and French diplomas. The British Medical Association immediately ruled out that holders of foreign degrees could not be allowed to practice medicine [London, 1859].

[...] a single woman could not attend classes [...] Sophie Jax-Blake organized a group of seven women [...] their male classmates placed a sheep in the anatomy room explaining that now «inferior animals» were no longer to be excluded from the classroom [Edinburg, 1869].

[...] The faculty of medicine opened classes for 90 women with so extreme conditions that only 25 graduated. Twelve died, two from suicide and seven from drugs consumption [Russia, 1872].

In the 60s, 90% of the candidates were male and the American doctor profile was a white man, protestant, medium-high class and a doctor' son. The gender balance was achieved on the 80's in many European countries (Kvaerner KJ et al; McManus IC) as in Portugal (1983) but in American and Canadian universities (Beagan BL), only in 2001, half of the medical students were women.

As astonishing as it can be, papers/editorials with titles such as *Women want opportunity in macho medical world* (BMA, *News Review,* 1994) or *Women in medicine: still a long way to go, baby* (*Tennessee Medicine,* 1999), could yet be found in medical journals.

Along the 21th century, medicine is fast becoming a women's domain. In Portugal, women account for 64,8% of all medical students, however in the largest Portuguese Medical School (Faculdade de Medicina de Lisboa) the feminization has diminished from 56,8 (1990) to 53,8% (2018). (Lisbon Medical School)

The Portuguese Medical Association has 30664 (54,4%) women out of the 56 364 medical doctors registered in all specialities but surgical ones remain male fields (Portuguese Medical Association).

The increasing admission of female students in medical schools all over the world can be the result of facilitating/promoting policies in schools and global policies from governments but it really does not seem so.

Probably, medicine is a less attractive career for men who are opting for finance and technology fields instead, professions with more visibility and autonomy and better salary opportunities which are found on the enterprise market. The female boom would be a kind of *ex vacuo occupation!*

Jorge Gaspar advocates the theory of mobility. Along the history, in great male moves as wars or the actual globalization, women take care of properties and local power. Once more, a negative misappropriation?

Another theory is that teaching models and the submission exams to universities are the most determinant factors of this recent unbalance, promoting feminization. Actually, primary and secondary school teaching has been a feminine area since long time ago, with 90% of female teachers. This could be a source of gender consequences on the way of learning, judgement and to get good assessment marks (Maria Ceu Machado, 2003).

Although the proportion of women in science, and in medicine in particular, has substantially increased over the last century, women remain underrepresented in academia, especially in higher ranks and decision-making bodies while men are still more likely to be promoted to full professorships (Bates C et al.2016).

The cohort effect should lead to highest representation in female leadership but the success in faculty can be a positive factor to be a doctor, but it does not reflect the probability of a tenure or a leader position.

The Association of American Medical Colleges (AAMC) stated that in 2014 women are only 21% of full professors and 15% of department chairs. (AAMC)

In Portugal, recent data (2017) from the Ministry of Education shows 58,7% women with a university diploma (within medical school graduates) but among those whom entered PhD programs, only 44,1% finished their doctoral thesis, 42% became professors in universities and figures fall dramatically with just 22,6% as full professors (DGEEC).

In the Lisbon Medical School, there is a gender balance on PhDs programs and on associate professors, but only 30% of women are full professor and less than 20% are discipline's chairs.

However, despite the gender equality policies implemented in academia and society, the chances of women achieving professorships have hardly improved over the past 20 years (Danell Rr, 2013)

Actually, after making their dream come true, to become a medical doctor, women face barriers to climb the career ladder, with less social and professional role models and less opportunities and struggling to conciliate family and work.

The barriers start with the pursuit of a research program or career and a higher academic degree. There is evidence of lack of research funding and opportunity to publish and of promotions have slower and lower rates as talent and benefits are less recognized. Women face considerable barriers in accessing mentors and sponsorship seen as the action of key leaders to advocate for opportunities (to sponsor emerging women leaders) are more difficult to pursue (Bates C et al.2016).

Gender bias in academia affects female scientists, resulting in their underrepresentation in academic institutions, particularly in higher ranks (Cislak A et al., 2018). They are also less praised for their work and success, what McManus calls *Salieri effect.*

Even though the fact that when looking at the conference halls or the departmental staff of many universities, at least half of them are women, the average proportion of invitations addressed to women is significantly lower than the current baseline (32% women). Few women are in editorial boards and, it is ten times more common for female authors to be incorrectly cited as males than for male researchers to be misattributed as female (Krawczyk M, 2017). Some authors propose to hide the name when female on the submission process!

Articles on gender discrimination are less often funded or published in prestigious journals than papers about racial discrimination. So, what are the possible causes of this effect?

External and internal forces have yet to be identified to explain this trend. The threats (external forces) are real barriers to a career degree and leadership but the weaknesses (internal forces) are inherent to feminine/masculine particular features.

The first ones are the lack of role models, mentorship and inadequate mentoring, no knowledge of promotion criteria, active discrimination, more time consuming on care than research, less papers published and different access to funding. Some of these are linked or due to family responsibilities (Reed V et al., 2001).

A study run in Canada, concluded that more men are married and have more children, with similar amount of weekly professional work (58 vs 52 hours), but women spend 2,5 more time with the husband, children and home work (36 *versus* 14 hours; $p < 0{,}01$). Professional joy is also similar but when comparing personal and professional life, it is much lower in women (Cujec B et al., 2000).

Maternal and paternal concepts are still mistaken with feminine and masculine ones. Feminine and masculine are identities, maternal and paternal are functions, parenting tasks and responsibilities. Male identity is acknowledged as aggressive, obstinate, powerful and self-sufficient but there are no adjectives to define a father.

Concerning internal forces, the intrinsic motivation, the need of success and peer recognition are equally important (Burkley) but for male doctors, visibility, academic degrees and leadership are much more valued.

For women, less ambitious, caring their patients and having tutors and local colleagues respect and recognition are enough to feel fulfilled, but men wish a national or even international appreciation. (Buckley L et al., 2000)

In the early 90s, the feminine population felt that they want the same opportunities and jobs, but this scenario is no longer important (Nonnemaker L, 2000), maybe because it is not necessary for women anymore, to prove that they have the same qualities and abilities.

Under the title «Women physicians in academic medicine», Nancy Lawless, Leslie Safer, Julia Gates, Lynn Nonnemaker e Catherine De Angelis exchanged aggressive letters with the editor of the *New England Journal of Medicine* (June 2000), rejecting specific strategies for career progression for women. Opportunities must be equals but the promotion should respect qualifications.

It is not so simple. Publishing in high impact medical journals as grants and awards are of the most important items as progression factors, and female multitasking generates less focus and less papers.

In summary, nowadays, there is a better balance and control of internal and external factors including stereotypes, and success is more often attributed to skills and less related to gender. Medicine practice requires intelligence, human qualities and continuous work and learning for men and women.

However, in a perspective of family and professional competition, women still choose the family and postpone power and influence. They are more resilient to frustration, they are more aware of family frailty and they project their career as they consider that it will be attainable. Let women choose their options!

Therefore, in Portugal as everywhere else, it looks like an anonymous inscription found in a tale in a Saturday Cambridge market is quite adequate:

To be a chief, a woman has to:

Think like a man
Work like a horse
Behave like a lady
And take care of herself like a teen.

GENDER EQUITY IN THE MEDICAL PROFESSION AS A MANAGEMENT STRATEGY

The presence of women in Portuguese medicine does not differ much from their past or current presence around the world. When Portuguese history is reviewed, the author finds reference to four women in medicine from the late nineteenth century, who distinguished themselves not only as doctors but also by their role in society, for which they deserve a special note. Domitília de Carvalho (1871-1966), the first woman to attend the University of Coimbra obtained three degrees in philosophy, mathematics and medicine. She worked in a Tuberculosis Care unit, and she was also a teacher at a high school that stood out the most; Carolina Beatriz Ângelo (1878-191), a medical doctor and Republican, fought for women's rights, and was the first woman in Portugal to vote in legislative elections. A Gynaecologist by training, she stood out during the movement of implementation of the Republic in Portugal; Adelaide Cabete (1867-1935), began her school education very late, after her marriage, to help support her husband. As an obstetric physician she intervened in favour of the protection of maternity and support to woman. She wrote several papers on the subject and promoted the construction of a maternity, which was decisive in the creation of the Maternity Alfredo da Costa in Lisbon in 1932. Also, part of the group of women with an active role in the implantation of the Republic was Sofia Quintino (1878-1964), the first woman to serve as director of physical therapy services at the Civil Hospitals of Lisbon. She was also an activist for women's (Wikipedia)

These women, with the exception of Domitília de Carvalho, were publicly recognized for their women's rights defence work as with feminist with republican ideals, all with great civic sense of responsibility.

Throughout the twentieth century the number of women with degrees in medicine rose, but it was not until the arrival of democracy in Portugal that women became increasingly represented in medical schools.

The Portuguese Health system has become increasingly feminized in all health areas, and by 2017 women represented 76.3% of national health workforce, with the highest percentage in the nursing sector. In 2017, doctors account for 21.7% of all professionals and of these, female doctors constituted 62.3% (ACSS, 2017) (Pordata, 2018) .

Another interesting aspect is the average age of the medical specialists in the national health system, not counting doctors in training. The average age is 50, however 53.6% of medical specialists are over the age of 50. When we look at the evolution of the distribution of women and men over the years, we observe a greater percentage of men in the groups over 60 years, in agreement with the changes in female access to medical school starting in the mid - 1970s (ACSS, 2017).

In another health ministry report (2005-2007) the feminization rate of professionals in general ranges between 74.2 and 74.7%. However, it is pointed out that in the same period the rate of feminization of the managerial staff is between 49.4 and 47.3%. These figures relate to the overall managerial staff and the report does not give more details about the professionals or institutions to which the data refer, but this difference also exists in the medical profession (ACSS web site).

Since the medical profession in Portugal has such a high rate of women, it would be expected that, in a similar proportion, leadership positions would also be occupied by women, but the numbers do not point to that.

If there is no incentive for women to take leadership positions, we may reach a managerial shortage given the disproportionate distribution between women and men in the medical profession (Santana, P, 2013).

Access to medical training is now free and there are more women than men completing medical school.

In Portugal, in parallel to what happens in other European countries, the completion of the medical degree poses some challenges. The choice of a specialty is free but subject to ranking in national competitions and vacancies assigned by the Ministry of Health. The choice of specialties is not homogeneous between women and men, with asymmetries in the surgical specialty options where men are predominant, such as urology or orthopedics. A study carried out in 2013, "Study of the Prospective Evolution of Physicians in the National Health System", referring to years 2002-2011, reports that of the 47 existing medical specialties, in 33 of them (58%), the number of women is over 50%; the specialties in which the difference between women and men is greater are Legal Medicine, Childhood and Adolescence Psychiatry, Immuno-hemotherapy and Radiotherapy. The specialties in which the gap between genders is higher with a higher percentage of men are Urology, Sports Medicine, Clinical Pharmacology and Orthopedics (Santana, P, 2013).

Some specialties are very time consuming not only during the training but also during practice, conditioning the option.

Portugal has legislation to support maternity, placing it among the most protective countries. It supports maternity leave up to 4 months, or longer, but with reduction of maternity. This important legislation gives the mother the opportunity to spend more time with the baby, which is so decisive in the development and growth of the child and the future of healthier adults. In a country that needs birth support measures, it is important to manage these absences so that services can be kept efficient without jeopardizing the rights of children and women. The feminization of the health professions, in medicine poses problems in the management of the services in which they work (Rego, 2012).

Women often complete their medical studies later in life, if they choose to have children. The maternity leave of at least 4 months must be compensated; which is on average a year of extension for each child born during medical training. Despite this delay in obtaining the title of specialist, this has not been a difficulty in career progression, other than obtaining the title.

The Portuguese society, despite having made a huge progress promoting equality of rights and responsibilities between men and women, still relays mostly on women for many of the activities related to family, children, and support to parents.

Portuguese society is still deeply rooted in gender-based division of labour, where women may face unique challenges, and where the right balance between work and life is not always easily found by women.

Female availability for career progression and to assume leadership and management roles requires making difficult choices, unless they have extra nuclear family support (Rego, 2012).

Women often refuse the challenge placed on them to take up leadership positions.

Today, among younger couples, the sharing of tasks, traditionally attributed to women, is more common and legislation to support parenting has strengthened. But assistance to young children is still often assumed by mothers, which can lead to frequent absences from work, conditioning task performance, and there may be penalties in some organizations (Arrizabalaga, P, et al., 2014).

Society as well as health institutions do not have structural support for families who work and intend to have children, such as nursery and schools with flexible schedules and adapted to the needs of the parents' professional life.

Hospitals and other workplaces should be organized to provide and promote accessible, flexible childcare services for working parents, recognizing the need for a better work-life balance.

A diverse and motivated workforce is beneficial to the health system and to patients.

As of now, the workplace schedule is not organized to be compatible with satisfactory family and social life. It is known that every individual is a better professional when private life and work are balanced.

The medical profession, by excellence, needs people who are attentive and available to listen to others, and a greater empathy it is important in a doctor.

The schedules of traditional practice are not compatible with a life with small children if there is no extra nuclear family support. The practice of medicine is not isolated from the rest of society and measures that promote gender equity in general have repercussions on the facilitation of resource management.

In a profession where the percentage of women is increasing, the changes that the society undergoes towards gender equity will certainly facilitate the lives of women doctors.

THE ROLE OF GENDER TO THE NETWORKS IN RESEARCH AND MEDICAL EDUCATION

Participation of women in networks of medical research, practice of medicine and medical education in different domains of medicine is being increased in the last decades in Portugal, aligned with similar evolution identified worldwide (Bickel et al., 2002; Cardoso, Carvalho, & Videira, 2018; Greenhill et al. 2015; Noronha, & Ferreira, 2016; OECD, 2017; United Nations, 2002).

A couple of years before "The April Revolution", which occurred in 1974, female students were already well represented as medical students, namely in undergraduate medical education. The scenario of change in social values after the revolution period, allowed the increase of the intervention of women in the academic life, their integration in research groups and in the teams of clinical practitioners, providing the enrichment of the few research groups and research networks that were starting growing research programs in Portugal.

The emerging created opportunities in the global scientific networks for development of scientific research programs and the increased funding for medical research from different public and private agencies, has promoted the involvement of women in these activities. A set of well recognized women in Portuguese Science can be identified now (Noronha, & Ferreira, 2016), with a significant presence of members in Health Sciences.

Nowadays, in Portugal, we have good examples of women who lead important research institutions as are examples the Instituto Gulbenkian da Ciência, Instituto de Medicina Molecular João Lobo Antunes of the Universidade de Lisboa and the Direction of PORDATA. However, it is known that women still often do not accept the challenge to take up leadership positions, due to several social factors that make this difficult choice (Borges, Navarro & Grover, 2012; Carr, et al., 2018; Edmunds et al., 2016).

This alignment is similar for medical practice where, although the number of female medical students and residents surpass that of men, they are not still – as well – reaching significant relevance in leadership positions, due to a variety of social factors reducing their potential of reaching high faculty positions or achieving tenure, as examples. However, in both fields – research and medical education – number of women in leadership positions is still scarce (Bickel et al., 2015; Bismark et al., 2015), despite a rapid increase in the proportion of women in the medical profession demonstrated in research studies, focusing gender differences in indicators as career duration, number of publications and research funding (Diamond, et. al., 2016; Holliday, Jagsi, Wilson, & Choi, 2014).

The work published by Elsevier (2017) - Gender in the Global Research Landscape - provides a detailed analysis of research indicators through a gender perspective "along 20 years, 12 countries (Portugal included), and 27 subject areas". The results of the work show an increasing proportion of women researchers *vs* men researchers in the field of Health and Life Sciences. This shows that some progress has been made towards gender equity in research based that, in Portugal, women constitute 49% of the researcher population. This represents an improvement as compared with the period 1996–2000 when only Portugal had about 40% women involved in scientsific research (41%). The effort made by the Portuguese institutions in order to promote the equality of women has been recognized by the United Nations (2002). New data show that between 2004-2016 the percentage of women with PhD increased from 48,2% to 55% (PORDATA, 2018) and medical professionals in Portugal in 2017 also showed a higher number of women (28.413 women *vs* 23.524 men) (PORDATA, 2018).

Very recently, the Portuguese situation in the academic world has been analysed in the general areas of women perceptions about academic representation, social recognition and employment conditions. It is interesting to observe that despite evidencing the deterioration and lack of insurance in employment, academics maintain a positive view regarding the academic profession, at least to some extent (Cardoso, Carvalho, & Videira, 2018). This constitutes an opportunity to trigger a necessary change both for the research activity and also for involvement of women in medical education, when a very close future is taken into consideration.

Medical Education: Research and Educational Involvement of Women

Gender equity and equality have been focused in different reports, where education and professions are of paramount importance (OECD, 2017). Medical Profession, Medical Education and Research in Medicine, are important issues within the global agenda of gender equity. The Portuguese situation was presented in a detailed quantitative work that provides national data concerning different indicators related to demography, health, education, science, and work (Santos, Amâncio, & Roux, 2015; Comissão para a Cidadania e Igualdade de Género. Presidência do Conselho de Ministros. Igualdade de Género em Portugal. Boletim Estatístico, 2017)

The international literature also focuses on indicators that are aligned with the Portuguese situation. As an example, the under-representation in academic surgery, conducting towards a poor representation of women in surgical leadership (Carpenter et. al., 2018; Webster, et.al. 2016; Weiss et al. 2014), emergency (Choo et al., 2016), Pediatrics (Rotbart, et al., 2012) dermatology (Shah, 2018) are just few examples. As well, gender differences in publication productivity were also identified in academic faculty (Diamond et al. 2016). There is also a differential time for tenure in leadership positions in academic medicine, as compared with males, due to institutional and personal conditions (White, McDade, Yamagata, & Morahan, 2012).

Although in the last decades, analyses from different metrics demonstrated that women have made great achievements in reducing the gender gap, female scientists continue to face major challenges namely due to differential salaries income, to disparities in access to funding opportunities as demonstrated in published work (AAMC, 2014; Shen, 2013) and their unquestionable roles in family, and effective existence of inequalities (Shen, 2013).

As far as Medical Education and role of women involvement, this relates with personality traits that make a differential approach in a profession where caring is at the very basis. Furthermore, adaptation to the rapid societal and professional paradigms is better accomplished by women, where they play relevant roles in training, informing and educating.

This leads to the situation that women often choose academic medicine not as an active decision but due to influence by the professional environment and compatibility with family life (Borges, Navarro & Grover, 2012; Edmund et al., 2016), which leads to disparities in their representation in some academic specialties, as previously reported.

However, women bring new perspectives to science, not only as researchers but also as subjects of research. They also bring new perspectives to Medical Education (Thibault, 2016) through the differential role of female personality and the caring condition of the gender (Carpenter et al. 2018).

Proposals to Improve Gender Equity in Research and Medical Education

Based on the state-of-the art of this issue, it is possible to identify and advance several social and institutional guidelines that can overcome the societal disparities in gender equity related to research and medical education, where Portuguese women are obviously included.

- To listen to women researchers and medical professionals, understand their experiences, consider their concerns and celebrate their successes;
- To increase the number of women in the national and international networks of research and medical education;
- To focus on special personal characteristics of females as leaders: authenticity, persistence, honesty and generosity, among others;
- To improve women interventions to address the needs of other women physicians and medical students and to help their progress to leadership positions and "climb the ladder" (Bickel et. al., 2002; Downs, Reif., Hokororo, & Fitzgerald, 2014; Moharan, et al., 2011);
- To implement strategies for overcoming conflicts between traditional gender roles and involvement in higher positions in academic medicine, by identification of barriers and establishing a strategy of intervention (Yedidia and Bickel, 2001);
- To attenuate tensions between career and family responsibilities (Downs et al., 2014), promoting institutional changes to support female faculty;
- To support active involvement in the process of authorship roles instead of remaining with contributorship roles (Macaluso, Lariviere, Sugimoto, & Sugimoto, 2016);
- To try to overcome gender differences in salaries (Willett et al., 2015);
- To implement projects like MedGoFem (Hasebrook Et. al., 2017), keeping the goal to facilitate implementations of gender equity processes in medical school for women if research and academic profession and promote more active role in research and places in academic medicine;
- To develop practice recommendations to support hiring, recruitment and advancement of women physicians (Choo et al., 2016), increasing the number of women in academic programs of research and medical education;
- To try to close the gender equity gap in our lifetime by bringing men into the gender equity conversation and breaking out the "Man Box".

CONCLUSION

The data existing in the role and involvement of women in research and medical education allow to conclude that national and international strategies will need to be reinforced by effective interventions in culture and organizational scenarios before women and men are equally valued for their contributions in networks of research and medical profession, including medical education (McKimm, da Silva, Edwards, Greenhill, & Taylor, 2015; Valentine & Sandborg, 2013).

Medical practice and science are far from evaluating their investment in women, where the humanistic and personalized roles of most women continue to be wasted.

REFERENCES

AAMC (2014). The State of Women in Academic Medicine: The Pipeline and Pathways to Leadership.

Abrantes, A., & Simões,, J. (2017). Thinking Ahead: Portugal's Health in 2027. Port. *J Public Health, 35*, 141–144. doi:10.1159/000488336

ACSS. (2017). *Relatório Social do Ministério da Saúde e do Serviço Nacional de Saúde.* Retrieved from http://www.acss.min-saude.pt

ACSS. (2005-2007). Relatório Social do Ministério da Saúde e do Serviço Nacional de Saúde, 2005-2007. Retrieved from http://www.acss.min-saude.pt

Arrizabalaga, P., Abellana, R., Vinas, O., Merino, A., & Ascaso, C. (2014). Gender inequalities in the medical profession: Are there still barriers to women physicians in the 21st century? *Gaceta Sanitaria, 28*(5), 363–368. doi:10.1016/j.gaceta.2014.03.014 PMID:24889702

Association of American Medical Colleges, Annual Report 2014.

Author's note (Machado MC): Many years later, he was my role model to enter the medical school and he was the most supportive within my family

Bates, C., Gordon, L., Travis, E., Chatterjee, A., Chaudron, L., Fivush, B., ... Moses, A. (2016). Striving for gender equity in academic medicine careers: A call for action. *Academic Medicine, 91*(8), 1050–1052. doi:10.1097/ACM.0000000000001283 PMID:27332868

Beagan, B. L. (2000). Neutralizing differences: Producing neutral doctors for (almost) neutral patients. *Social Science & Medicine, 51*(8), 1253–1265. doi:10.1016/S0277-9536(00)00043-5 PMID:11037215

Bickel, J., Wara, D., Atkinson, B., Cohen, L., Dunn, M., Hostler, S., & Stokes, E. (2002). Increasing Women's Leadership in Academic Medicine: Report of the AAMC Project Implementation Committee. *Academic Medicine, 77*(10), 1043–1061. doi:10.1097/00001888-200210000-00023 PMID:12377686

Bismark, M., Morris, J., Thomas, L., Loh, E., Phelps, G., & Dickinson, H. (2015). Reasons And Remedies For Under-Representation Of Women In Medical Leadership Roles: A Qualitative Study From Australia. *BMJ Open, 5*(11). doi:10.1136/bmjopen-2015-009384 PMID:26576814

Borges, N., Navarro, A., & Grover, A. (2012). Women Physicians: Choosing a Career in Academic Medicine. *Academic Medicine*, *87*(1), 105–114. doi:10.1097/ACM.0b013e31823ab4a8 PMID:22104052

Buckley, L., Sanders, K., & Hampton, C. (2000). Obstacles to promotion? Values of women faculty about career success and recognition. *Academic Medicine*, *75*(3), 283–288. doi:10.1097/00001888-200003000-00021 PMID:10724319

Cardoso, S., Carvalho, T., & Videira, P. (2018). Is It Still Worth Working In Academia? The Views from Portuguese Academics. *Higher Education Policy*. doi:10.105741307-018-0123-7

Carpenter, A. M., Tan, S. A., Costopoulos, K., Cooper, L. A., Sarosi, G. A., & Shaw, C. M. (2018). Gender Diversity in General Surgery Residency Leadership. *Journal of Surgical Education*, *75*(6), e68–e71. doi:10.1016/j.jsurg.2018.07.021 PMID:30177356

Carr, P., Raj, A., Kaplan, S., Md, M. P. H., Terrin, N., Breeze, J., ... Md, M. P. H. (2018). Gender Differences in Academic Medicine: Retention, Rank, and Leadership Comparisons from the National Faculty Survey. *Academic Medicine*, *93*(11), 1694–1699. doi:10.1097/ACM.0000000000002146 PMID:29384751

Ceu Machado, M. (2003). A feminização da Medicina. *Analise Social*, *166*, 127–7.

Choo, E. K., Kass, D., Westergaard, M., Watts, S. H., Berwald, N., Regan, L., ... Nobay, F. (2016). The Development of Best Practice Recommendations to Support the Hiring, Recruitment, and Advancement of Women Physicians in Emergency Medicine. *Academic Emergency Medicine*, *23*(11), 1203–1209. doi:10.1111/acem.13028 PMID:27286760

Cislak, A., Formanowicz, M., & Saguy, T. (2018). Bias against research on gender bias. *Scientometrics*, *115*(1), 189–200. doi:10.100711192-018-2667-0 PMID:29527071

Comissão para a Cidadania e Igualdade de Género. Presidência do Conselho de Ministros. *Igualdade de Género em Portugal*. Boletim Estatístico, 2017

Cujec, B., Oancia, T., Bohm, C., & Johnson, D. (2000). Career and parenting satisfaction among medical students, residents and physician teachers at a Canadian medical school. *Canadian Medical Association Journal*, *162*(5), 637–640. PMID:10738448

Danell, R., & Hjerm, M. (2013). Career prospects for female university researchers have not improved. *Scientometrics*, *94*(3), 999–1006. doi:10.100711192-012-0840-4

Diamond, S., Thomas, C. Jr, Desai, S., Holliday, E., Jagsi, R., Schmitt, C., & Enestvedt, B. K. (2016). Gender Differences in Publication Productivity, Academic Rank, and Career Duration Among U.S. Academic Gastroenterology Faculty. *Academic Medicine*, *91*(8), 1158–1163. doi:10.1097/ACM.0000000000001219 PMID:27144993

Downs, J., Reif, L., Hokororo, A., & Fitzgerald, D. (2014). Increasing Women in Leadership in Global Health. *Academic Medicine*, *89*(8), 1103–1107. doi:10.1097/ACM.0000000000000369 PMID:24918761

Edmunds, L., Ovseiko, P., Shepperd, S., Greenhalgh, T., Frith, P., Roberts, N., & Buchan, A. M. (2016). Why do Women Choose or Reject Careers in Academic Medicine? A Narrative Review of Empirical Evidence. *Lancet*, *388*(10062), 2948–2958. doi:10.1016/S0140-6736(15)01091-0 PMID:27105721

Elsevier. (2017). *Gender in the Global Research Landscape.* Available at Elsevier.com/ research-intelligence/resource-library/gender-report

Estatísticas - Direção-Geral de Estatísticas da Educação e Ciência. Retrieved from www.dgeec.mec.pt/np4/estatisticas

Faculdade de Medicina de Lisboa (Lisbon Medical School) – Relatório. (2017). Retrieved from www.medicina.ulisboa.pt/wp-content

Gaio Alves, M. & Lopes, P. (2012). Ensino Superior em Portugal: retrato sociográfico. Gabinete de Estudos da SNESUP, Dezembro 2012. Retrieved from www.snesup.pt/htmls/_dlds/relatorio-retrato-sociografico-af.pdf

Gomes, A. (2004). (in press). O primeiro congresso feminista em Portugal realizou-se há 80 anos. O Público 4 May 2004. Retrieved from https://www.publico.pt/2004/05/04/sociedade/noticia/

Greenhill, J., McKimm, J., Da Silva, A. S., Taylor, C., & Edwards, S. (2015). Women and Leadership in Medicine and Medical Education: International Perspectives. In Gender, Careers and Inequalities in Medicine and Medical Education: International Perspectives (pp. 69-98).

Hasebrook, J., Hahnenkamp, K., Buhre, W., de Korte-de Boer, D., Hamaekers, A., Metelmann, B., & Pfleiderer, B. (2017). Medicine Goes Female: Protocol for Improving Career Options of Females and Working Conditions for Researching Physicians in Clinical Medical Research by Organizational Transformation and Participatory Design. *JMIR Research Protocols, 6*(8), e152. doi:10.2196/resprot.7632 PMID:28768613

Helitzer, D., Newbill, S., Morahan, P., Magrane, D., Cardinali, G., Wu, C.-C., & Chang, S. (2014). Perceptions of Skill Development of Participants in Three National Career Development Programs for Women Faculty in Academic Medicine. *Academic Medicine, 89*(6), 896–903. doi:10.1097/ACM.0000000000000251 PMID:24871241

Holliday, E., Jagsi, R., Wilson, L. D., Choi, M., Thomas, C. R. Jr, & Fuller, C. D. (2014). Gender Differences in Publication Productivity, Academic Position, Career Duration, and Funding Among U.S. Academic Radiation Oncology Faculty. *Academic Medicine, 89*(5), 767–773. doi:10.1097/ACM.0000000000000229 PMID:24667510

Isabel, L. (2010). *Adelaide Cabete (1867 - 1935). Comissão para a Cidadania e a Igualdade de Género.* Lisbon, Portugal: Presidência do Conselho de Ministros.

Janz, O. & Schonpflug, D. (Eds.). (2014). Gender History in a Transnational Perspective: Networks, Biographies, Gender Orders, (pp. 53, 61–62). New York, NY: Berghahn Books. doi:10.2307/j.ctt9qcxnt

Krawczyk, M. (2017). Are all researchers male? Gender misattributions in citations. *Scientometrics, 110*(3), 1397–1402. doi:10.100711192-016-2192-y PMID:28255187

Kvaerner, K. J., Aasland, O. G., & Botten, G. S. (1999). Female medical leadership: Cross sectional study. *BMJ (Clinical Research Ed.), 318*(7176), 91–94. doi:10.1136/bmj.318.7176.91 PMID:9880281

Macaluso, B., Lariviere, V., Sugimoto, T., & Sugimoto, C. (2016). Is Science Built on the Shoulders of Women? A Study of Gender Differences in Contributorship. *Academic Medicine*, *91*(8), 1136–1142. doi:10.1097/ACM.0000000000001261 PMID:27276004

McKimm, J., Da Silva, A. S., Edwards, S., Greenhill, S., & Taylor, C. (2015), Women and Leadership in Medicine and Medical Education: International Perspectives. In Maria Tsouroufli (Ed.), Gender, Careers and Inequalities in Medicine and Medical Education: International Perspectives (International Perspectives on Equality, Diversity and Inclusion, Volume 2). Emerald Group. doi:10.1108/S2051-233320150000002005

McManus, I. C., & Sproston, K. A. (2000). Women in hospital medicine in the United Kingdom: Glass ceiling, preference, prejudice or cohort effect? *Journal of Epidemiology and Community Health*, *54*(1), 10–16. doi:10.1136/jech.54.1.10 PMID:10692956

Miller, C. A. (1994). What's a woman doing in a place like this? *Surgical Neurology*, *42*, 171–176. doi:10.1016/0090-3019(94)90383-2 PMID:8091297

Morahan, P., Rosen, S., Richman, R., & Gleason, K. (2011). The Leadership Continuum: A Framework for Organizational and Individual Assessment Relative to the Advancement of Women Physicians and Scientists. *Journal of Women's Health*, *20*(3), 387–396. doi:10.1089/jwh.2010.2055 PMID:21351872

Nonnemaker, L. (2000). Women physicians in academic medicine: New insights from cohort studies. *The New England Journal of Medicine*, *342*(6), 399–405. doi:10.1056/NEJM200002103420606 PMID:10666431

Noronha, A. (Coord.),& Ferreira, A. P. (Fotogr.) (2016). Mulheres na Ciência. Lisboa: Ciência Viva.

OECD. (2017). *The Pursuit of Gender Equality: An Uphill Battle*. Paris, France: OECD. doi:10.1787/9789264281318-

Pordata. (2018). Retrieved from https://www.pordata.pt/Portugal

PORDATA, INE. Last update: Aug. 8, 2018.

Portuguese Medical Association. (2019, January)

Reed, V., & Budderberg-Fischer, B. (2001). Career obstacles for women in medicine: An overview. *Medical Education*, *35*(2), 139–147. doi:10.1046/j.1365-2923.2001.00837.x PMID:11169087

Rego, M. do Céu da Cunha. (2012). *Gender equality policies in the European Union and in Portugal: Influences and inconsistencies.* Ex aequo [online]. 2012, n. 25, pp. 29-44.

Rotbart, H., McMillen, D., Taussig, H., Daniels, S., & Md, P. (2012). Assessing Gender Equity in a Large Academic Department of Pediatrics. *Academic Medicine*, *87*(1), 98–104. doi:10.1097/ACM.0b013e31823be028 PMID:22104061

Santana, P. (2013). *Estudo da evolução prospetiva de Médicos no Sistema Nacional de Saúde*. Universidade de Coimbra.

Santos, M., Amâncio, L., & Roux, P. (2015). Numbers do not tell the whole story: Gender and medicine in Portugal. *Women's Studies International Forum*, *53*, 73–82. doi:10.1016/j.wsif.2015.08.005

Shah, A., Jalal, S., & Khosa, F. (2018). Influences for Gender Disparity in Dermatology in North America. *International Journal of Dermatology*, *57*(2), 171–176. doi:10.1111/ijd.13875 PMID:29330932

Shen, H. (2013). Inequality Quantified: Mind the Gender Gap. *Nature*, *495*(7439), 22–24. doi:10.1038/495022a PMID:23467149

Thibault, G. (2016). Women in Academic Medicine. *Academic Medicine*, *91*(8), 1045–1046. doi:10.1097/ACM.0000000000001273 PMID:27306968

United Nations. (2002). Committee Experts Praise Portugal's Efforts to Promote Equality of Women [Press release]. Retrieved from https://www.un.org/press/en/2002/WOM1309.doc.htm

Valantine, H., & Sandborg, C. (2013). Changing the Culture of Academic Medicine to Eliminate the Gender Leadership Gap: 50/50 by 2020. *Academic Medicine*, *88*(10), 1411–1413. doi:10.1097/ACM.0b013e3182a34952 PMID:23969359

Webster, F., Rice, K., Christian, J., Seemann, N., Baxter, N., Moulton, C., & Cil, T. (2016). The Erasure of Gender in Academic Surgery: A Qualitative Study. *American Journal of Surgery*, *212*(4), 559–565. doi:10.1016/j.amjsurg.2016.06.006 PMID:27640905

Weiss, A., Lee, K. C., Tapia, V., Chang, D., Freischlag, J., Blair, S. L., & Ramamoorthy, S. (2014). Equity in Surgical Leadership for Women: More Work to Do. *American Journal of Surgery*, *208*(3), 494–498. doi:10.1016/j.amjsurg.2013.11.005 PMID:24933664

White, F. S., McDade, S., Yamagata, H., & Morahan, P. S. (2012). Gender-Related Differences in the Pathway to and Characteristics of U.S. Medical School Deanships. *Academic Medicine*, *87*(8), 1015–1023. doi:10.1097/ACM.0b013e31825d3495 PMID:22722362

Wikipedia. Retrieved from https://www.wikipedia.org/

Willett, L. L., Halvorsen, A. J., McDonald, F. S., Chaudhry, S. I., & Arora, V. M. (2015). Gender differences in Salary of Internal Medicine Residency Directors: A National Survey. *The American Journal of Medicine*, *128*(6), 659–665. doi:10.1016/j.amjmed.2015.02.002 PMID:25731136

Yedidia, M., & Bickel, J. (2001). Why Aren't There More Women Leaders in Academic Medicine? The Views of Clinical Department Chairs. *Academic Medicine*, *76*(5), 453–465. doi:10.1097/00001888-200105000-00017 PMID:11346523

Chapter 14
Gender Equity in the Medical Profession as a Democratic Culture:
The Portuguese Experience

Helena Alves
Instituto Nacional de Saúde Dr. Ricardo Jorge, Portugal

ABSTRACT

Gender Equity is still a challenge 45 years after establishment of democracy in Portugal. The author makes a historical framework of gender equality in the context of democracy and brings together demographic and statistical data on education, science, women's political participation in governments, parliament, and local power levels, the medical profession, and medical specialties. Also focused are the governmental structures to promote gender equality and the way of recruitment/appointment for public administration leaders. A comparison is made with other countries, using data from the OECD. The conclusion is that although there is a high rate of feminization in medicine in Portugal, this is due to the great competitiveness, work capacity, and dedication of women, which guarantees the entry of more women into medical schools. It remains to be seen that men are better represented in top positions and women are clearly overlooked, although the best performance of women in financial management is known. There is a lot of work to do until achieving a true gender equality in Portugal.

INTRODUCTION

Portuguese laws concerning Gender Equity had the most important modifications in the 1970´s, following "carnation´s revolution" of 25 April 1974. From a regimen of fascism to democracy, beyond global freedom of expression, improvements in women's rights were one of the most impressive effects of democracy. In 1974 women could vote and be elected for the first time in a free and universal way. In 1976, a husband's right to open the postal mail of his wife was abolished. Other equity rights were given to women in the Civil Code revised in 1978. In 1974 new Laws opened to women the opportunity to become magistrates, diplomats and to have a local administrative career.

DOI: 10.4018/978-1-5225-9599-1.ch014

Traditionally the Portuguese woman is an important pillar within the family. She is the Mother, the educator, the manager of the family economy, the holder of ancestral knowledge in the art of cooking, feeding, dressing the children, creating the basic agricultural and farmer resources for the support of the family, caring for disease, teaching ethical and religious principles and basic school knowledge. This central position of women in the family is widely, highly respected and recognized by the Portuguese men, and it is even expressed in the popular saying that men like to remember as a joke: "In home, she is in charge, but I am her boss".

Even before "April Revolution" in 1974, many girls were students in the Portuguese Medicine Faculties. In the years post revolution, the political crisis and the democratic values of the Universal Right to Health positively influenced the role of female physicians in the community.

The project of a National System of Health was a challenge and one opportunity for the young female physicians in the building of a new country. In the first 10 years of democracy, one of the most important political decisions was to spread medical services to the small cities in the country.

To promote equal access to medical services was a democratic objective. At that time, the first democratic governments sent young doctors to work for one year in small cities as a civic service. The experience of working in rural areas attracted young physicians; this helped to develop small Charity Hospitals from the local charity associations named "Misericórdias" and fixed physicians in the less developed regions of the country.

This spread of General Practitioners and family doctors was the basis of primary care that still today has an impressive impact in many health indicators and improved the wellbeing of Portuguese population.

Infant mortality rate decreased from 38.9 in 1975 to 3.2 in 2016 (Children who die less than one year old for 1,000 births) and the Maternal mortality rate decreased from 42.9 in 1975 to 7.3 in 2014 (women who die because pregnancy or after delivery per 100,000 births).

Women were a significant proportion of physicians who chose to be General Practitioners at that time (1980's). Not because they could not compete with men in the national examination of access to the specialty, but because it was easier to reconcile the medical profession with maternal and family duties.

At a time of financial crisis post revolution, which brought the International Monetary Fund to Portugal for the first time, it was also easier and cheaper to start a new family, buy a home and live, in the country regions, than it was in the big cities. All these factors influenced many women in the 80s, to choose Primary Care and be General Practitioners.

The proportion of female Medical Doctors in research also increased after this revolution period. The political change opened the country and opened the frontiers to Portuguese people. The training exchange with other countries created opportunities and developed scientific research.

The Portuguese are creative and curious people. The interest in "discovery" has remained in the Portuguese DNA longer than the time of the Discoveries in the 15th- 17th centuries. Democracy brought to Portuguese women the opportunity to contribute as researchers and physicians to develop medical careers in Public hospitals and democratise the National System of Health.

Considerable data were obtained and analysed and are presented in the rest of this chapter, with links that have not previously been correlated. The limitations were the availability of some data.

COUNTRY EVOLUTION IN DEMOGRAPHY

Population

In the year 1974, the resident population in Portugal was 8,630,000.

In 2017, the resident population was 10,300,300 (52.7% were women) (INE, 2019.).

Family

At familial level and maternity responsibilities, from 1974 until 2016 there was also a change of woman's age at birth of the first son/daughter that has increased from 24.1 years old in 1974 to 30.3 years old in 2016. (CIG, 2017.)

COUNTRY EVOLUTION IN EDUCATION AND SCIENCE

Education

Equal access to Education and equity of opportunities were also values from the young democracy. From 1974 a great effort was made to finance Education and free Health for all citizens.

In 1978 there were 81,582 men and women attending University and polytechnic education (34,065 were women, 41.75%). In 2018 there were 372,753 men and women (200,518 were women, 53.79%). (INE, 2019)

A study published in February 2019, about Portuguese women found that 84% of those women had a higher school level than their mothers had. (FFMS, 2019)

Considering graduates, by gender, in Portugal (scholar year 2000/01 to 2016/17) in 2000/01 scholar year, women were 41,048 in a total of 61,140 representing 67.1% and in the scholar year 2016/17, women were 52,937 in a total of 90,889 (58.2% were women) (DGEEC, 2018)

At education professionals, teachers are women for the most part in all the teaching levels (rates of 99.1% to 71.6%) with exception of the university level, where there are mainly men (55.5% men versus 44.5% women). Even so, when looking at heads of departments in universities, just 22.4% are women and 77.6% are men (CIG, 2017,)

PhDs

Concerning PhD degrees, women accounted for 6.7% in 1970 and 53.5% in 2017.

Concerning all those who have completed the doctoral degree between 1970 and 2008, a total of 19,876 doctorates were identified, being 12% in Medical and Health Sciences, with a similar number of men and women.

While in the decade of 1970s, women accounted for only 18% of the total number of PhDs performed, this percentage was about 50% in 2000-2008. In total, 7,783 women were identified with the doctorate completed or recognized by Portuguese universities between 1970-2008 in a 2009 publication. (GPEARI, 2011)

Publications

The evolution considering number of publications (sciences area) per million inhabitants in the various countries of the European Union comparing 2005 and 2015: In 28 countries, Portugal has the 11th position (510 in 2005 and 1,298 in 2015). Denmark was the country with higher number of publications (1,661 in 2005 and 3,050 in 2015), followed by Sweden, Finland, Netherlands and others as UK (1,241 in 2005 and 1,603 in 2015), Germany 12th position, Spain has the 15th position, France 18th position (856 in 2005 and 1,085 in 2015). (DGEEC, 2015)

The number of Portuguese publications indexed in the Web of science, by scientific area: 2005, 2010 and 2015, Medical and Health Sciences: 1,784 in 2005, 4,573 in 2010 and 6,415 in 2015 (DGEEC, 2016)

Women in Politics and Companies

Parliament

Despite a higher proportion of women in higher education, this seems not to matter when power and decision-making is the subject. As an example, participation in Parliament. In 1975 women were just 7,6% and it was necessary to create the Parity Law in 2006 to increase opportunities for women be more represented in the Parliament. In 2015 women were 33% against 67% for men. It took 9 years to attain the 33% defined by Law. (CIG, 2017; Pordata, 2018)

Even so, Portugal evolved quicker than other European countries. Comparing with UK data (proportion of female members of Parliament in the United Kingdom (UK)), in 1979 there was just 3% women in the UK Parliament and in 2015 there was just 29%. (Statista 2019)

Governments, Presidency, Supreme Court of Justice

The evolution of women´s participation in the composition of governments has been increasing from 1.9% in 1976 to 30.5% in 2015. (CIG, 2017)

Although women are even more represented in governments, when comparing levels of power and responsibility, there is a systematic deviation in favour of men. As an example, just 22.2% women were Ministers.

The same occurs in the Heads of governmental bodies and Public Administration, where high positions are mainly for men (just 24.8% women in 2016).

The most impressive deviation can be seen in the Council of State that works near the President of the Republic that has just 1 woman (5.3%) in 2016 and 2 (10.5%), in 2018.

No better is the Supreme Court of Justice with 17% of women. (CIG)

Local Power

Although since 1974 there is an effort to increase numbers of women in political positions, when looking for participation of women in local power, there were just 7.5% women mayors of municipalities in 2013. (CIG, 2017)

Companies

The proportion of women and men in the largest listed companies' board members was 14% against 86% men, in 2016. In the EU28 the average was 23% for women and 77% for men. The presence of women in the administration boards of firms PSI 20, in Portugal is lower than the UE28 average, but has increased since 2008 from 3% to 15.5% in February 2017. (CIG, 2017)

MEDICAL HUMAN RESOURCES

Medical Doctors in Portugal

According to data provided by the National Institute of Statistics INE: In 1991 there were 28,326 Medical Doctors, 16,941 men and 11,385 women. In 2017 there were 51,937 Medical Doctors, 23,524 men and 28,413 women (54.7%). (DGEEC/MEd-Mctes, Pordata, 2018)

Considering all the medical doctors, it was in the year 2010, that the relationship between men and women was reversed and the number of women became higher than the number of men, 20,652 males, 20,779 females. Probably this change occurred because female students got better grades than males when competing to enter in the university, mainly in courses that have higher grades, as Medicine. The same phenomenon is seen in courts, where Prosecutors of the Public Prosecutor's Office, Magistrates and Judges are mainly women.

This tendency of increasing number of females between physicians is in accordance with the tradition of have higher number of women in health-related professions. Comparing females versus males graduates in the years 1994 and 2017, in higher education in health, including medicine, nursing, pharmaceutical sciences or other areas of health, there are 2,177 females versus 547 males (3.97) in 1994 and 8,881 females versus 2,808 males (3.16) in 2017. (DGEEC/MEd-Mctes, Pordata, 2018)

Medical Specialties in the National Health System

According to data provided by the Central Administration of the Health System (ACSS) in its Social Report of the Ministry of Health and the National Health System 2017 (ACSS, 2017), 53.6% of the medical specialists are older than 50 years and for each age the predominance is of the female gender, except for ages over 61 years, in which physicians are mostly males.

This age of 61 at 2017 corresponds to the medical course 1973-1979, that began functions in the first years of democracy, at year 1980, indicating clearly that the beginning of the feminization of the medical profession in Portugal coincides with the beginning of democracy.

Since then the rate of feminization has been growing. At the age of 47 years, corresponding to the course that initiated functions in the year 1994 the rate of feminization was accentuated and in the ages between 31 years and 36 years, women specialists in the NHS are more than twice the men. Overall, the rate of feminization of medical specialists in the National Health System is 62.3%, the highest rate in Immuno-haemotherapy (74%) and the lowest rate in Urology (4,6%).

Looking at the distribution of females in several specialties (Graphic 1), women remain far behind in many specialties, being over represented in others. The difference is clear if the specialties are grouped in surgical/clinical-surgical specialties (26%), clinical specialties (49%), and laboratory/Clinical-laboratorial specialties (62%).

In **surgical/clinical-surgical specialties,** the female proportion average is 26%, the 5 with lowest female proportion are Urology 4.6%, Orthopaedics 10.1%, Cardiothoracic Surgery 11.9%, Neurosurgery (16.9%) Angiology and Vascular Surgery (17.9%), Maxillofacial Surgery (19%). The top five: Plastic reconstructive and aesthetic surgery (27.8%), Otorhinolaryngology (28.6%), Ophthalmic (37%), Paediatric Surgery (44.6%), Gynaecology-Obstetrics (64%).

In **Clinical specialties**, the female proportion average is 49%, the 5 with lowest female proportion is seen in Clinical Pharmacology 11%, Sports Medicine 11%, Tropical Medicine 22%, Cardiology 30%, Occupational medicine 40%. The top five: Internal Medicine 59%, General and Family Medicine 61%, Immuno-allergology 62%, Anaesthesiology 67%, Paediatrics 70%.

The higher female representation is seen in **laboratory/Clinical-laboratorial specialties** with 62% females, being the lower percentage in Radiodiagnosis with 43.7% and the higher in Immuno-haemotherapy/Transfusion Medicine with 74%.

Management of Health Services has 39% females.

Comparing these data with Australian data from 2015 about surgical specialties, published in Level Medicine.org.au, (Seebacher, 2017), the feminization rate in Portugal is clearly higher, with the exception of Urology (Table 1).

GOVERNMENTAL MECHANISMS FOR PROMOTING GENDER EQUALITY

The Commission for Citizenship and Gender Equality (CIG)

Mainstreaming Gender Equality at all levels of the Public Administration is a political commitment, a strategy for achieving Gender Equality and is considered a requisite for good governance by the Portuguese Government. The governmental mechanism for promoting gender equality is the Commission for Citizenship and Gender Equality (CIG), established by Regulatory Decree in 2012 under the Office of the Presidency of the Council of Ministers (PCM) (EIGE, 2015)

The Presidency of the Council of Ministers, is the central government department that has the mission to provide support to the Council of Ministers, the Prime Minister and the other members of the Organically integrated Government and promote inter-ministerial coordination of the various governmental departments (D-L nº 202/2006, Diário da República)

The tasks of the PCM are the design, implementation and coordination of public policies in the following areas of intervention: a) administrative modernization; b) Citizenship and gender equality; c) Immigration and Intercultural Dialogue; d) Youth; e) Sport; f) Media. (D-L nº 202/2006, Diário da República)

The Commission for Citizenship and Gender equality is one of the central services that are included in the direct administration of the State under the Presidency of the Council of Ministers.

In 1977 was institutionalized the Commission on the Status of Women (D-L nº 485/77, Diário da República)

Figure 1. Feminization rate in Medical specialties and sub-specialties in Portugal ACSS data, 2017 (ACSS, 2017, http://www.acss.min-saude.pt)

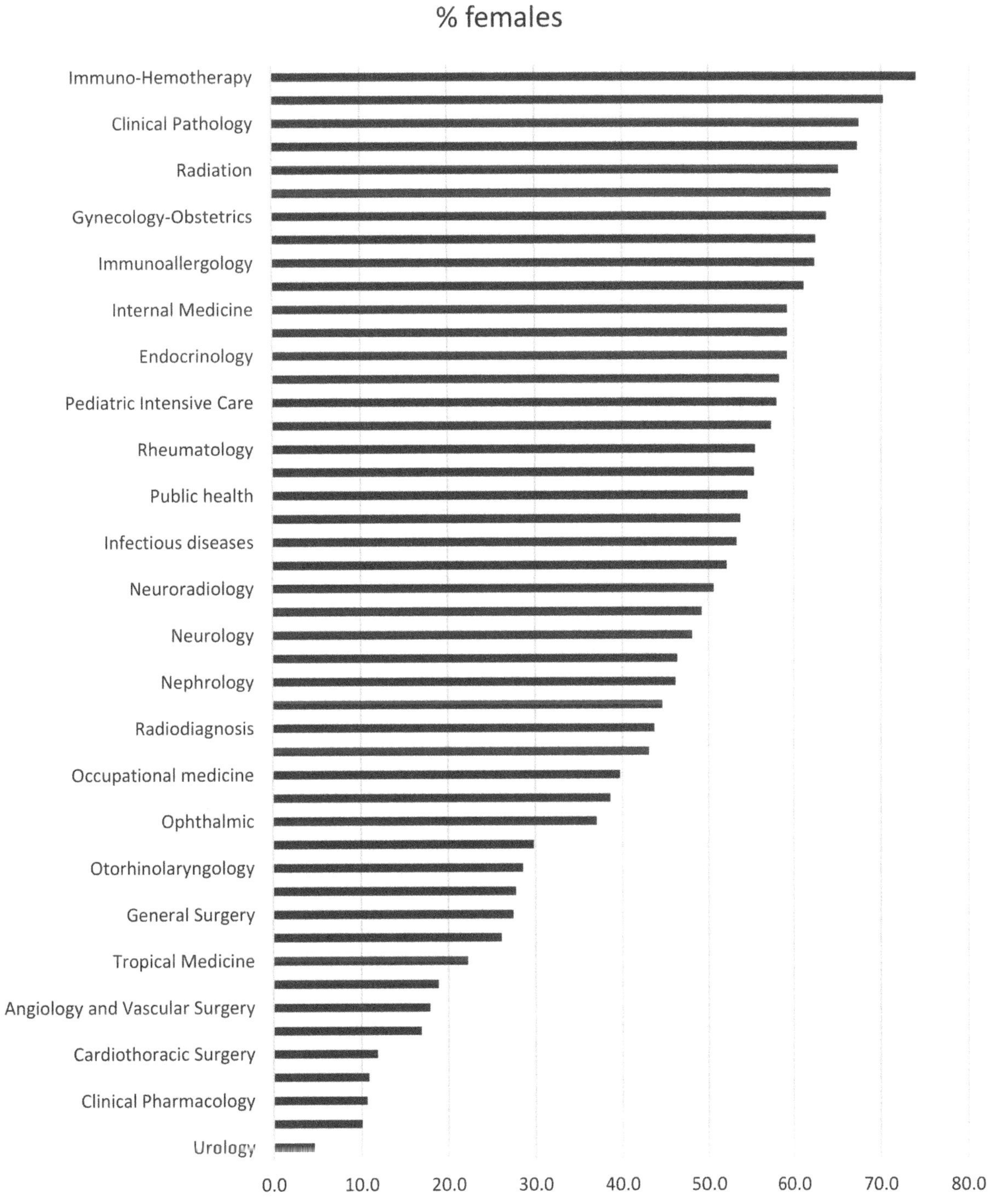

Table 1. Feminization rate in surgical specialties in Australia 2015 and Portugal 2017

	%Female	
	Australia	Portugal
Cardiothoracic surgery	5.6	11.9
General Surgery	11.6	27.5
Neurosurgery	10.9	16.9
Orthopedics	3	10.1
Otolaryngology	9	28.6
Pediatric Surgery	20	44.6
Plastic Reconstructive	12.1	27.8
Urology	6.9	4.6
Vascular Surgery	7.3	17.9

Twenty years later, in 1997, the integration of a gender perspective at all policy levels became more visible in the Global Plan for Equal Opportunities, approved by the Council of Ministers. Since then, several National Plans for Equality were issued. The most recent is the V National Plan for Gender Equality, Citizenship and Non-discrimination 2014-2017. (EIGE, 2015, https://eige.europa.eu)

CRESAP: Recruitment and Selection Committee for Public Administration

Law n.° 64/2011 22 December (Diário da República, 1ª série-N°244- 22 December 2011), modifies the procedures of recruitment, selection and provision in the positions of higher management of the public administration, proceeding to the Fourth Amendment to Law No. 2/2004, of 15 January, that approves the status of the Directors of the services and bodies of the Central, Regional and Local Administration of the State, and the Fifth Amendment to Law No. 4/2004 of 15 January, which establishes the principles and standards to which the organization of the direct administration of the State must comply.

In the Article 2, changes to the 18°,

1. The holders of higher management positions shall be recruited, by a concursal procedure, in accordance with the following articles and 19a, of between individuals with a degree completed at the opening date of the tender for at least 12 or 8 years, depending on the positions First or second degree, linked or not to the public administration, which possess technical competence, aptitude, professional experience and training appropriate to the performance of their duties.
2. The initiative of the procedure referred to in the preceding paragraph shall be for the member of the Government with the power of direction or superintendence and guardianship on the service or organ in which the office is incorporated, competing in this context to define the profile, Professional experience and management skills required of applicants...etc (Law n.° 64/2011, Diário da República)

CReSAP makes selection of candidates by concursal procedures, but also evaluates profiles of public managers nominated by the government or supervisors of Public (or public/private partnerships) companies and bodies.

Considering all the Ministries, in the years 2015, 2016 and 2017 CReSAP concluded 102 concursal procedures.

In the same 3 years 2,819 candidates registered in the platform, 984 did not finish the register, 22 were excluded, 73 gave up, 1,740 were evaluated (1,150 men (66.1%) and 590 women (33.9%)). (CRESAP, n.d.)

From these 1,740 evaluated, were proposed 300 as possible nominates (216/300 men (72%) and 84/300 women (28%)). Finally, government provisioned in 101 positions 61 men (60.4%) and just 40 women (39.4%). (CRESAP, n.d.)

Considering years separately, 2017 was the first year that had more women (12 women) than men (8 men) provisioned.

These numbers should not be expected because they are not in accordance with the higher rates of women graduated. The author's view is that there are factors acting as a bias that deviates women from the centers of power and decision. The first factor is the woman's role inside the family, that prevents many women from running for a position as head of an institution. The second factor is the general belief that there is not clean competition, that public recruitments are often preceded by political appointments, usually men, who gain curricular advantage by being nominated for positions that come to recruitment just many months or years later.

The general belief is that such men thus become artificially favorite candidates for a place they would lose if the competition were done cleanly and transparently at the beginning of the need for placement. As this practice is known, many potential candidates, especially women, give up running for public places, as they believe the nominee is defined at the outset.

The actual weight of this bias is not known, it may be overvalued in the public opinion, but being a common belief, it removes credibility to the contests and decreases the number of competing women.

For the sake of transparency, officials should not be temporarily appointed to positions that should go to public competition, because this is seen as a way arranged within democracy to circumvent the democratic rules and laws that democracy produces.

Another work done by CRESAP is the issuance of opinions on "political appointments".

Opinions for public managers asked in 2017**:** The opinions to be issued by CReSAP are triggered by the necessary request for the evaluation of the curricula and the adequacy of the competencies of nominated personalities. The initiative of the proposal is from the member or members of the Government responsible for the supervision of the company or body.

In the same 3 years (2015, 2016 and 2017), CReSAP was asked to evaluate the suitability profile of 674 personalities (424 men and 250 women), nominated for public management positions. Considering the years separately, from 2015 to 2017, the number of women nominated increased, being 74/218 (33.9%) in 2015, 93/250 (37.2%) in 2016 and 83/206 (40.3%) in 2017. (CRESAP, n.d.)

In 2017 CReSAP was asked to evaluate the suitability profile of 206 personalities (123 men, 83 women), nominated for public management positions.

The Permanent Technical Committee assigned 199/206 adequate opinions (96.6%), 4/206 adequate opinions with constraints (1.9%) and 3/206 unsuitable opinions (1.5%).

119 (58%) of all opinions issued were asked by the Ministry of Health, being asked 67 for men (56.3%) and 52 for women (43.7%).

This does not mean that those women are Medical Doctors.

Considering concursal procedures, in 2017 CReSAP received 83 requests, being just 10 (12%) from the Ministry of Health. (CRESAP, n.d.)

Parity Law

The "Parity law" appeared in 2006, has been revised, at the beginning asking for 33% women in the director boards of public bodies and listed companies on bourse and now in the revision that is being done, it is also asking for 40% of women in the electoral lists to Parliament.

COMPARING PORTUGAL WITH OTHER COUNTRIES

When Education is Considered

Young women in OECD countries now often obtain more schooling than young men, but continue to be less likely to study in the lucrative science, technology, engineering and mathematics fields.

Portugal has the 13th position in Female share of graduates from bachelor´s programs, %, 2014 or latest

Portugal has the 10 position in Female share (%) of bachelor´s graduates in STEM, %, 2015 or latest (27)

When Employment is Considered

Women's labour force participation rates have moved closer to men's over the past few decades, but in every country, women are still less likely than men to engage in paid work. When women do work, they are less likely to advance to management positions and continue to earn less than their male counterparts.

Gender Gap in the labour force participation rate (15-64 years-old), p.p. 2015 or latest, Portugal has the 37th position

Female share of managers (all ages), %, 2015 or latest, Portugal has the 22nd position (OCED, n.d.).

When Entrepreneurship is Considered

Women are still much less likely to be self-employed than men, and are less likely than men to employ staff. Reflecting the size of their companies, the sectors in which women operate, and a variety of other factors, self-employed women earn less than their male peers – at least a fifth less, in almost all OECD countries

Gender gap in the self- employment rate (15-64 years-old), p.p. 2016 or latest Portugal position is 19th

Gender gap in the share of employed who are employers (15- 64years-old),p.p 2016 or latest, Portugal position is 23th (OECD, n.d.)

Generally, women are less likely to be involved in businesses, it may be more likely that high-flying women would apply to public service roles.

When Public Life is Considered

Gender inequalities pervade public life, as well. Across OECD countries, women remain underrepresented in political office and in government management positions.

Female share of seats in Parliament, %, 2016: Portugal position is 12nd

Female share of employment in senior management in Central Government, %, 2015 or nearest. Portugal position is 17th. (OECD, n.d.)

Females as Managers

A recent publication from the International Monetary Fund named "Women in Finance: A case for closing gaps" written by Ratna Sahay, Martin Cihák, and other IMF staff (IMF Staff discussion note, September 2018 SDN/18/5) analyse women performance in finance. The paper found large gaps between the representation of men and women in leadership positions in banks as well as in banking-supervision agencies worldwide. Women accounted for less than 2 percent in the group of financial institutions' chief executive officers and less than 20 percent of executive board members.

The higher presence of women on bank boards appears associated with greater financial resilience and greater bank stability.

In the IFM paper, because of literature review, the authors found numerous studies that had highlighted the small share of women in senior corporate management. Either in the government or the private sector, in many countries and industries, female representation in senior positions is low (International Labour Organization 2015; Credit Suisse, 2012, 2014; Catalyst 2014; Wolfers 2006; Elborgh-Woytek et al 2013).

Several authors refer that women constitute 8 - 10% of directors over the period 1990 to 2009. (20-22) (Adams and Ferreira 2009; Farrell and Hersch, 2005; Catalyst, 1999)

Catalyst (2003) finds that the proportion of board seats women held in the Fortune 500 rose from 9.6% in 1996 to 13.6% in 2003 (23). When there are women in the boards, the majority of firms with female directors have only one woman and this pattern has not changed much over time. The differences between proportions of women and men got contestation actions worldwide in the last decades and some firms have increased women in the boards by tokenism. Although female directors may be chosen because of tokenism, Adams and Ferreira results show that women are able to impact board governance.

Meta-analyses from Post and Byron (2015) and Pletzer et al. (2015) on corporate boards and company performance, suggest that female board representation is positively related to accounting returns.

Adams and Ferreira 2009, Women in the Boardroom and Their Impact on Governance and Performance (Journal of Financial Economics 94 (2009) 291-309) studied the relationship between board effectiveness and gender diversity using the fraction of female directors on the board and show that female directors have a significant impact on board inputs and firm outcomes.

Companies with more women board directors experience higher financial performance, according to latest Catalyst bottom line report (n.d.)

The study looked at three critical financial measures: return on equity, return on sales, and return on invested capital, and compared the performance of companies with the highest representation of women on their boards to those with the lowest representation. The study concludes that diversity, well managed, produces better results, lead more independence, better innovation, good governance and better performance.

CONCLUSION

Democracy recognized to Portuguese women the right to achieve Gender Equality early after revolution, increasing in 1975 the rate of females in the Parliament and creating in 1977 the Commission on the Status of Women.

Gender Equality was a "*non grato*" subject for the dictatorship, since the 1920s.

2 years after creating this Commission, was held the 1979 UN Convention on the Elimination of All Forms of Discrimination against Women (CEDAW).

Although there was at that time some European countries more committed with Gender equality, the first European Parliament resolution on gender mainstreaming, was published just at 13 March 2003.

And just in 2011 was adopted by the European Council the European Pact for Gender Equality (2011-2020)

In Portugal, in 2012 and after, several National Plans for Equality were issued, and governments introduced permanent governmental mechanisms for promoting Gender Equality.

The direct dependence of the Commission for Citizenship and Gender Equality (CIG), under the Presidency of the Council of Ministers has been important to promote inter-ministerial coordination of public policies in gender equality.

Over the years after April Revolution, Gender Equality was assumed as part of the Democratic Culture.

Comparing concordance of CRESAP with Political decisions, CRESAP agreed in 96.6% of nominated personalities previously chosen by political power, whatever the gender, meanwhile in concursal procedures, CRESAP nomination proposals disagreed with political power in 11,4%. CRESAP proposed as possible nominates just 28% women, being the political decision 39.4% of provisioned positions to women, tending more to gender equality.

From this work the author concludes that important changes were introduced by democracy in a short time-scale, but although mainstreaming Gender Equality at all levels of the Public Administration is a political commitment in the law, there is a gap between laws and reality, reflected also in the Commissions work created by democracy to promote gender equity.

Portuguese female doctors still face challenges related with political appointments to leadership where professional merit is secondaries, what means fewer female doctors in leadership positions.

There is still a lot to do to achieve gender equity in Portugal, as well as to mature democracy. Medical organizations and social associations still have a role to continue this work.

The appointment to leadership positions should be more transparent and the appointment of "personalities" should be based on professional merit and healthy competition, independent of political affiliations.

Patients, institutions and the economy will benefit from women's commitment in positions of leadership and high management of hospitals and health institutions.

REFERENCES

ACSS. (2017). Relatório Social do Ministério da Saúde e do Serviço Nacional de Saúde. Retrieved from http://www.acss.min-saude.pt/

Adams, R. B., & Ferreira, D. (2009). Women in the Boardroom and Their Impact on Governance and Performance. *Journal of Financial Economics, 94*(2), 291–309. doi:10.1016/j.jfineco.2008.10.007Catalyst Report. (1999). Catalyst Report: 1999 Catalyst Census of Women Corporate Officers and Top Earners. Retrieved from https://www.catalyst.org/

Catalyst Report. (2003). Catalyst Report: 2003 Catalyst Census of Women Board Directors of the Fortune 500. Retrieved from https://www.catalyst.org/

CIG. (2017). Comissão para a Cidadania e Igualdade de Género. Boletim estatístico 2017. Retrieved from https://www.cig.gov.pt/2018/02/igualdade-genero-portugal-boletim-estatistico-2017/

CIG. (2017). Comissão para a Cidadania e Igualdade de Género (2017). Igualdade de Género em Portugal, Indicadores-Chave 2017. Retrieved from https://www.cig.gov.pt/2017/07/igualdade-de-genero-em-portugal-indicadores-chave-2017/

CRESAP. (2017). Comissão de Recrutamento e Seleção para a Administração Pública, "Relatório de Atividades 2017". Retrieved from http://www.cresap.pt/

Decree-Law nº 202/2006 of 27 October, Diário da República, 1ª série—Nº 208— 27 October 2006.

DGEEC. (2015). *Portuguese scientific production: Statistics series 2005-2015.* General Direction of Statistics in Education and Science. Retrieved from http://www.dgeec.mec.pt/

DGEEC. (2016). Direção Geral de Estatísticas da Educação e Ciência. InCitesTM, Clarivate Analytics. Data updated in November 2016. Retrieved from http://www.dgeec.mec.pt/

EIGE. (2015). European Institute for Gender Equality, about Portugal. Retrieved from https://eige.europa.eu/

<eref>DGEEC. (2018). Direcção-Geral de Estatísticas da Educação e Ciências - Data updated in October 2018. Retrieved from http://www.dgeec.mec.pt/ DGEEC/MEd-Mctes

<jrn>Farrell, K. & Hersch, P. L. (2005). Additions to corporate boards: The effect of gender. Journal of Corporate Finance, 11(1-2), 85–106. doi:10.1016/j.jcorpfin.2003.12.001</jrn>

<eref>FFMS. (2019). As mulheres em Portugal, hoje. Retrieved from https://www.ffms.pt/publicacoes/grupo-estudos/3584/as-mulheres-em-portugal-hoje</eref>

GPEARI. (2011). *Fluxos e situação profissional dos doutorados em Portugal – 2009.* Ministério da Ciência e Ensino Superior, Estatísticas Oficiais. Junho 2011. Retrieved from http://www.dgeec.mec.pt/np4/208

INE. (2018). Health personnel statistics. Source: Pordata. Last update: Aug. 8, 2018. Retrieved from https://www.pordata.pt/

INE. (2019). *População.* Instituto Nacional de Estatística. Retrieved from https://www.ine.pt/

Decree Law Nº 485/77, Diário da República n.º 266/1977, Série I, 1977 11-17.

Law n.º 64/2011 22 December, Diário da República, 1ª série-Nº244- Dec. 22, 2011.

OECD. (2017). The Pursuit of Gender Equality. Retrieved from http://www.oecd.org/gender/the-pursuit-of-gender-equality-9789264281318-en.htm

OECD. (2019). Retrieved from https://www.catalyst.org/media/companies-more-women-board-directors-experience-higher-financial-performance-according-latest

Pletzer, J. L., Nikolova, R., Kedzior, K. K., & Voelpel, S. C. (2015). Does Gender Matter? Female Representation on Corporate Boards and Firm Financial Performance-A Meta-Analysis. *PLoS One*, *10*(6). doi:10.1371/journal.pone.0130005 PMID:26086454

Pordata, I. N. E. (2018). *Portugal: Mandatos nas eleições para a Assembleia da República deputados do sexo feminino por partido político.* Last update: Nov. 6, 2018. Retrieved from https://www.pordata.pt/

Pordata. (2018). Graduates in year, in higher education in the area of health: total, by area of education and training and sex. Last update: Sept. 24, 2018. Retrieved from https://www.pordata.pt/</eref>

Post, C. & Byron, K. (2015). *Women on Boards and Firm Financial Performance: A Meta-Analysis, Academy of Management Journal, 58, 5.* Thematic Issue on Gender in Management Research.

Sahay, R., Cihák, M., & other IMF staff. (2018). *Women in Finance: A case for closing gaps.* (IMF Staff discussion note, September 2018 SDN/18/5)

Seebacher, N. (2017). Gender Equity in Medical Specialties. Retrieved from http://levelmedicine.org.au/resources/completed-fellowship-papers/gender-equity-in-medical-specialties/

Statista. (2019). *Proportion of Female Members of Parliament in the United Kingdom (UK) from 1979 to 2017.* Retrieved from https://www.statista.com

Chapter 15
Gender Equity in Medicine in Sweden

Elizabeth Lorraine-Lichtenstein
Uppsala Akademiska Hospital, Sweden

ABSTRACT

This chapter is about gender equity in medicine in Sweden. It is a descriptive chapter starting with a historical overview of women´s situation in Sweden, and a short history of Swedish women in medicine and academia. It describes the Swedish system and what enhances the possibilities of gender equality. Although there are structural mechanisms working towards gender equality and equity, there are still a lot of problems. Some are accounted for and described. Among other things browsed are healthcare issues where inequity is occurring, medical students and researchers, sexualised violence, and the #metoo-movement which had a big impact in Sweden.

HISTORICAL BACKGROUND OF WOMEN IN SWEDEN

In the old days…

During the Viking age, women in Scandinavia held a strong position and were in many ways men´s equal. Free women were allowed to practice any guild, they were independent and active on many levels in society. They had the right to choose their spouse and were sexually liberated. Women who married with a dowry had a right to keep it if they later wanted a divorce (Ingelman-Sundberg, 2009). Economically, women did not inherit if there was a male sibling, but if there was no such - or they were widowed, women could be land-owners and have their own business. The Viking woman was known to be self-sufficient and strong-headed. With the introduction of Christianity (900-1200 A D) and other values, women lost most of their freedom and independence. They became part of a religion where male dominance and male rights took over. Through the supremacy of the church, old ways of conflict resolution on a local (often familiar or clan) level, were abandoned. The new ways meant more control over female sexuality and women were submitted to a secluded life within the family or sometimes the church. This meant that from medieval times towards the end of the industrialization women in Sweden were not entitled to practice a guild or a profession, with few exceptions. If they had children or sexual relations out of wedlock this was regarded

DOI: 10.4018/978-1-5225-9599-1.ch015

as shameful and with time also punishable The practice of birth-control was sinful, and eventually also regarded as witchcraft, for which many women lost their lives in Sweden - the last one in 1704. As from the middle of the 19th century things started changing. Women started to advance in society as it became more apparent that they were needed in the workforce. Even with this, despite women being part of family business and agricultural life, they were not recognized as part of the official workforce until very recently.

Towards a Modern Society

Even through the development of today's modern society (as from industrialization and onwards) women were not always allowed to access higher education. Women born into upper classes could sometimes gain theoretical knowledge through private tuition. In the 19th century this changed quite remarkably as economic growth and social interactions developed. A lot of patriarchal laws, which earlier had ensured that women were kept out of higher education and (therefore) leading posts in society, were changed. This was not an easy task as society, and even the state, were of the opinion that women´s education was a family matter and not a state matter. Allowing women access to higher education was against nature´s laws as the main opinion was that women were meant to breed and take care of the family. If girls were to be allowed to educate themselves, this ought to be within professions that enhanced their femininity (Kvinnsam – National Library for Gender research, 2019). Women that entered into men´s sphere of occupations were perceived as threats. With the growth of industrialization educated women were needed first in the workplace and eventually took place in society as well.

Unmarried women could apply to court to gain majority from 1858, before that they had to apply to the Majesty. As from 1864 unmarried women attained majority at the age of 25 (men at 21), married women gained majority first in 1921, which was also the first year women could vote in Sweden. Sweden was the last Scandinavian country to give women this right. In 1864, women gained rights to open their own private business (a right women in Scandinavia had had during the Viking age). Women did not inherit on an equal basis as men before 1845. In 1873, women were allowed to study at university, with the first woman gaining access to higher education in 1871 when Betty Pettersson studied philosophy at Uppsala University, gaining permission from the Majesty´s royal court.

Women in Academia and the First Female Doctors

The first female doctor to graduate in Sweden was Karolina Widerström in 1888 (Andreen,1988, Bjurman & Paul,1988). She was however not the first female doctor in Scandinavia but had two predecessors. Rosina Heikel from Finland managed to pass the final exam in 1878 after having to make an individual application for every course in the curriculum (Bjurman & Paul,1988, Gustavson-Kaddaka, 2010). Her graduation was not officially acknowledged - but she was eventually allowed to practice medicine in Helsinki after a special resolution was taken by the Finnish senate regarding her qualifications. In Denmark, Nielsine Nielsen graduated from the University of Copenhagen in 1885. She was not to allowed to continue her specialization in Gynecology and Obstetrics in her hometown and moved to Switzerland and England to fulfil her dreams. There were also other women who attempted to study medicine in Sweden but for various reasons (illness or decisions to complete their studies elsewhere) never graduated from a Swedish higher education institution (Hedvall, 1974). The first woman to do a Ph D in medicine was Anna Stecksén in 1900 (in Pathology), but she died in 1904 at the age of 34 having given up her research 2 years earlier due to illness (Bjurman & Paul,1988, Gustavson-Kaddaka, 2010, Hultcrantz et al,1998).

Between 1888 and 1914 47 women doctors finished their medical studies at universities in Sweden. Many of them worked in Gynecology and Obstetrics, others in Pediatrics and Dermatology. Women did not officially have access to posts in university or public employment before 1925, which meant that the private sphere was the only one accessible to women with higher education. In 1901, thirty-one female doctors and medical students signed a petition that they sent to the Majesty to open up the possibilities of public employment. Their demands were met, and from 1903 and onwards, unmarried female doctors were allowed to work in local hospitals, as town physicians and prison doctors. Senior posts were not accessible to female doctors, nor were municipal appointments. Women with university degrees of all kinds were mainly confined to working within the private sector or in their own business. Among others, judicial and legal practices were very late in letting women into their profession. Elsa Eschelsson became a PhD in 1897 at Uppsala University having written a highly praised dissertation. She was recommended for an Assistant Professorship immediately due to the high quality of the dissertation but not granted by the faculty. She was openly campaigned against, all through her career and obstructed from teaching at the university. She was repeatedly passed over by less competent men and when she was finally allowed to teach, which was on a very basic level her class was referred to as the Kindergarten class. Legislation was eventually changed, but Elsa continued to face opposition to the position of Professor (despite the fact that she had the relevant competencies for 20 years) The head of the faculty finally agreed to that all the chairs were openly accessible to women but still exempted the Chair in Elsas field. She had become very depressed during this time and was found dead the day after the decision to open the Professorships to women she was actively opposed and the head of faculty agreed to that all the chairs were accessible to women except the one that was in her field. By then she had become very depressed and was found dead the following day (in 1911) after this decision, after fourteen years of open harassment. The cause of death was attributed to an overdose of sleeping pills. No woman attempted to break the male barriers within the legal faculties of Swedish universities until 1958 when the next woman defended her dissertation at the university of Lund. Today the President of the Lawyer's Guild is a woman.

It was not easy being a female doctor at this time as both society and legislation were opposed to the concept. Women were not permitted to work in Public Hospitals nor allowed into all specialties and therefore were compelled to work in their own private practice, very often within Gynaecology. The first female doctors were very aware of the barriers they had overcome to attain their positions in society. Firstly they acquired formal scientific knowledge and then had to overcome the societal norm of acceptance of the woman´s understanding of the human form. They continued to push the boundaries regarding female awareness of the body and bodily functions. For example, this meant informing and educating the public about sexuality, teaching hygiene and the importance of physical empowerment went hand in hand with their deeds as medical doctors.

Karolina Widerström the First Female Doctor to Graduate in Sweden

Karolina Widerström was an only child and was supported by her parents in her striving to become a doctor. She was one of four women at this time at the University of Uppsala (Andreen,1988, Bjurman & Paul, 1988). She finished her studies at the Karolinska Institute in 1888. After graduating, she started her practice in her own apartment, and though many were of the opinion that people would not have confidence in a female doctor, her practice was a success and women from all over Stockholm queued for hours in her waiting room. Karolina was among those who took a strong stand for women´s health and hygiene. She was opposed to the clothing that forced women bodies into corsets and uncomfortable shoes. She did not only treat women and their ailments, she worked hard at educating women in reproductive health and sexual hygiene, among other activities; educating teachers in girl´s schools and as a school doctor. 1898 she wrote an article in a famous Swedish paper - Idun -about menstruation (Bjurman & Paul,1988). This was extremely controversial at the time and did not enthuse the editors of Idun who officially took a stance against the article. Karolina was of the opinion that if God had created man and woman, the reproductive organs were also part of this. Karolina also took a stand against prostitution and the laws that forced women prostitutes, or just women suspected of leading a promiscuous life, to be controlled and registered in an attempt to hinder venereal diseases. Men who used prostitutes were above suspicion and did not have compulsory check-ups. Karolina agitated towards a legislation where men and women should have check-ups regarding venereal disease before marriage to minimize the spread. Karolina Widerström founded two female societies, one being the Female Academic Club (1904) and the other the Female Doctors Club (1916). The Female Doctor´s Club was founded together with six other female doctors and their first task was to fight for the right to employment within the public sector, the right to specialize in any field of their choice and equal pay. Two of these have been accomplished, equal pay is still not apparent. These two associations are still active. The Academic Association has inherited Karolina's flat which is completely intact as it was at the time of her death (1949) and is today used for gatherings and lectures. The Swedish Medical Women´s Association is still very active and has today about 1500 paying members and over 7000 group-members on Facebook.

More Female Role Models

Eventually the path was forged for more female doctors. In 1901 there were 14 female doctors in Sweden. The first female surgeon in Sweden was Ada Nilsson (Lundgren, 2014, Nilsson, 1963) who was also very active in the petition to Parliament in 1901 about women gaining access to hospital employment and other public faculties. Ada Nilsson experienced the disadvantages of being a female medical student. Amongst many incidents she recalled one, whilst undergoing an anatomy oral examination together with two male students. She was far more knowledgeable and could answer to more questions than her fellow male students but at the end of the exam they were all granted the same mark of pass and no one passed with distinction. When she asked the Professor why she had not received higher marks the answer was that her male contemporaries were not up to a higher mark and he could not give a female student a higher mark than a male. On another occasion she was refused employment at the last moment in a hospital on the grounds of her gender which led her to her persistence in bringing the petition to Parliament in 1901.

In 1923, unmarried women could finally be appointed as civil servants, with the exception of posts associated with a risk of violence (e.g. military service), or to work as priests or judges. Until 1939 married women had to apply to the Majesty to gain access to employment as civil servants (Kvinnsam – National Library for Gender research, 2019).

In 1937, the first female Professor in Medicine was appointed; Nanna Svartz who specialized in Internal Medicine at the Karolinska Hospital in Stockholm (Bjurman & Paul, 1988, Hultcrantz et al., 1999). Her research within Gastroenterology and Rheumatic disease resulted in (among others) in the development of Sulfasalazine which is still in use. It was not until 1964 that a second female professor in Medicine was appointed in Sweden; Dora Jacobson (a Jewish doctor from Berlin who fled the Nazis in the 1930´s). She spent her professional life in Sweden at the University of Lund where she made epoch-making discoveries within Endocrinology.

The first pioneer women doctors were not only engaged in women´s health and hygiene, but also social problems in society. They were also active in the struggle for women's right to vote, many were also engaged in local politics and some were even active in Parliament.

THE SITUATION OF GENDER EQUITY AND EQUALITY IN SWEDEN TODAY

Today Swedish society and official life is said to be one of the most equal in the world. Women are represented in all aspects of public life and there are no professions where women are not allowed. Even so, the Swedish labor market is one of the most horizontally segregated in OECD. Among the 30 largest occupations, only three have an equal number of men and women (range 40 – 60%). These are cooks, high school teachers and store managers (Central Bureau of Statistics Sweden, 2018). Only 15% of the workforce are found in professions that are gender-equal. Women are overrepresented in traditional caregiving areas such as healthcare, childcare and cleaning jobs. Men are overrepresented in technical areas such as factory workers, truck drivers and maintenance. Women in academia are well represented and there are more women today with university degrees than men. Medicine however is one of the few professions that are more or less gender-equal even though the choice of specialty is not (Sveriges Läkarförbund, 2016).

THE SWEDISH WELFARE SYSTEM

Sweden has a highly developed welfare system which applies to all subjects and over the complete life span. Many of the social reforms and welfare systems that have been developed over time in Sweden are incomparable to other countries although there are many similarities among the Nordic countries.

Laws Regarding Labour

The holiday laws in Sweden guarantee 5 weeks of paid holiday annually (Arbetsdepartementet, 1977). The first law about annual holidays came in 1938, agreeing two weeks annually, which increased in the sixties to four weeks (Kvinnsam – National Library for Gender research, 2019). Since 1978 five weeks are agreed although many professions and their unions have agreed an increase in the number of days dependant on seniority. The maximum working day is normally eight hours, passed in 1919, and it was only in 1971 that Saturdays were no longer included in the working week. The European Working Time Directive (2003) has now changed the length and numbers of hours worked especially on call for the better.

Student Life

Since the 1960s, in Sweden higher education has been tuition-free (Swedish National Agency for University Studies, 2017). Students have been offered a combination of government grants and student loans with favorable interest to enable everybody to higher education without private financial means. The system is applicable to all students whatever their financial background and is used by a vast majority of students today. This means that the student borrows money from the state for a low interest and pays back after completion of studies. About 70% of the financing are loans and 30% are grants. For students with family and children the grants are raised to cover the cost of living. There is also the possibility of applying for other state grants to cover part of housing or rent costs as these are suspected to be higher if you have a family. Student organizations and public landlords offer cheap accommodation for students in student corridors and small one-room apartments - but also larger accommodation such as flats for families and couples. Besides financing University studies with state supplied grants and loans the students are allowed to have a certain annual income from employment. If the income is too high the loans and grants are diminished, depending on how high the income.

In 1977 Universities underwent a reform to strengthen the role of the student and expand the access to higher education to groups that historically had not attempted to pursue higher education (Swedish National Agency for University Studies, 2017). This resulted in more students from lower socioeconomic classes and also more female students. Female students have since become the majority attending Swedish Universities. Today 48% of Swedish women and 37% of men have gained University education (The University and College Council, 2018). During the last 40 years more women have applied to study medicine and at least 50 per cent have been women since the 90's, according to some even since the 70's. 65% of all university graduates are women. On the next level (doctorate) 46% are female. What happens to the women when they graduate? Why don´t they take the next step in an academic career? This will be discussed further on in this chapter.

Reproductive Health and Parental Rights

The prohibition against the use, information and sale of contraceptives was abolished just before the beginning of WWII. In 1964 the contraceptive pill was approved (Kvinnsam - National Library for Gender research, 2019). Sweden was the first country to legislate against rape within marriage (1965). In 1975 the new abortion act was passed where women are entitled to abortion up to the 18th week of pregnancy without having to explain why. Between the 18th until the 22nd week of pregnancy one can apply to have an abortion under special circumstances and this is currently under debate.

Prenatal care for mothers is free and constant during pregnancies. Expectant mothers having strenuous or physically heavy jobs can get paid leave (80% of their salary) through the Swedish social insurance agency, during the last part of the pregnancy. After giving birth, both parents are given the opportunity to stay in the maternal ward (or adjoining patient "hotels") for the first two or three days. Becoming parents entitles access to parental leave from work, which is usually initially taken by the mother, but also to ten days, in connection to the birth, for the other parent to spend with the newborn family member and the mother.

Sweden has a long history of letting parents take time off with their new family members. In 1901 women gained the right to four weeks unpaid maternity leave (Kvinnsam - National Library for Gender research, 2019). In the late thirties several acts on motherhood and childcare came into force. Employed women could no longer be discharged due to marriage, pregnancy or childbirth. In the early 50s women could become legal guardians of their children. In1974 maternal leave was exchanged for parental leave and fathers could also take part. In 1980, 5% of fathers took the opportunity to stay at home with their little ones. As from 1979 the right to work a six-hour day for parents of small children was established. In 1995 the paternity month was included in the parental insurance, implying that 30 days of the parental leave must be used by the father (a similar arrangement for the mother is included). Parental leave is today 480 days where 390 days are payed by the state on the same level as sick leave which is approximately 80% of the income. The last 90 days are reimbursed on a minimum level of at the moment 180 Swedish crowns per day. As from 2014 parental leave must be shared between the parents with a minimum of three months to each parent. Apart from these three months parents can decide on who takes more leave according to their personal situation. This has resulted in more fathers being engaged in their children even though the bulk of parental leave is still left to the mother (72%). As it is possible to take your parental leave up to the child´s eighth year men tend to take more of the parental leave with older children (over the age of 2 years). With more than one child, and working part-time, parents can make the parental leave last for quite some time. Taking parental leave is on paper today not a problem in Sweden even during surgical training or training in other specialties. As more male doctors see the benefits of having good contact with their children, they are also taking parental leave to a higher extent. Many of them have also partners with careers which means that they share responsibilities for household and children.

Swedish parents are entitled to temporary parental leave up to the age of twelve when their children are ill. This is more equally divided by parents, 62% women and 38% men.

Swedish families have a monthly allowance from the government for their children. This allowance continues up to the age of sixteen. Families having more than one child get an extra supplement besides the monthly allowance per child. As from the age of 16 children attending high school are entitled to a student's allowance.

Nurseries and Day-Care

Due to the parental insurance most children spend their first year in the home with one of their parents. From the age of about 18 months the majority of Swedish children attend a daycare institution where qualified teachers supervise them daily Monday to Friday. 84% of children between the ages of one and four attended nurseries and 95% of five-year-olds in 2017 (Sveriges kommuner och landsting, 2017). School starts from the age of 6 years where the first schoolyear has not been compulsory until recently. As parents are entitled to a shorter work-day most parents try to reduce the numbers of hours their children spend at the nursery.

Health Care

In Sweden, responsibility for health and medical care is divided up into three administrative levels, the National Government, regions and municipalities. The aim of the healthcare system is to achieve good health and healthcare on equal terms for the entire population. The government establishes overall principles and guidelines. The regions are responsible for organizing and providing health care for the individuals in the 21 different regions that constitute the backbone of Swedish medical care. These must comply with the laws and terms regulated on national level by Government even if they are autonomous. The regions are just like government and municipalities represented by vote in national elections. Municipalities are responsible for care of the elderly and those with special needs.

Private health care accounts to approximately 2% of the total spending on health care in Sweden. Private health care insurance via work was previously reserved for executives in bigger organizations, but today over 650 000 Swedes have private health care insurance (13% of the workforce in 2017)(Central Bureau of Statistics Sweden, 2018). The areas covered via private insurances are normally minor - not emergent - surgery, out-patient care and health check-ups.

Equity and equality are strong incentives in the Swedish health care and medical system. In spite of tis there are lots of examples of gender inequalities and inequities.

GENDER INEQUITIES IN SWEDEN

Despite all laws and regulations to secure the equal rights of the individual, Sweden is one of Europe´s most gender-divided workplaces. The overall aim of Sweden's gender equality policy is for women and men to have the same opportunities, rights and responsibilities in all areas of life. This implies among others; an equal distribution of power and influence between women and men, the same opportunities for women and men to achieve economic independence, equal conditions and opportunities, equal access to education, shared responsibility for children and the home and freedom from sexual (gender-related) violence

Every third woman in Sweden works part-time compared to every tenth man (Central Bureau of Statistics Sweden, 2018). Many times, the part-time work is not a choice but compulsory as these people are not offered the possibility of working full-time.

Women as a group do more unpaid work than men in Sweden. With the pay gap between sexes it is estimated that women´s work is unpaid for the last 56 minutes of the eight-hour workday (2019). This gap has decreased with a few minutes every year. (A museum in Stockholm took this into account and for a while had different entrance fees for men and women – this was experienced (by some men) as extremely unfair.) This becomes even more apparent when time outside work is taken into consideration, women spend more hours doing household work than men and even more so if they have children. Even these differences are diminishing yearly and with the younger generation.

Sexualised Violence

Rape within marriage is illegal in Sweden since 1965 (Kvinnsam – national library for gender research, 2019). Even so, this law was not tried in court until 1984. Sweden is one of a few countries where buying sexual services is illegal. The act of prohibition against the purchase of sexual services came into action 1999 (The Swedish Government, 1999). This means that the illegal act in contact with a prostitute is committed by the client and not the seller. In 1999 13.6% of Swedish men between the ages of 18 and 74 said they had bought sexual acts (Häggström, 2016). In 2008 this had diminished to 7.9%. 90% of those buying sex had no earlier police record. Criminalizing the purchase of sexual services can make a big difference in the way people (men) perceive prostitution and what it really incriminates. (Sex buyers are found in all social classes and all professions, they have two things in common, they are men and they consume pornography (Häggström, 2016).) Thanks to this law women in prostitution in Sweden do not fear the police as they did earlier, are in less risk of being raped and assaulted and can also be helped to come out of prostitution. What drives prostitution is poverty and many of the women caught in prostitution in Sweden are from other countries (mainly south-eastern Europe and Africa) and brought to Sweden under slave-like conditions (Häggström, 2016). There are enormous profits for organizations behind these women and there is no other black-market product that is so easy to transport, market, cover-up and sell repeatedly. (Compare with weapons and drugs, which you can only sell once). Thanks to the prostitution law from 1999, the police have a better chance of getting at trafficking and the organizations exploiting these women who are at the bottom of society.

Every year an average of 10 -15 women are killed in close relationships in Sweden (Central Bureau of Statistics Sweden. 2019). This is a figure that has not changed much for the last twenty years but lately seems to have increased, (in 2018 there were 22 women killed in close relationships (Brottsförebygande rådet, 2019)). The culprit is often known as violent and threatening, not only by the victim but also by the authorities. Yet very little is done to protect these women. This can be compared to the millions that are invested in police actions during football matches, where during the last twenty years one person has lost his life.

Since July 2018 Sweden has legislated against sex without consent, it is no longer possible to rape (i.e have sex without mutual consent) somebody whilst, sleeping or unconscious and claim that you didn´t know they didn´t want to have sex.

Female genital mutilation is prohibited in Sweden since 1982, yet due to immigration there are women who are mutilated and turn up in the health care system when seeking hospital care for for example pregnancy. There have been cases where families have travelled to their country of origin and girls have undergone mutilation there. This is also prohibited by law, and the guardians can be charged on their return to Sweden. So far only three people have been charged according to this law, whereof two were sentenced to prison. Women who have undergone female genital mutilation need extra resources and care, especially when giving birth. Swedish doctors have very little education in this area and it is not approached at all in the medical curriculums at the different medical schools.

Health and Illness

Women in Sweden have a higher rate of illness during their lifespan and are also perceived to be less healthy, yet women live longer. This is the health paradox to which we have very few explanations today. Women in Sweden have more depressive and anxiety disorders and are also more prone to work-related stress. Men on the other hand are overrepresented when it comes to alcohol-related disease and suicide (Central Bureau of statistics, 2018).

Increase in effectivity and financial cut-downs has affected the Swedish health-care system. Not only does this mean difficulty in access to care (out-patient surgery within gynecology for example) where many patients today experience increased waiting times. Among other parts affected is maternity care where there today is a lack of mid-wives. This has medical consequences as increased amount of vaginal injuries (perineal tears) during childbirth in which Sweden for the moment has the highest incidence of the Nordic Countries (Sveriges kommuner och landsting, 2018).

In Sweden the system for reimbursing costs in hospitals from the state is funded via charts stating exactly what a diagnosis or operation is worth. For example; if you have your appendix out, the doctor will add such a code (DRG – diagnose related groups) and the cost for it will be calculated. Within this system there is a bias which has yet to be evaluated to the full. A urinary tract infection will give a certain point, but if it occurs simultaneously with a pregnancy (which is a complicating factor) the amount of points it scores is significantly less (Socialstyrelsen, 2014). Cancer in the lower part of the abdomen is valued lower if it is an ovarian cancer than cancer of the colon. Abdominal pain during pregnancy is valued lower than other abdominal pain (Schwartz, Elin, 2015). Not only is this the system for calculating costs but also the system for allocating resources. If diagnosis and DRG-points are systematically lower when it comes to ailments specific for women, it also lowers the future resources directed to women´s health. As from 2014 sex is now included in the statistics and hopefully such errors will be discovered and rectified.

Even when it comes to treatments of the same ailment there are gender biases, for example, men treated for AMI (acute myocardial infarction) are given more costly treatment than women. Men are more likely to be submitted to PCI than women. When looking at costs for AMI in the ages 25-44 men´s costs were more than twice that of the women on an average. Women under the age of 45 had a higher risk of dying of their AMI than men, 7,5% versus 4,5% (Mättä, Sylvia, 2015). The same study showed that even the costs of appendicitis differed. Men´s appendectomy was more expensive than women´s. This may be attributed to the fact that laparoscopic methods were more often used in operating in women than men to rule out gynecological reasons for acute abdominal pain.

Intensive Care Units in Sweden have a high standard, but beds are scarce, patients admitted to the ICU are either acutely ill or have undergone major planned surgery such as transplants or large cancer surgery. ICU units in Sweden treat more males than women. This is more significant in the ages 45 to 80 (more than 60%) and the up to the age of 4 (children), but occurs all over the age-span (SIR, 2019). Swedish women on the whole have longer life expectancy than men, 84 versus 80. Why do men inhabit more of the ICU-beds in Sweden? Are they more often subjects to major surgery, are they more ill from the beginning? This has yet to be determined.

There are more examples of gender-biases in healthcare (Mannberg-Zackari, 2015). Men are more likely to get dialysis, hip operations, eye-operations, light treatment for psoriasis. When parents call to health services for advice, the advice is very different depending on if the caller is male or female. Women patients and callers are on the whole demanded to take more active steps regarding their health (diets, skin care, children´s care) than men who on the whole tend to get more technical and more expensive solutions.

In a dermatological ward, men were more likely to get light therapy and in-ward treatment for psoriasis and eczema, whereas women were instead subscribed self-treatment and ointments for the same conditions (Osika, 2005).

According to a study in Gothenburg women have to wait longer in the Emergency room than men, this was ascertained after all other factors such as among others illness, symptoms and socioeconomic status were taken into account (Robertson, J., 2014).

Even though statistics are plentiful there are few papers identifying the factors behind the gender bias in Sweden. One exception is a paper describing the differences in waiting times in eye clinics for men´s and women´s access to cataract extractions (Smithwaite, 2017). Through focus-group interviews the authors were able to establish that the way gender was constructed had impact on the waiting time cataract extraction. Gender is constructed in the ways people (in this case doctor´s) react in accordance to norms and notions of one´s sex category. In this paper, where women overall had to wait longer for eye operations than men, two clinics were compared where one had a bigger than average gender gap with another with a less than average gender gap. At the clinic with the larger gender gap traditional male occupations were described as more demanding for visual acuity while the need for good eyesight in women´s working life was questioned. This included driving as a traditional male occupation. Awareness of gender equity and bias was low in the clinic with the larger gender gap. There was also an atmosphere where misogynic jokes and racist connotations were present. Not surprisingly the clinic with the larger gender gap was dominated by men. The clinic with the lower than average gender gap (but there was still a gender gap) reasoned in terms of safety as men with poor eyesight were considered a safety risk regarding driving and hunting. It was assumed that older women with bad eyesight stopped driving whereas men didn´t. Assertiveness among men to get treatment was explained in legitimizing ways. Supposedly the medical gender bias and the way of reasoning when it comes to treating patients can apply to more fields in medicine than eye operations.

Female Doctors of Today

As we already have concluded there are more and more female physicians in Sweden. According to the latest statistics, 51% of the medical work force is female. There are more and more women within all specialties. Among younger doctors closer to 60% of the workforce are women. Even so, different specialties in medicine are very biased. Heavy surgical specialties such as Neurosurgery, Thoracic Surgery and Orthopedics are strictly male-dominated with about 85% men. Women dominate specialties like Child Psychiatry, Dermatology, Gynecology and Geriatrics (Sveriges Läkarförbund, 2016).

Women are overrepresented both by numbers of employees in the healthcare sector and are also reportedly more ill than men working in healthcare. This is not only significant among nurses and sub-nurses but also among doctors. 30% of female physicians reported work-related health problems compared to 17% among male physicians. Long-term sick-leave among doctors is twice as common among women doctors compared than men, largely related to psychiatric diagnosis such as burn-out and depression (Holmberg, 2017). Several theories attempt to explain this. Female physicians and male physicians are treated differently in the work-place and expected to do different tasks that are not always in line with their job-description. Women are more often expected to do part of the caregiving work around a patient. Secretarial tasks and services are automatically provided to male doctors – not always so to female. With an increasing demand of efficiency an increase in the invisible work (most often performed by women) occurs. This type of work – not being formalized – is not visible and can therefore not always be taken into account when you compare workloads. Examples of such invisible work is back-ground support - to let the organization run smoothly, empathy work such as building relationships and intervening crisis and even emotional labour such as encountering sadness, aggression and fear. This type of work has traditionally been performed by women in private life and is of vital importance in healthcare (Kosny &MacEachen, 2009). To not recognize it and see its importance can be a co-founding factor to the larger numbers of illness in healthcare among women. In a gender-equal workplace such work might have a higher recognition. Women´s higher degree of sick leave can in other words be a sign of an unequal work environment (Wänje, 2015). This has not altogether been proved but there is research that shows that an unequal work organization and discrimination enhances negative health and conflicts. Gender equity will bring out creativity and productivity in employees.

Male doctors in Sweden have on an average a higher salary during their career. In 2018, a male doctor earned an average of 4382 Swedish Crowns more per month than his female colleague. During an entire career, it is estimated that a male doctor will earn roughly the equivalent of 70.000 Euro more than his female peer, all other factor´s taken into consideration. Are male doctors more skilled than female? There are few studies that take gender into account as to comparing patient outcome. There is one however that shows that fewer patients treated by female surgeons died, were readmitted to hospital, or had complications within 30 days than those treated by male surgeons (Wallis, 2017). If this is the case it suggests that male doctors (surgeons) should not be higher ranked or better paid than female doctors (surgeons).

Students in Medicine

Today there are more women than men applying to go to medical school. It has been suspected that some medical schools favour male applicants to even out the sexes as there are more female applicants than male. Recently (Autumn 2018), applications to study medicine at the Karolinska institute were 38% male but accounted for 53% of those admitted (Swedish national agency for university studies, 2017). These numbers are consistent where roughly 40% of the applicants have been male but 50% of the admitted during the last decade. This is to be compared with the overall admittance to higher studies in Sweden where 65% of the applicants are female and 65% of students admitted are female. After finishing the compulsory schooling (which ends after year nine and at about the age of sixteen) in Sweden 87% of the girls continue to a higher level of education and 82% of the boys. Girls have also, for at least the last twenty years, on an average had statistically significant higher grades than boys. Are the male applicants to the Karolinska Institute more qualified than their female contenders? – in contradiction with the rest of the university world, or is history repeating itself, a100 years after Ada Nilsson, where male students are judged by different standards than female? There does seem to be a gender bias favouring male applicants when it comes to medical studies at the Karolinska Institute in Sweden. As for the rest of the university world 65% of the graduates are women.

Girls have an average of higher marks from high school than boys (The university and college council, 2018). As there is no other marking of grades in medical school other than pass or fail it is difficult to determine if this difference continues throughout medical school. Even when writing exams to get their doctor´s license (which is done in Sweden after 5 1/2 years of medical studies and 20 months of compulsory clinic work as an intern) less women fail and they also have better results than men. Later when male doctors get higher salaries, have they become better than their female counterparts? Do they surpass their female colleagues with increasing age and experience – or is this just another expression of male homosociality?

Within the field of gender and medical careers, there is the underlying question whether women have the same rights as men and have access to all medical specialties. A thesis published in 2017 looked at choices of specialty within the medical profession among young doctors and medical students (Diderichsen, 2017). This was done by interviewing medical students and young doctors. The medical profession being more or less gender equal as a whole still shows big differences when it comes to specialties. Is the choice of specialty gender neutral or are there other forces that determine how male and female doctors choose? Men continue to be predominant in specialties with high prestige, mainly by male homosociality and exclusionary practices. Many of these become apparent to medical students already in medical school as they are included or excluded in practical training and limited possibilities of receiving supervision.

It is virtually only female students who experience sexual harassment and discrimination during their education. According to a report by the Swedish Junior Doctors'Association, 26% of the female and 3% of the male junior doctors have experienced gender discrimination. When it came to choosing specialty female junior doctors spoke more of workplace cultures where hierarchical and macho jargons with sexistic jokes ruled out some specialties. Men spoke more of the actual job and were dissuaded by boring work tasks rather than the work-culture. The conclusions in this study was that the largest difference between men and women was that women were dissuaded by negative cultures and exclusion (Diderichsen, 2017). More than half of the women in the study were discouraged by macho cultures in comparison to 14% of the men, whereas half of the men were deterred by boring tasks compared to the women where only 25% were discouraged by this. Women also experienced more problems with their professional identity when it§ was inconsistent with a male-chauvinistic work-culture. Young male doctors seem to have the privilege of choosing specialty according to their interests rather than young female doctors who experience exclusion in traditional male dominant areas. Gender awareness in medical education among clinical teachers and supervisors needs to increase.

Women in Research

In 1997 two Swedish researchers proved that to be granted a post-doc post a woman had to be more than twice as productive as a man (Wennerås & Wold, 1997). Ten years later another study showed that men had a 40% higher possibility of being granted funds for research than women (Norström, 2009). Men had an overall average lower score than women but were valued higher than women both by men and women.

More women than men in Sweden have university degrees (64% in 2015/16), this has so been since over 30 years, yet women are underrepresented at the next academic level (46%).

This is what some call the “leaking pipe-line” – women drop off at a disproportionate rate at every level of an academic career (Norström, 2009). Looking back on statistics, men who did their dissertation in 1980 - 1991 were twice as likely to become a Professor within 12 years compared to their female peers. Why? You can look at the problem in two ways; women disappear during academic careers due to family and/or psychological factors or men are allocated. The former explanation focuses on women being the cause, this could be managed by for example mentor programmes. The latter brings into consideration the perspective that homosocial factors contribute to how merits are assessed and how funding and appointments are granted. The aspect of having a family is often used as making excuses for why women don´t advance in academia. Figures show that women with a family and children are not less productive than single women without. On the contrary in some cases they are even more productive. Single women with no children do not have a more successful career than married women with children. Why then do women not prosper like men in academia? Hypothesis have been put forward that expectations of brilliance might underlie gender inequities. In sciences supposed to require talent (mathematics, music and philosophy for example) women are underrepresented. Where talent or brilliance and not hard work or productivity count, women tend to disappear. Are women not talented? How do you judge talent or brilliance? That there exists a gender inequity has been very apparent in how research funds have been distributed since the so called “excellency billions” were instituted in 2000 (Sandström & Wold, 2010). The idea was to promote excellent research and strong environments/networks with very large sums to enhance their academic work. Less than 15% of the funding has gone to women researchers. When examined only 55% of those granted funds through the excellency project were among the top ten % in their field (according to quotation index). Every sixth researcher receiving these grants were among the 50% least quoted. There was only one woman among the 25 top grants. Not only do these grants give huge sums to researchers and net-working projects, the idea that the home institution is to give the same amount as the state excellence grant takes resources form other researchers too. This becomes a double backlash as other researchers get the signal that they are not excellent, do not partake of these funds and also have to see their faculty funds go to somebody already well financed.

How can we battle the gender inequity in academia? We know for a fact that female and male papers are judged differently both by males and females. When judging excellency and brilliance these seem to be most partial judgments and pure meritocracy ought in many cases be more objective and efficient. It is time to see over and change the system rather than blaming the victim (telling women where they fail/lack).

#Metoo

In November 2017, 100 years after women began to gain rights in the modern society such as the right to have a profession, study, vote and so forth, came the next big step in women´s liberation. Women started to share their stories of sexual harassment and abuse. What has been going on for centuries where the shame has been put on the culprit and every woman who has ever suffered abuse, harassment and assault has more often than not kept quiet knowing what the consequences are if you tell. The women not only keep it to herself but also blames herself for what has happened. This changed at the end of 2017 when people started adding #metoo on their profiles in social media. Just grasping how big the problem of sexual harassment and abuse is, meant that women who earlier never talked to anyone about their experiences opened up and started telling. This was/is not an isolated phenomenon in certain socioeconomic classes or in specially exposed environments but frequent incidents occurring everywhere, anytime. Sweden too had it´s #metoo movement; women in a number of different professions told their stories to the public for the first time. Many of these resulted in women signing petitions dressed to authorities and employers asking for actions and regulations against harassment. The biggest #metoo movement with over 10400 signatures (signed by women doctors and medical students) began on the Swedish Medical Women´s Associations Facebook page. Together with the signatures horrifying stories of sexual abuse by senior colleagues towards younger female doctors and students came to light (Lundbäck & Trysell, 2017, Testimonies from #metoo-victims). Suspicious voices were - and are - in such cases nearly always raised saying that the victim is lying, especially when the witness is anonymous. Regarding the magnitude of the #metoo movement it was and is more difficult to neglect the problem and imply that witnesses are lying.

The National Centre for men´s violence against women (98% of violent acts are committed by men) has spent decades discussing and researching this area (Nationellt centrum för kvinnofrid, 2018). The figures that were exposed in the #metoo movement where 65% of all women throughout their lifespan were in some way exposed to sexual harassment, abuse or assault came as no news to them. The difference today is that they now can show those figures without being questioned about their validity. 42% of women are sometime during their life-time victims of minor sexual violence such as unwanted kissing, caresses or physical restraint. One out of five women are during their life subject to rape. It is most common that the victim and the perpetrator know each other and that there is a hierarchical structure where the victim is in a situation of dependence. This does not differ within the medical world and among the countless histories of sexual assault and abuse that emerged thanks to the #metoo movement some these stories have come to light. Incidents ranging from verbal sexistic abuse in teaching situations, medical rounds, and social gatherings to rape have been reported. What characterizes most of these testimonies is the exploitation of seniority to harass, and sometimes even pressure women into sexual acts (Testimonies from #metoo-victims). The second thing that hits you reading the testimonies is the lack of support and actions to stop harassment once victims pick up the courage to tell. Not surprisingly many of the testimonies that came forth derive from specialties with strong male dominance such as Neurosurgery and Orthopedics. The world of medicine being very hierarchic, junior doctors being for years in a dependent situation towards their senior colleagues, secure employment often not established until you become a specialist (which today takes about 12 years in Sweden from the beginning of medical school), paves the way for such behavior. With the #metoo petition, signed by 10400 Swedish female doctors and medical students demanding plans to stop and programs to prevent harassment at hospitals and universities, hopefully this culture within medical faculties and hospitals will come to an end. A lot of hospitals and universities have started working towards this and are now employing programs to enhance the work against harassment and abuse.

Sexual harassment is not confined to the medical world but exists all around. Even at school, statistics show that girls are up to 5 times more exposed to sexual harassment as boys. Assaults against women are more common in the home by someone you know, assaults against men are more likely to occur outside by someone unknown. This implies that the place that ought to be a safe haven in fact is the most dangerous place to be for some women.

CONCLUSION

This has been an attempt to describe the situation of gender equity in medicine in Sweden. In spite of being one of the world's most gender equal countries there are still big differences between males and females in our country such as lack of equal opportunities, work related health issues and segregation within professional life. Legislation and formal contracts are gender-neutral but actual life seldom is.

It is obvious that we still construct gender and our presuppositions in a non-neutral way where gender, race and other factors play bigger parts than we would like to admit. The first step is to recognize that that is the fact. Transparency and challenging our traditional views and preconceptions ought to be mandatory in working towards an equal society. The next is to find ways to combat inequities. Obviously, this is not done over-night. The situation is better than it has been, but there is also a tendency towards back-lash and strong forces today thinking that the revolutionary idea of feminism; that men and women should have the same rights and opportunities has gone too far. Let us hope that we can continue to work for a better world where the first amendment of the Universal Declaration of Human Rights (Roosevelt, 1948) stating that all human beings are born free and equal in dignity and right is not just a recommendation but an actual fact.

REFERENCES

Andreen, A. (1988). *Karolina Widerström, En levnadsteckning*. Norstedts.

Arbetsdepartementet/Swedish government. (1977). Retrieved from www.riksdagen.se/sv/dokument-lagar/dokument/svensk-forfattningssamling/semesterlag-1977480_sfs-1977-480

Bjurman, A. & Paul, U. (1988). I Karolina Widerströms Fotspår. 100 år med kvinnliga läkare i Sverige, särtryck av föreläsningar.

Brottsförebyggande rådet, BRÅ. (2019). Statistics March 2019. Retrieved from https://www.bra.se/om-bra/nytt-fran-bra/arkiv/press/2019-03-28-slutlig-brottsstatistik-2018

Central Bureau of Statistics Sweden. (2018). Women and men in Sweden. Facts and figures.

Wallis, C. J., Ravi, B., Coburn, N., Nam, R. K., Detsky, A. S., & Satkunasivam, R. (2017). Comparison of postoperative outcomes among patients treated by male and female surgeons: A population based matched cohort study. *BMJ (Clinical Research Ed.), 2017*, 358. PMID:29018008

Diderichsen, S. (2017). *It's just a job, a new generation of physicians dealing with career and work ideals.* (Dissertation, Umeå University).

Smirthwaite, G., Lundström, M., & Swahnberg, K. (2017). Doctors doing gender at eye clinics – Gender constructions in relation to waiting times for cataract extractions in Sweden. *NORA*, *25*(2), 107–125. do i:10.1080/08038740.2017.1345006

Gustavson-Kaddaka, E. (2010). Om kvinnliga medicine vid Karolinska Institutet i slutet av 1800-talet. Retrieved from https://issuu.com/ki200/docs/evi_g_kadaka_om_karolina_widerstrom

Häggström, S. (2016). Shadow's Law. Bullet point publishing.

Hedvall, G. (1974). *Särtryck ur Nordisk Medicinhistorisk årsbok*. Fingraf Tryckeri.

Holmberg, K. (2017). Statistics from SLF and AFA, lecture April 22, 2017.

Hultcrantz, E., & .... (1998). *Läkare doktor kvinna*. Studentlitteratur.

Ingelman-Sundberg, C. (2009). *Boken om vikingarna*. Norstedts.

Kosny, A. & MacEachen, E. (2009). Gendered, invisible work in non-profit social service organizations: Implications for worker health and safety. *Gender, Work & Organization, 17*(4), 359-380.

Kvinnsam- National Library for Gender Research. (2019). Notable years, Gothenburg university library. Retrieved from http://www.ub.gu.se/kvinn/artal

Läkarförbund, S. (2016). Läkarfakta, statistik över medlemmar, Sveriges läkarförbund. Retrieved from https://slf.se/app/uploads/2018/04/laxxkarfakta-2016.pdf

Lundbäck, A, & Trysell, C. (2017). 10 400 läkare skriver under uppropet # utantystnadsplikt, Läkartidningen.se Nov. 30, 2017.

Lundgren, K. (2014). *Barrikaden valde mig. Ada Nilsson. Läkare i kvinnokampen*. Wahlström & Widstrand.

Mannberg-Zackari, C. (2015). Män får dyrare sjukvård. Tidningen Curie. Retrieved from https://www.tidningencurie.se/nyheter/2015/08/27/man-far-dyrare-sjukvard/

Mättä, S. (2015). Män kostar mer än kvinnor vid hjärtinfarkt och appendicit [DEYT]. *Lakartidningen, 2015*, 112.

Nationellt centrum för kvinnofrid. (2018). Kriminalstatistik och våldsutsatthet, Sexualbrott. Retrieved from https://www.nck.uu.se/

Nilsson, A. (1963). Glimtar ur Mitt liv som läkare. Natur och kultur.

Norström, T. (2009). Män har större chans att få forskningsanslag. *Lakartidningen*, *79*, 1290–1326.

Osika, I. et al. (2005). Tvättsäcksprojektet – genusskillnader in på bara skinnet, Läkartidningen 2846-2851, 40, 2005, 102.

Robertson, J. (2014). Examensarbete, Väntetider på akutmottagningen ur ett jämställdhetsperspektiv, Institutionen för medicin, Sahlgrenska akademin, Göteborgs universitet

Roosevelt, E. (1948). Universal declaration of The human rights, UN.

Sandström, U., Wold, A., Jordansson, B., Ohlsson, B., & Smedberg, Å. (2010). Hans Excellens: om miljardsatsningarna på starka forskningsmiljöer. Retrieved from https://www.forskningspolitik.se/files/dokument/Hans_Excellens.pdf

Schwartz, E. (2015). Läkare kräver genusanalys av sjukvårdens ersättningar. Retrieved from http://www.fria.nu/artikel/117029

SIR (2019). Swedish Intensive Care Register Jan. 2019.

Socialstyrelsen. (2014). DRG-statistics, Socialstyrelsen.se

Sveriges kommuner och landsting (2017). Öppna jämförelser. Retrieved from https://skl.se/skolakultur-fritid/forskolagrundochgymnasieskola/forskolafritidshem/forskola/faktaforskola.3292.html

Sveriges kommuner och landsting. (2018). Vården i siffror. Retrieved from https://vardenisiffror.se/report/view?id=592d2150d4475b02dc29887d

Swedish National Agency for University Studies. (2017). Åren1900-2000. Retrieved from http://www.uka.se/fakta-om-hogskolan/den-svenska-hogskolans-historia/aren-1900-2000.html

Testimonies from #metoo victims. (2018). Confidential mail from victims.

The Swedish Government. (2017). Sexualbrottslagstiftning. Retrieved from https://www.riksdagen.se/sv/dokument-lagar/arende/betankande/en-ny-sexualbrottslagstiftning-byggd-pa_H501JuU29

The University and College Council. (2018). Statistics regarding universities in Sweden. Retrieved from https://statistik.uhr.se/

Wänje, A. (2015). Sick leave—A signal of unequal work organizations? *Nordic Journal of Working Life Studies, 5*, 4.

Wennerås, C., & Wold, A. (1997). Nepotism and sexism in peer-review. *Nature, 387*(6631), 341–343. doi:10.1038/387341a0 PMID:9163412

Chapter 16
Women in the Medical Field in India:
A Developing Economy – A Dichotomous Picture

Monica Sivakumar
Apollo Gleneagles Hospitals, India

ABSTRACT

There is a vast difference in the status of women in the medical field in India as compared to the West. However, much progress has been made in the past two decades at least in the urban areas. There is a tremendous disparity in the rural and urban areas when it comes to the number of women who enter this field. The urban areas are almost on par with the western standards at present. Despite having so many women who are leaders in the field, the situation in rural India remains desolate. Many hopes are dashed and much talent is wasted as societal interference, early marriages, and poor socio-economic status make it extremely difficult for the women in the semi-urban and rural areas to enter this lengthy and endurance-testing field. The patriarchal nature of the society, ancient customs, and inability to adapt to modern times are some of the common reasons that so few women enter this field.

INTRODUCTION

Currently, India is considered the fastest developing economy in the world. With its high population, it has an abundance of human resource. The utilization of this bountiful human resource is however highly improper and mismanaged. It is well known that the development of any country is directly linked to the education of females in the country. Kofi Annan once said, "There is no tool for development more effective than the empowerment of women" (Annan, 2005). In this chapter, we take a look at the aspects of gender equality and quality of education and the treatment of females especially in the medical profession and where this country stands in comparison to its more developed western counterparts.

DOI: 10.4018/978-1-5225-9599-1.ch016

A DICHOTOMOUS PICTURE

When we speak of the education of females it is necessary that we understand the extremely dichotomous picture presented by this country. On one hand we have pioneers who have etched a name for themselves in the history books. Dr Kadambini Ganguly, wife of the renowned social reformer Dwarakanath Ganguly, the first woman physician of India, Dr SI Padmavati, the first woman Cardiologist of India, Dr Indrani Hinduja who has bought the Gamete Intrafallopian transfer technique (GIFT) to this country, which subsequently led to the birth of the first GIFT baby on January 1988 and (Chandramouli & General, 2011), Dr Jayashree Mondakar who was the founder of Asia's first Human Milk Bank are some notable names. There are many more inspiring stories of parents encouraging their daughters to take up this noble profession and become free-thinking, independent, strong and holistic individuals. On the other hand, we have stories of crushed hopes and sacrifices. Let us start by taking a look at the statistics.

THE STATISTICS

For every 1000 males, there are 943 females in India. However, the gender ratio is not uniform in all the 28 states. States like Kerala and Tamil Nadu have a near 50:50 gender ratio whereas states like Haryana and Jharkhand have the lowest sex ratio averaging around 700 females for every 1000 males. Female infanticide and child marriage are still an on-going practice in many parts of these states. The gender ratio is an indicator of the attitude that the people have towards the female sex and is directly proportional to the higher educational standards of girls in the respective states.

More relevant to this chapter, the average female literacy in the world is currently around 79.7 percent. Per the census 2011 report, the average female literacy in India is 65.46 percent (Chandramouli & General, 2011). These numbers obviously speak for itself. The rates of school dropouts amongst the adolescent females in India, particularly in the rural areas is staggering indeed. The National Commission for Protection of Child Rights reports that 39.4% of the girls aged 15-18 dropout of schools and colleges (Singh, 2018). Meanwhile, the percentage of boys not attending any educational institution in the same age group is 35 per cent quoted by the same study. According to an article By Nisha Bala written in 2014, the top three reasons for high dropout rates are expectations of domesticity, safety and infrastructure barriers (Bala, 2014).

A LOOK INTO THE PAST

Much of the progress in the medical field happened in the end of the 19th century and beginning of the 20th century, when India was a colony under the British Government. Cross-cultural exchanges between India and her colonial rulers laid the foundation for scientific allopathic medicine in this country as which was previously ruled by various indigenous systems like Ayurveda, Siddha and Unani. The emergence of females in the medical field also happened due to the colonial influence. The Countess of Dufferin Fund established in India during 1885 provided scholarships for medical education to women. Notably Dr Anandibai Joshi was India's first female to qualify as a doctor in 1886, although she had a very untimely death. Two physicians, Dr Charlotte Ellaby and Dr Edith Peachy, British graduates, collaborated and established the first women only hospital in India in 1886. In 1883, Calcutta Medical college had the distinction of accepting the first female candidates into the medical sciences. In 1907, the Association of Medical women in India was set up marking a landmark achievement. There was a gradual increase in women entering the medical field in the 1930s-40s. The 1990s, the glorious age of television and mass media communications, witnessed the fastest rise in the percentage of women doctors in India. According to an article published in the *Indian Anthropologist* journal, the enrolment of women in graduate medical school was 50% in the 2010 (Bhadra, 2011) . However, the post-graduate as well as doctorate fields still tend to be male dominated. Female doctors represent a third of the doctorate field. An article published in a leading daily newspaper claims that only 17% of all allopathic doctors in India are females (Times of India, 2016). Administrative positions in the medical also tend to be dominated by men.

THE PRESENT SCENARIO

Enrolment has improved vastly in the last 3 decades as evidenced by the above statistics and is definitely one of the positive effects of globalization and westernization. The challenge is to understand the progression of female doctors once qualified. Is there evidence of parity and independent choice within specialties?

It appears that many women do not practice or progress with post graduate degrees once qualified. A major factor is the societal and familial pressure of marriage. The average Indian female is married by the age of 22-25 (Statista, 2014) . In fact, majority of the ladies get married soon after the completion of or even in the midst of their graduate degrees. Any progression once married is dependent on the desire of the husband and family. There is an expectation that any career aspirations must fit with the husband's career and family plans. Some women are made to study medicine to improve their marriage potential especially into a medical family which to an outsider may appear positively Victorian.

THE RURAL VS. URBAN SETTINGS

There is a stark contrast between the urban and rural settings within India. There are talented female leaders in the urban areas but the situation in rural India remains desolate at present. Many hopes are dashed and much talent is wasted as societal interference, early marriages and poor socio-economic status make it extremely difficult for the women in the semi-urban and rural areas to enter this lengthy and endurance-testing field. The patriarchal nature of society, ancient customs and inability to adapt to modern times are some of the common reasons challenging women to flourish in this field. There are instances where having entered medicine, women are forced to leave, so that they can switch to a shorter degree allowing them to become breadwinners earlier. The most important drawback is that people in the rural areas are very set in their customs and highly reluctant to change despite the logical evidence provided to the contrary.

HINDERANCES TO FEMALES IN THE MEDICAL FIELD

Most female doctors are encouraged to choose specialties that enable them to work office hours as they have family responsibilities. In India, women are primary caregivers for their husband, children and often by extension to their in-laws. The societal expectation is that the professional life is auxiliary to the role as a homemaker and carer. Therefore, women working in specialties such as Orthopaedics or Surgery with long irregular hours and shift work, face a tough time both professionally and personally. This results in very few women entering these fields (Sikdar, 2016).

A paper on women in medicine published by Dr Rakesh Chadda and Dr Mamata Sood of the All India institute of Medical sciences (AIIMS) says the there is a preponderance of women in the pre-clinical subjects like anatomy, physiology, pharmacology, pathology and microbiology (Chadda & Sood, 2010). According to this study, in basic and non-clinical sciences, women held 48 per cent of the faculty positions. The department of internal medicine had 22 per cent of women faculty, the figure reaching 35–50 per cent in other medical specialties like endocrinology, neurology, haematology, psychiatry and paediatrics. If one excluded the disciplines of obstetrics and gynaecology (66 per cent) and ophthalmology (32 per cent) from surgical branches, only 5 per cent of faculty positions in surgery were occupied by women (Chadda & Sood, 2010). This study also claims that the percentage of women faculty goes up if the department is headed by a woman (49% percent in departments headed by women versus 19% in department headed by men) (Chadda & Sood, 2010).

There are no published reports which suggest the actual percentages of the females enlisted in surgical fields in India. There are many situations where female surgeons have faced discrimination amongst their peers, superiors as well as the supporting staff. Recent literature published in the British Medical Journal and done in Canada has suggested that the outcomes of surgeries performed by female surgeons are better when compared to the males (Wallis, Ravi, Coburn, Nam, & Detsky, 2017). Despite this, archaic beliefs of surgeons being male figures still dominates the nation.

Sexual harassment and innuendoes are common day to day events in the life of female surgeons. The concept of gender equality and equity appears to be a distant dream in the surgical field with harassment and bullying being business as usual without challenge. Female doctors are thought to be unable to become surgeons due to an inability to make 'good' surgical decisions and due to reduced mental resilience. Current female surgeons are to be lauded in excelling in such a negative environment.

In many medical specialties, one would be expected to move to train and work. This is a major hindrance in India. In this country, a female should not live alone. A single female is at risk of both sexual harassment as well as injury. India is geographically large and there are 28 States and 7 Union territories. Each State has its own regional language and culture and Hindi may not be used by everyone which caused barriers to patient doctor relationships. It is also difficult for families to relocate but the trend is changing, and female doctors are now travelling both for further training as well as practice.

VIOLENCE AGAINST DOCTORS: AN EPIDEMIC IN INDIA

The most recent hinderance to gender equity has been the resurgence of violence against doctors in India. An ongoing study by Indian Medical Association (IMA) reports that 75 per cent of doctors in India have faced violence at some point of time in their life, and most of the time, it is verbal abuse (Ghosh, 2018). Certain local factors such as mob mentality and politicians play an important role in inciting violence which frequently develops into crisis in hospitals. Death of a loved one is often used by the local politicians as a show of strength by ransacking and damaging hospitals' property. This problem is very common in small primary health centres which lack facilities and where even trivial problems cannot be dealt with properly. A study done by Indla Ramasubba Reddy revealed that female doctors are more likely to face violence and that majority of the violent incidents arose from the Department of obstetrics and Gynaecology, which usually consists of a high percentage of female staffs, followed by the medicine department with allied specialties, and surgery with allied specialties (Reddy, Ukrani, Indla, & Ukrani, 2019).

STRATEGIES TO PROMOTE GENDER EQUITY IN THE WORK FORCE

Although progress has been made to develop gender equity, there is still a long way to go and the hurdles remain challenging. The Indian Department of Women and Child Health has suggested several strategies. Developmental policies and programmes, both in the women-specific and women-related sectors, that have been put into action through various Five-Year Plans, have brought forth a perceptible improvement in the socio-economic status of women in the country. `Empowerment of Women' being one of the nine primary objectives of the Ninth Plan, every effort is being made to create an enabling environment where women can freely exercise their rights both within and outside home, as equal partners along with men. This will be realised through early finalisation and adoption of the `National Policy for Empowerment of Women' which laid down definite goals, targets and policy prescriptions along with a well-defined Gender Development Index to monitor the impact of its implementation in raising the status of women from time to time (Government of India).

Although a lot of legislation does exist and numerous policies have been made to protect the interests of women in this country, a majority of the beneficiaries are not even aware of these. For India to maintain its position as a global growth leader, more concerted efforts at local and national levels, and by the private sector are needed to bring women to parity with men. Hence, the author recommends that out-reach strategies must be improved by the government so that maximum benefit may be availed. The Rashtriya Mahila Kosh (RMK) is a remarkable success story of reaching credit to the poor and asset-less women in the informal sector, through the medium of NGOs. The RMK has been networking with 170 NGOs to reach about 2 lakh women.

Leaving alone the government policies, a lot of strategies can be adopted by any individual and/or a small group in order to promote gender equity at the workplace.

The first and most important strategy is creating an awareness of female Indian, Asian and Global role models. Female leaders also serve as role models and raise educational and career aspirations for adolescent girls and their parents. This requires a digital and social revolution highlighting the current problems and possible solutions. It also engenders a support network so that stories can be shared. These stories #MeToo may reveal unknown problems that will need their own rapid solutions.

The second strategy is the need for female colleagues to support other women to become successful in their own rights. If women aid and assist each other, demonstrating that they are not on their own, a revolution will be created where there is benefit and improvement to the society as a whole. Prolific speaker Iyanla Vanzant said it best “The way to achieve your own success is to be willing to help somebody else get it first”. Who but a woman can better understand the predicament of another woman? Mentorship programs may be started in which female head of departments and in fact any other female in a position of authority can be taught how to be effective mentors.

The third and most important strategy is tackling the problem at the grassroot level. This can only be achieved by empowering the mothers and the other female family members of a girl child. After all, a mother knows what is best for her children.

STRATEGIES TO PREVENT VIOLENCE AGAINST DOCTORS

The need of the hour in this country, is to swiftly curb the rising trend of violence against doctors. Violence is particularly high in the states of Maharashtra and West Bengal with many doctors suffering grievous injuries that threatened their life as well as careers (Outllok Magazine, 2019). Protests are being made, rallies are being conducted in order to bring awareness on this issue and to violence against doctors a criminal offence with high penalty. Zero tolerance for violence against doctors is a must. Importantly, our public health system needs to be strengthened and made accountable. There needs to be open communication between patients and doctors on treatments and expected outcomes. There is need to give undergraduate and post-graduate doctors some grounding in behavioural sciences, to predict better patient behaviour. Almost every doctor is worried about violence at his/her workplace, and very few doctors are trained to avoid or deal with such situations.

CONCLUSION

The exposure of the issues above will increase the profile of female doctors and require further National strategies which at present are sadly lacking. Women specific interventions in all policies, programs and systems needs to be launched as national policy is influential both in terms of resetting societal norms as well as embedding the funds required strategies to improve early schooling of girls is in place but emphasis needs to shift to higher education especially in STEM fields.

G.D. Anderson states "Feminism isn't about making women strong. Women are already strong. Its about changing the way the world perceives that strength". The perception in India is slowly but surely changing. Increasing the visibility of Women leaders will only accelerate this change. It is essential that women come to the fore-front of the medical profession. The continued development of this profession demands women at its helm. Though India lags behind western standards with regards to gender equity, the fact remains that the past 60 years has been eye-opening and this country is fast on its way to a force to be reckoned with.

REFERENCES

Annan, K. (2005). Empowerment of Women is the Most Effective Development Tool.

Bala, N. (2014). The 3 Biggest Reasons that India's Girls Drop Out of School.

Bhadra, M. (2011, January). Indian women in medicine: An enquiry since 1880. *Indian Anthropologist*, *1*, 17.

Chadda, R., & Sood, M. (2010, June). Women in medicine: A perspective. *Indian Journal of Gender Studies*, *17*(2), 277–285. doi:10.1177/097152151001700204

Chandramouli, C., & General, R. (2011). *Census of India 2011*. Provisional Population Totals.

Ghosh, K. (2018, August). Violence against doctors: A wake-up call. *The Indian Journal of Medical Research*, *148*(2), 130. doi:10.4103/ijmr.IJMR_1299_17 PMID:30381535

Government of India . (n.d.). 9th Five Year Plan (Vol-2).

Outlook Magazine. (2019). *Bengal doctors' strike enters day 4*. Healthcare services hit in Delhi, Maharashtra too.

Reddy, I. R., Ukrani, J., Indla, V., & Ukrani, V. (2019). Violence against doctors: A viral epidemic? *Indian Journal of Psychiatry*, *61*(10). PMID:31040474

Sikdar, P. (2016). Women surgeons a vanishing tribe. Retrieved from https://timesofindia.indiatimes.com/life-style/health-fitness/health-news/Women-surgeons-a-vanishing-tribe/articleshow/51303079.cms

Singh, A. (2018). 39.4% of adolescent girls do not attend schools: NCPCR study.

Statista. (2014). Average age at marriage across rural and urban India in 2013-14, by gender.

Times of India. (2016). More women study medicine, but few practise.

Wallis, C., Ravi, B., Coburn, N., Nam, R. K., Detsky, A., & Satkunasivam, R. (2017). Comparison of postoperative outcomes among patients treated by male and female surgeons: A population based matched cohort study. *British Medical Journal*, *359*, j4366. doi:10.1136/bmj.j4366 PMID:29018008

Chapter 17
Gender Equity in Surgical Academia in Kuwait and the Arabian Gulf Region

Asmaa Al-Rashed
Al-Amiri Hospital, Kuwait

Maha Al-Gilani
Zain Hospital, Kuwait

ABSTRACT

Gender equity has been a topic of interest in medicine for decades; however, it has extended to include surgery, a field that has been dominated by men for centuries. Nowadays, gender inequity in surgery is a worldwide issue that needs to be addressed since significant disparities exist in the surgical field compared to the medical one. In this chapter, authors introduce the current status of Kuwait and the Gulf region regarding gender equality, and outline the history of women surgeons in the region. The evolution of medical education in surgery and the evolution of the healthcare system and how these relate to gender equity in surgical academia is presented. Challenges related to the uniqueness of the Arabic and the Islamic culture and the future directions of where the field of surgery is headed in relation to gender equity is discussed.

INTRODUCTION

Gender equity has been a topic of interest in medicine over the past decades; however, it has extended to include surgery, a field that has been dominated by men for centuries. Nowadays, gender inequity in surgery is a worldwide issue that needs to be addressed since significant disparities exist in the surgical field compared to the medical one.

In this chapter the authors will introduce the current status of Kuwait and the Gulf region regarding gender equality, and outline the history of women surgeons in the region. The evolution of medical education in surgery and the evolution of healthcare system and how these relate to gender equity in

DOI: 10.4018/978-1-5225-9599-1.ch017

surgical academia will be presented. Challenges related to the uniqueness of the Arabic and the Islamic culture and the future directions of where the field of surgery is headed in relation to gender equity will be discussed in this chapter.

BACKGROUND

The Arabian Gulf Region is located in the Middle East, and includes six countries; The State of Kuwait, The Kingdom of Saudi Arabia (KSA), The Kingdom of Bahrain, The State of Qatar, The United Arab Emirates (UAE) and Sultanate of Oman with a population of 54.6 million in 2017. These countries share religious and social bonds that are rooted into the Arabic and Islamic culture for centuries. In 1981, a Charter was signed as these countries have formed a political and economic alliance called the Gulf Cooperation Council (GCC) (GCC, n.d.); in realization of the unique global power this region holds with its strategic geographical location and its wealthy oil and natural gas resources and revenues. On the other hand, this region is situated in the center of the Middle East neighboring regions of conflict and facing ongoing challenges related to the regional and global struggle of power.

Where do the Gulf Countries Stand in Gender Equity Globally?

To appreciate gender equity in surgical academia in the Gulf region, we should start by clarifying where the Gulf countries sit compared to the rest of the world in gender equity in general. According to the United Nations Development Program (UNDP) report of 189 countries and territories in 2017, the Gulf countries have very high Human Development Index (HDI), with the UAE topping the Gulf countries in the 34th position, followed by Qatar in the 37th, KSA in the 39th, Bahrain in the 43rd, Oman in the 48th and Kuwait in the 56th position; however, when it came to gender equality, the Middle East and North Africa regions remained to rank last globally as measured by the Gender Inequality Index (GII) and the Gender Development Index (GDI). The GII reflects gender-based inequalities in three dimensions; reproductive health, empowerment, and economic activity; and the GDI measures gender inequalities in achievement in three basic dimensions of human development: health, education; and command over economic resources (UNDP, 2018; UNDP Human, 2018). In that report, the UAE continued to be the highest among the Gulf countries, ranking in the 120th position globally, as it has made remarkable improvement on gender parity in ministerial positions and wage equality for similar work and has closed the overall gender gaps by 65%; while Bahrain, ranked in the 126th position and have closed 63% of the overall gender gaps (Gulf Business, n.d.) Kuwait, Qatar and KSA ranked 126th, 130th and 138th, respectively. It is worth mentioning that in 2015, Kuwait has pledged to meet the UN Sustainable Goals including Gender Equity by 2030 and Bahrain, UAE and Qatar have resembling stands (UNDP, n.d.; UNDP "Kingdom of Bahrain", n.d.; Cookman n.d.; "Qatar UN Goals", n.d.). In the light of this report, it is imperative to appreciate that some political, legislative and cultural variations exist among the Gulf countries and that may have resulted in discrepancies in relation to the progression of gender equity in the medical profession and that the Gulf countries require more work to improve gender disparities overall.

THE JOURNEY OF WOMEN IN THE EVOLVING SURGICAL PROFESSION IN THE GULF REGION

History at a Glance

In the Middle Eastern, ancient Egyptian, Sumerian and Babylon historical explorations have revealed evidence of women practicing medicine and performing surgical procedures. In the Gulf region specifically, the Islamic history recognized Rufaida Al-Aslamia, who came from a family of physicians, as the first woman Muslim who practiced nursing and surgery treating soldiers in battles around 620 AD (Miller-Rosser et al., 2006). During the middle ages, women were pushed out of the medical profession in Europe up until the era of modern medicine, when women fought their way back into this profession relentlessly (Wynn et al., 2000).

In the western world, the first woman physician has graduated medical school from Geneva Medical College in New York in 1849, and then followed by the first woman to be recognized as a surgeon in the United States Army in 1863 (Wirtzfeld et al., 2009). While, pioneer women in the Middle East were recognized for the first time as women doctors in the 1930s. The first Arab women pioneers were from Egypt, Tunis and Lebanon, attaining their qualifications from the United Kingdom (UK), France and Lebanon, respectively, and then specializing in gynecology ("Coptic Medical Society", n.d; Beltaib et al., n.d.; "The Khalil Gibran", n.d.). The American University of Beirut Medical College in Lebanon, established in 1867, was the first university in the Middle East to enroll and graduate a female doctor in the region in 1931 (Ghossain et al., 2003).

Evolution of Medical Education

The development of medical education and healthcare systems began as the Gulf countries were influenced by the British and American missionaries in the region in the beginning of the late 19th century to the early 20th century. These missionaries have introduced the concepts of modern medicine, surgery, anesthesia and preventive medicine that led to the construction of health centers in some Gulf countries ("Ministry of Health Kuwait" n.d.). Back then, some of the Gulf countries have sent high school graduates on scholarships to pursue medical education in neighboring countries such as Egypt, Lebanon, Iraq and then later to Europe, until the establishment of local medical schools and the construction of health care facilities. Kuwait and KSA have trail blazed the evolution of the healthcare systems and the medical education in the region. Evolution of civil law with the Health Act and legislations has expedited this process in Kuwait. In 1969, the first medical school in the Gulf region was opened in King Saud University in KSA (Al-Awami et al., 2000) but women medical students were accepted in 1975 (Baqi et al., 2017). On the other hand, the Faculty of Medicine in Kuwait University was established in 1973 ("Kuwait University", n.d.) and has accepted women and men in its first batch of students making it the first university in the Gulf to enroll women on its first batch at that time.

In 1979, the General Convention of Arab Education for the GCC decided to establish the Arabian Gulf University (AGU) in the Kingdom of Bahrain. The College of Medicine and Medical Sciences in the AGU has accepted it first batch in 1982. More medical schools have opened in KSA and the first in UAE and Oman in 1984 and 1986respectively. By the late 1980s, the Gulf countries had local medical schools for undergraduate medical education, except for Qatar, which had its first medical school in 2001 ("Arabian Gulf University" n.d.; "Oman Med School", n.d.; "Qatar Med School" n.d.). Today, there are a total of 37 public and private medical schools in the Gulf region enrolling both genders ("Wikipedia Medical School List," n.d.).

The Evolution of Postgraduate Education in Surgery in the Gulf Region

The region has encountered a rapid evolution in the postgraduate medical education (PGME) between the late 1970s to the mid 1980's that offered variable routes to new medical graduates to develop their professional career. These routes were (1) scholarships to Europe or North America for residency programs, or (2) local clinical training (in mentorship style) and then entrance to the fellowship of the Royal Colleges of Surgeons (England and Ireland) for qualifications or (3) enter a local PGME program.

Pioneer Local Surgical Programs in the Gulf

Arab Board

The first PGME program in the Gulf region has started with the foundation of the Arab Board of Medical Specializations by the Council of Arab Health Ministers in 1978 ("Arab Board Web", n.d.) This board accepted candidates from all the Arab countries. The first batch accepted for surgical training was in 1982. The surgical program was structured over 5-year period, instruction languages were English, Arabic or French, and it required written and oral examinations and logbook completion prior to certification. Examinations centers were located in many Arab countries.

King Faisal University Fellowship

The first postgraduate general surgery program in KSA was in King Faisal University in Dammam and has started to accept trainees in surgery in 1983 and it was structured for 5½ years with academic and clinical rotations. In 1993, the Saudi Council for the Health Specialties was established to supervise and regulate all aspects related to the PGME programs, Continuous Medical Education (CME) and accreditation in KSA.

Kuwait Boards of Surgery (KBS)

The foundation of the Kuwait Boards of Surgery was with the Kuwait Institution for Medical Specialization (KIMS) establishment in 1984 ("Kuwait Institute", n.d.). The board was structured over 5 years period. The first admission of female in this board was in 1987.

It is worth mentioning that in 1990, the Iraqi militant invasion to Kuwait has destroyed the infrastructure and disrupted the medical education and training in the country. This has adversely affected the relationship between some of the Arab countries and that has reflected on all forms of collaborations including the medical education and training. Rebuilding and restoring the educational and health care system in Kuwait has required many years. Today, KIMS supervises and regulates the PGME programs, CME and accreditation, and the Arab Board programs are not present in Kuwait. However, the Arab Board training programs remain to run in some Arab and Gulf countries such as Bahrain, UAE and Qatar.

Women in Surgery in the Gulf

Pioneer women from the Gulf region entered the surgical arena as early as 1984 and then have earned their qualifications from the Royal College of Surgeons in 1987 (KSA), 1988 (Kuwait), 1992 (Bahrain) and 1993 (UAE), while their men counterparts had earned their qualifications in the late 1960s. Ever since, more women followed suit and pursued their surgical training locally in their homeland as well as internationally.

Scholarships Programs

By the end of the millennium and the start of a new one, scholarships to surgical programs have accepted many applicants and opened the doors to women to explore surgery in different parts of the world in all surgical specialties. Women surgeons in the Gulf have obtained qualifications in many surgical specialties from North America, Europe, Asia and Australia and have returned home bringing back refined surgical expertise and diverse culture to the surgical profession in the Gulf.

The Current Status of Gender Equity in Surgery in Kuwait and the Gulf

Undergraduate Medical Education

Kuwait has one Faculty of Medicine in Kuwait University and Health Science Centre and since the abandoning of the 50:50 gender-seat-allocation rule in 2011, the enrollment of female to male ratio has increased and 60% of the medical student graduates were females by 2018. Similar increase in numbers of women medical students was noticed across the Gulf countries. In one article titled Growth in the Number of Female Medical Doctors in Oman, What are the reasons? the author mentioned that Oman Medical College has admitted 86% women medical students in 2010 (Goveas et al., 2012). The Arabian Gulf University, located in the Kingdom of Bahrain, reported female medical graduates constitute 74% of all graduates in 2012. The rest of the Gulf countries have similar rates of women entering and graduating medical schools that matched those rates of the developed world. The authors could confidently state that a significant progress in gender equity in the undergraduate medical education in the Gulf countries has been made.

Training Surgical Programs

In 2018, Kuwait Institution for Medical Specialization (KIMS) reported women in surgical training constitute 21.6% of all surgical trainees, while the Saudi Council for Health Specialties (SCHS) data reported numbers of women in surgical training in KSA to be 27% in the same year ("Saudi Council" n.d.). Data from the Department of Surgery at Salmaniya Medical Complex in Bahrain showed that women in surgical training counts for 39.2% of all trainees in 2019. Interestingly, in 2019 women residents' graduates were 46.6% from general surgery program, 63% of residents in-training and the new candidate accepted for 2019-2020 were 70% in Omani Boards of Surgery.

A basic fact such as the numbers of residents/fellows in surgical training programs will help appreciate the status of gender equity. However, as discussed earlier, the training through local postgraduate surgical programs is only one route in the Gulf, and some doctors go on scholarship abroad. Many institutions in the Gulf are permitted to sponsor these scholarships, such as universities, ministries of health, ministries of defense and private hospitals and in the absence of centralization of the data of these doctors; acquisition of the numbers is difficult. Although women medical students and surgical residents from the Gulf region on scholarships abroad were not included in this chapter, the overall numbers of women in training in the surgical specialties has shown a growth comparable to the current numbers of women surgeons in practice as will be discussed later in this chapter.

Enrollment in Surgical Programs

The authors have inquired about enrollment rates in the PGME surgical programs in KIMS. Information about the number of applicants from both genders and the number of accepted candidates from both genders over the last five years was requested. Based on the above information, it is unclear if biases related to gender are present in candidate selection into surgical programs and further information is needed. No data from the Gulf countries available.

Completion of Training and Examination

In 2018, KIMS data showed that the pass rates of the surgical programs candidates were 100% for the first takers of Kuwait Board of Surgery, Kuwait Board of Urology and Kuwait Board of Otorhinolaryngology examinations, and women graduates represented 30%, 50% and 50% of the candidates in these programs respectively. No further data available about the rates of completion of training and examination in previous years by the time of writing this chapter; however, we are aware that the data exists and requires time to be obtained. No data from the Gulf countries available.

WHAT'S OUT THERE FOR WOMEN SURGEONS IN ACADEMIA?

Faculty Positions

Kuwait has only one College of Medicine with a total of only 20 faculty members in the department of surgery ("Kuwait University Health Sciences Center", 2018-2019). This has posed a challenge to those interested in academic positions, as the number of full-time faculty members is small. Women surgeons represent 10% of the faculty members and are in the positions of assistant and associate professor. One female surgeon has held two faculty positions in two universities in KSA prior to moving to Kuwait. She also has held a Chairperson of Department of Surgery position in Kuwait between 2009-2014.

The Kingdom of Saudi Arabia has the largest numbers of medical schools in the Gulf region (a total of 25 medical schools and many PGME programs) and that potentially offer various academic opportunities to men and women.

In the Gulf region, many women surgeons are holding academic positions such as assistant, associate and professor of surgery, researcher and chairperson of surgical departments; as the authors will show in a survey conducted later in this chapter; however, the precise numbers of those faculty positions are not available.

Directors of Surgical Board Programs

In Kuwait, there are six surgical residency programs (excluding gynecology), general surgery, otorhinolaryngology, urology, orthopedics, neurosurgery and ophthalmology. All surgical program directors were men except for the years 2014-2015, when there was a single woman program director. The surgical foundations program has a single woman assistant program director since 2017 to date.

The authors are aware that there are women surgeons holding the positions of program director and assistant program director in Bahrain, UAE, Qatar, KSA and Oman; however, the exact data is not available at the time of writing this chapter. Similarly, the numbers of women surgeons in roles such as clinical site coordinators, clinical tutors and clinical lecturers are not available in KIMS or in the Gulf.

The Clinical Practice

Kuwait laws and regulations permit physicians and surgeons to work in the government and part-time in the private sector concurrently. With that in mind, the Medical Licensing Administration reported that Kuwaiti women surgeons working in the private sector represented 12% compared to 88% of their men counterparts; whereas, the total women surgeons (Kuwaitis and Non-Kuwaitis) represents only 7.3% of all the surgeons in the private sector in 2019 [32]. Moreover, data from the Ministry of Health (MOH) estimated that women surgeons working in the government sector to be 9.3% in 2018. Bearing these rules and regulations in mind, conclusion about which sector maybe more appealing to women surgeons can't be withdrawn.

In Bahrain, the Department of Surgery at Salmaniya Medical Complex, a government hospital, data showed qualified women surgeons to count for only 10.7% of its surgeons in May 2019, while the Saudi Council for Health Specialties (SCHS) data reported 20% of qualified women surgeons in practice in 2018 ("Saudi Council for Health Specialties", 2019).

Looking at the numbers of women in surgery then and now, Kuwait has 9.3% women surgeons in practice and 21.6% in training, KSA has 20% in practice and 27% in training ("Saudi Council for Health Specialties", 2019) and Bahrain has 10.7% in practice and 39.2% in training. These numbers demonstrate that perhaps Bahrain seems to show the highest growth rate of women training in surgery; however, the authors are aware that both KSA and Kuwait send doctors abroad for training in higher numbers than Bahrain does, which most likely dilute the presented numbers of the residents/fellows in training compared to Bahrain, and that the numbers were only from one health centre in Bahrain. Overall, when comparing the numbers of women surgeons in practice today and the numbers of women in surgical training, the authors found that the numbers have increased but the question remains if these numbers add-up to be considered as a significant growth that will tighten the gender gap in surgery, further studies and transparency of data is needed to be able to answer that question.

Administrative Roles

Many women surgeons hold administrative roles where they work, however, no published data available to date to address the issue of gender inequity in this area.

Leadership Positions

Although women remain a minority in the surgical field in the Gulf countries, many of those women surgeons have attained high ranks in the leadership positions in their countries and have achieved local, regional and international recognition and held international leadership positions. In May 2019, the authors have conducted a survey about pioneer women surgeons in the Gulf countries with a total of 51 responses from five of the Gulf countries. Surgical subspecialties represented were general surgery 29.4%, ENT 15.7%, ophthalmology 15.7%, gynecology 11.8%, pediatric surgery 9.8%, plastic surgery 9.8%, orthopedics 9.8%, urology 3.9% and neurosurgery 2%. About 68% had subspecialty qualifications in addition to their primary surgical specialties, 52% had one subspecialty, 26% had two, 6% had three and 2% had more than three additional subspecialties. When asked about holding a leadership position(s), 72.5% of the women surgeons surveyed mentioned that they have held leadership positions, whereas, 27.5% have never held any leadership position. The positions which were held by the women surveyed were: 21.6% department chairperson, 21.6% section/division chief, 33.3% program director/assistant program director, 13.7% hospital administration, 23% president or vice-president of national societies, 23% researcher and 17.6% have held others leadership positions. Those who held leadership positions were likely to hold more than one position with most of these leadership positions being academic and administrative. More data is necessary to objectively evaluate where women stands in leadership comparable to their counterparts in surgery.

Challenges in Gender Equity in Surgical Academia in the Gulf Region

As mentioned in the beginning of this chapter, the Gulf region is unique in its cultural roots and although the Islamic religion gave women their rights thousands of years ago, the culture and willingness to protect women has unfortunately been the reason that has delayed entrance of women in surgical fields in the region. Some of the challenges that face women in our region were perception of surgery as a male-dominated field, issues of society trusting a woman's abilities to be a surgeon, long hours and higher stress in the work environment along with concerns regarding family planning and social norms. On the other hand, some challenges identified in the western world may not hold true for women in our region, such as equal pay. In the Gulf, women are paid equally to men throughout their medical career.

Equal Payment

Let's talk about equal pay. In the Gulf region, there is a clear pay structure for physicians in all levels of their career and this does not discriminate women and men. So thankfully equal pay has been established since day one. However, in the private sector, there is much place for negotiation of pay at private hospitals and that lays on the surgeon's personality and their negotiation skills. The authors do not have exact data on pay disparities in the private practice so no comment on that can be made.

Attrition

Since no published data are available about attrition rates in surgical programs in Kuwait, the authors have inquired about attrition in a correspondance with KIMS. There have been 2 documented withdrawals from surgical programs; one male at PGY3 level and one female at PGY-1 level in 2015 and 2017 from different surgical programs. No further information is available about the destination of those residents after withdrawal such as change into another surgical or medical specialties or quitting the medical profession nor the causes for the withdrawal. Although the numbers of withdrawal were low, more information is required to better evaluate the reasons of attritions in the training and if gender inequity was a contributor.

Intimidation and Harassment

Intimidation and harassment are not uncommon in the surgical field and both genders can be affected or involved. In Kuwait, KIMS has strict policy on the professional conduct and the procedure of reporting and investigating these claims or actions during training("Kuwait Institute for Medical Specialities", 2016-2017). However, there are no published data about this area. Similar policies exist under the Ministry of Health and Kuwait law; however, no available data to comment if intimidation and harassment is a factor for gender equity in surgical academia.

Social Responsibilities, Culture, and Tradition

There is a common expectation that comes with tradition and culture that women are responsible for the 'home making'. Their responsibilities extend to taking care of the home, the husband and children whereas the man is the moneymaker. As this has been for years in the western countries prior to the women rights movements and the women suffrage in the USA, it holds true in the Gulf region. In the Gulf region, families used to live in large family homes where the women would live with their in-laws in a large extended family situation. This system is very helpful in the fact that the women in the household usually share responsibilities. However, there are social obligations that are expected from the daughter in law, other than the usual home making responsibilities. These social responsibilities include but not limited to attending social events for her in-laws and her own family, as well as help organize them. This is important to note, as these larger extended family homes don't exist in the same structure as they did in the past, but the social obligations still stand true. Most households in the Gulf countries are still very traditional, where the woman is expected to do all the home making and child caring responsibilities even if she had her own career, while men are in charge of working outside the home. Many younger couples are changing this concept by sharing responsibilities of the home but still most of the burden does lie within the women. This is uniquely a very cultural and non-Islamic way of living. Prophet Mohammed -peace be upon him- has always helped his wives in their household duties and has encouraged men to do so but these gender roles that have dominated after his passing have developed due to culture and tradition.

While most household responsibilities lie on the shoulder of the women, outsourcing some of these duties is feasible with the local domestic labor that is usually affordable for women in the Gulf regions. This may help reduce some of the household workload for working mothers; however, the supervision of these domestic workers still is considered a woman's duty.

Perspectives of Society

In addition, the society may have doubted the abilities of women surgeons and may have not chosen women as their physicians in the beginning. Although women physicians are sought in our society for obstetrics and gynecological problems, that may not hold true for other specialties. The authors do not have data comparing numbers and genders of patients attending women vs. men surgeon clinics at the time of writing the chapter. However, there is a common perception among physicians that patients will not pursue a woman as their surgeon from a survey that the authors have conducted and will be discussed shortly.

Perspectives Within the Medical Profession

To identify the perception of gender issues in surgery, an online anonymous survey was distributed to physicians in the Gulf region regardless of their specialty in June 2019. The researchers collected demographics as well as specialty and position information. They had 390 respondents. Majority of which were women (70.7%). The majority of the participants were surgeons (43.9%) and from Kuwait 66.9%). There were participants from Saudi Arabia, United Arab Emirates, Oman, Qatar and Bahrain as well. There were 53.8% married participants and 52% had children. It was noted that 80% of the men were married while 42% of the women were married. See tables for more details.

Table 1. Demographics of the participants in the gender equity in surgical academia in the Gulf survey

Demographics		%	Number
Gender	Female	70.7	276
	Male	29.3	114
Age (years)	20-29	37.9	148
	30-39	27.2	106
	40-49	22	86
	50-59	10.3	40
	60-69	2.6	10
Marital Status	Single	44.1	172
	Married	53.8	210
	Divorced	2.1	8
Profession	Surgical Specialty	43.9	171
	Medical Specialty WITH procedural	18	70
	Medical Specialty WITHOUT procedural	22	86
	Dental	11.5	45
	Medical students	3.8	15
	Nursing	0.8	3
Country	Kuwait	66.9	261
	Saudi Arabia	11.8	46
	Bahrain	5.9	23
	United Arab Emirates	4.9	19
	Oman	3.6	14
	Qatar	1	4
	Others	5.9	23

The majority of participants believed there was no gender discrimination in salary pay, recognition or financial reimbursement for extra work. This is very similar to another study conducted at a government university hospital of 1015 doctors in Kingdom Saudi Arabia in 2017.

The participants have been equivocal when asked about the likelihood of women being accepted in surgical programs, where approximately a third were pretty neutral about their opinion and a third felt women had equal chances of being accepted into surgical programs while a third believed women had less chances of being accepted into surgical programs.

When the issue of attrition of women in surgery was addressed, about 41% of participants believed that women were more likely to drop out of surgical residency than men. As discussed earlier, data about attrition are limited, till the time of writing this chapter. The surgical literature has found that women had higher rates of attrition compared to men (Alghamdi et al., 2014; Albakr et al., 2017).

The participants were asked whether they felt that lack of women role models in surgical academia could be a challenge for women in surgery. Results showed that 26% were neutral, 34% felt this was not a challenge while 40% did feel this is a challenge for women in surgery. In the survey, 40% of the participants felt that lack of mentors for women in surgery poses a challenge for women in comparison to their men counterparts.

Interestingly, 48% of the participants believed women had the required personality of a Surgeon. As well, 54% believed that women were as proactive as men. Regarding harassment, 55% believe that women are more subjected to harassment than men. With subgroup analysis, women were more likely to agree that women were more subject to harassment with 47% of men agreeing to that and 59% of women.

The researchers also asked whether society expectations of women to be mothers and wives could be a challenge. Surprisingly 59% have felt that this is truly a challenge with slightly more women (64%) agreeing to that than men (48%). In addition, 45% of participants believe patients will not seek a woman surgeon with 59% of women vs 49% of men agreeing to that, and 53% of the participants believed being a parent poses a challenge for surgical careers and that was similar amongst men (49%) and women (53%) as well as those who had children (55%) vs. those who do not have children (50%).

WHAT CAN WE DO TO CREATE GENDER-BALANCE IN SURGICAL ACADEMIA?

Shared Social Responsibilities

Despite the complexity of the region, there are many programs under way. As mentioned above, shared responsibilities in the household is becoming the trend among younger couples and that will be helpful in reducing the stress and burden on the working mother in general and the woman surgeon specifically. Raising awareness in the society is needed.

Institutional Level Changes Supporting Gender Equity

There are many legislative regulations that can support women in their surgical careers in Kuwait. KIMS has explicit policy and procedure on leaves during residency and fellowships. Female residents or fellows are allowed 30 days of maternity leave twice during residency and once during fellowship. Female widow grieving leave are allowed to Muslim female resident upon the spouse's death for 4 months and 10 days as per Civil Service Commission rules and regulations ("Kuwait Institute for Medical Specialties" 2016-2017) as this is based on religious grounds.

It's important to note that Kuwait Civil Service Commission rules and regulations has an excellent program by the government designed to support all working women. Pregnant women are allowed to work two hours less a day starting from the 7th month of pregnancy till its termination. In addition, Kuwaiti women are given 3 months of maternity leave with full pay and then an optional 3 months with half pay. Women are also given a 2-hour reduction in work hours till their child reaches two years of age. The decree clearly states that these reductions should not influence performance evaluations.

In KSA, women are given 2 months of maternity leave at full pay then can get up to three years at a reduced pay which is different according to the length of leave. Women are also given two hours of reduced work hours till their child reaches two years of age. It is important to note that these rules and regulations do not roll over to cover residents in KSA and that residents have only 4 weeks of leave.

In the view of gender equity in the Gulf region, the authors believe that paternity leave for residents, fellows and working men should be considered, as it will likely provide further support to female and male residents and fellows in the demanding surgical training and practice.

Professional Societies' Level Changes Supporting Gender Equity

In 2018, women surgeons in Kuwait have collaborated and established the Women Surgeon Committee (WSC) that aims to empower, aspire and support women surgeons in fulfilling their personal and professional potentials and they have the support of the Kuwait Association of Surgeons and the Kuwait Surgical Society. Oman Surgical Society shares similar vision with the appointing of the first president women surgeon in 2018.

Supporting women in those roles is essential to close the gap in gender equity in surgery in our region.

CONCLUSION

In conclusion, to be able to state where we stand in gender equity in surgical academia objectively in the Gulf region, it is important to better assess both genders' perspectives on the issue within the surgical and medical professions utilizing tools such as research, and then it is imperative to be able to identify the challenges and areas that necessitate improvement in surgical training and clinical practice, and lastly to support and empower institutions and professional societies to collaborate to implement solutions geared toward gender balanced environment nationally and regionally. The authors believe that the gaps in gender equity in surgery and surgical academia are still present today for women in the Gulf countries and the Middle East; however, these gaps are comparable to those in leading countries in the world. More work is needed to close these gaps and achieve gender equity in surgery.

Challenges to Writing the Chapter

Data about gender equity in surgery in the Gulf is scarce, additionally; obtaining data from six countries of the Gulf was challenging due to logistics of data sharing and time constraints.

ACKNOWLEDGMENT

Dr. Fayza Haidar, Dr. Abdulaziz Al-Saif, Dr. Zainab Al-Balushi, Saudi Council for Health Specialties (SCFHS), Kuwait Institution for Medical Specialization (KIMS).

REFERENCES

Al-Awami, S. M. (2000). Surgery in Saudi Arabia. *Archives of Surgery (Chicago, Ill.)*, *135*(3), 354–357. doi:10.1001/archsurg.135.3.354 PMID:10722041

Albakr, F., Bruce, E., Davidson, P., Schlaffer, E., & Kropiunigg, U. (2017). Empowered but not equal: Challenging the traditional gender roles as seen by university students in Saudi Arabia. *Forum for International Research in Education*, *4*(1), 52-66.

Alghamdi, T. (2014). Balance between career and family among female doctors at KAMC, Riyadh, Saudi Arabia. *International Journal of Medical Science and Public Health*, *3*(2), 203–211. doi:10.5455/ijmsph.2013.021220133

Arab board web. *About the Board.* Available at http://arab-board.org/en/content/about-board

Arabian Gulf University. *Homepage*. Available at http://www.agu.edu.bh/english/university/uni_facts.aspx

Arabian Gulf University. *University Facts*. Available at http://www.agu.edu.bh/english/university/uni_facts.aspx

Baqi, S., Albalbeesi, A., Iftikhar, S., Baig-Ansari, N., Alanazi, M., & Alanazi, A. (2017, October). Perceptions of gender equality, work environment, support and social issues for women doctors at a university hospital in Riyadh, Kingdom of Saudi Arabia. *PLoS One*, *12*(10). doi:10.1371/journal.pone.0186896 PMID:29073172

Beltaib, M. (n.d.). *Tunisia's First Female Doctor: The Life of Tawhida Belsheikh.* Available at https://raseef22.com/article/1068287-tunisias-first-female-doctor-life-tawhida-belsheikh

Gulf Business. (n.d.). *UAE, Bahrain, Saudi rise, Kuwait, Qatar fall in gender equality ranking*. Available at https://gulfbusiness.com/uae-bahrain-saudi-climb-kuwait-qatar-fall-gender-equality-ranking/

Cookman, L. (n.d.). *UAE ranks highest for gender equality in GCC, says Human Development Report.* Available at https://www.thenational.ae/uae/uae-ranks-highest-for-gender-equality-in-gcc-says-human-development-report-1.737261

Coptic Medical Society UK. (n.d.). *Dr. Helena Sidarous*. Available at http://copticmedical.com/dr-helena-sidarous/

GCC. (n.d.). *Population-STAT*. [Online].

GCC. (n.d.). *GCC Charter*. Available at http://www.gcc-sg.org/en-us/Pages/default.aspx

Ghossain, A., Freiha, F., & Geahchan, N. (2003). Surgery in Lebanon. *Archives of Surgery (Chicago, Ill.)*, *138*(2), 215–219. doi:10.1001/archsurg.138.2.215 PMID:12578423

Goveas, S. (2012, August). Growth in the Number of Female Medical Doctors in Oman. What are the reasons? *Sultan Qaboos University Medical Journal*, *12*(3), 380–381. doi:10.12816/0003159 PMID:23269954

Kuwait Institute for Medical Specialties. (2016-2017). Manual of Policies for postgraduate. *Medical Education*.

Kuwait Institute for Medical Specialties. About KIMS. Available at https://www.kims.org.kw

Kuwait University. *Faculty of Medicine Homepage*. Available at http://www.hsc.edu.kw/FOM/

Kuwait University Health Sciences Center. *Undergraduate Handbook*. 2018-2019.

Medical Licensing Administration at Ministry of Health. (2019). *Physician Statistics*. Kuwait.

Miller-Rosser, K., Chapman, Y., Francis, K. (2006). Historical, Cultural, and Contemporary Influences on the Status of Women in Nursing in Saudi Arabia. *The Online Journal of Issues in Nursing*, 2006, 11(3).

Ministry of Health Kuwait. *MOH website history: Historical Overview*. Available at https://www.moh.gov.kw/en/Pages/Aboutus.aspx

Oman medical school. *Homepage*. Available at https://www.squ.edu.om/medicine/About-College/About-CoMHS/History

Qatar med school. *Homepage*. Available at http://qatar-weill.cornell.edu/about-us/overview/weill-cornell-medicine-qatar

Saudi Council for Health Specialties. *SCHS document on Residents statistics*. 2019.

The Khalil Gibran Chair for Values and Peace. *Dr. Edma Abou Chedid*. Available at https://pioneersandleaders.org/women-pioneers/dr-edma-abou-chedid

UAE med school. *Homepage*. Available at https://cmhs.uaeu.ac.ae/en/index.shtml

UN. (n.d.). *Qatar UN goals Qatar: Taking Action for Sustainable Development*. Available at https://www.un.org/sustainabledevelopment/wp-content/uploads/2017/07/Qatar_Govt.pdf

UNDP. (2018). *Human Development Indices and Indicators: 2018 Statistical Update*. Available at http://hdr.undp.org/sites/all/themes/hdr_theme/country-notes.pdf

UNDP. (2018). *Human Development Indices and Indicators: 2018 Statistical Update, Kuwait*. Available at http://hdr.undp.org/sites/all/themes/hdr_theme/country-notes/KWT.pdf

UNDP. (n.d.). *Support Kuwait's implementation of SDG 5*. Available at http://www.kw.undp.org/content/kuwait/en/home/projects/support-kuwait_s-implementation-of-sdg-5.html

UNDP. (n.d.). *Kingdom of Bahrain. Sustainable Goals. Goal 5: Gender Equality. Bahrain UN goals* Available at http://www.bh.undp.org/content/bahrain/en/home/sustainable-development-goals/goal-5-gender-equality.html

Wikipedia. Medical Schools List. Available at https://en.wikipedia.org/wiki/List_of_medical_schools_in_the_Middle_East

Wirtzfeld, D. (2009, August). The History of women in surgery. *Canadian Journal of Surgery*, *52*(4), 317–320. PMID:19680519

Wynn, R. (2000). Saints and Sinners: Women and the Practice of Medicine Throughout the Ages. *Journal of the American Medical Association*, *283*(5), 668–669. doi:10.1001/jama.283.5.668-JMS0202-4-1 PMID:10665711

Chapter 18
Gender Inequity in the United States Surgical Workforce

Christine A. Heisler
University of Wisconsin, USA

Elizabeth H. Stephens
Ann & Robert H Lurie Children's Hospital Northwestern Medical Center, USA

Sarah M. Temkin
Anne Arundel Medical Center, USA

Pringl Miller
Rush University Medical Center, USA

ABSTRACT

Despite the consistently reported gender parity among accepted applicants to US medical schools, upstream parity in surgical training, academic promotion, leadership positions, pay equity, grant funding, and efforts to promote wellness specific to the needs of women surgeons is seriously lacking. Along with these known disparities, women surgeons disproportionally suffer from gender bias, micro-aggressions, bullying, discrimination, and harassment that together create an unjust, unsafe, undignified, intolerable if not hostile work environment. This chapter will explore these issues and offer a landscape that will set the stage for future initiatives to invoke change.

UNITED STATES SURGICAL LANDSCAPE

Looking at the historical tapestry of surgery, one expects to see a thick-woven carpet of rugged masculinity with a smattering of recently added fibers of feminine thread. However, the history of women in surgery extends back 170 years, with Dr. Elizabeth Blackwell matriculating first in her class in 1849 (Ali & McVay, 2016). One of the most well-known women in surgery, Dr. Mary Edwards Walker, graduated from medical school in 1855. Although a surgeon by training, Dr. Walker was referred to as a battlefield

DOI: 10.4018/978-1-5225-9599-1.ch018

nurse during the Civil War and was the only woman awarded a Congressional Medal of Honor (Rutkow, 2000). The pervasive misperception that surgery is a male profession led early women surgeons to disguise themselves as men in order to practice (de Costa, Chen-Xu, Bentounsi, & Vervoot, 2018). Many women have since followed in Dr. Blackwell's and Dr. Walker's footsteps, with the proportion of women entering medical school increasing to nearly 50% in 2008 (Sexton et al., 2012). Unfortunately, the journey to establish parity in surgical training programs has been slow and fraught with obstacles such that women remain a minority in most surgical specialities.

Surgical residencies have historically not attracted equal numbers of women. Although the proportion of women entering into general surgery residencies has increased for United States Medical Graduates (USMG) more recently to 32-40% (Davis, Risucci, Blair, & Schdeva, 2011), parity among the sexes is not anticipated until 2028 (Frangou, 2018). Despite more women entering surgical residency, the rate of attrition among women in their fourth year of residency is higher than for men (24% vs. 17%) (Yeo et al., 2018) and women surgical residents are less likely to reach board certification (Greenberg, 2017). Certain surgical specialties continue to have marked gender disparity, such as cardio-thoracic surgery (5% women), neurosurgery (5% women) and orthopedic surgery (6.5% women) (Stephens et al., 2016; Spetzler, 2011; Brown, Erdman, Munger, & Miller, 2019). The reasons for gender disparity vary slightly according to specialty but generally include work-life balance, lack of mentorship and role models, lack of support for childbearing and parenting, and culture not conducive to females (Donington, Litle, Sesti, & Colson, 2012; Reed et al., 2010; Vaporciyan et al., 2009).

Research focused on medical students has demonstrated that mentorship and role models are key factors in specialty selection (Schmidt, Cooper, & Guo, 2016). Women faculty mentors are limited to absent in many surgical specialties (Valsangkar et al., 2016), having the effect of dissuading even interested women students from choosing those particular surgical subspecialties. In addition, medical students most closely interact with residents while on surgical rotations. Since women surgical residents are 1.6 times more likely to experience burnout (Elmore, Jeffe, Jin, Awad, & Turnbull, 2016) or be clinically depressed and have higher attrition rates (Greenberg, 2017) than male peers, women medical students may be less likely to choose surgical specialties due to negative associations while on surgical services. Various minority organizations within specialties have sought to provide women students with exposure to and mentorship within their surgical specialty to counteract these issues.

Surgical Identity as Women

Women surgical trainees and faculty face a daily struggle to be recognized and respected as surgeons. #ILookLikeASurgeon is a social media movement started in 2015 designed to bring visibility to women in surgery. In just 3 months this prompted 128 million impressions and 40,000 individual tweets (Hughes, 2015). The related New Yorker magazine cover challenged women to replicate real life images of themselves in the Operating Theatre emulating the cover by artist Malika Favre depicting four female faces overlooking a patient and labelling their photo with #ILookLikeASurgeon (Mouly & Bormes, 2017). Both movements demonstrate the desire for women to be recognized as surgeons and the difficulty of developing a surgical identity as a woman. While successful, the hashtag itself highlights the fundamental problem that women have to prove that they *look like* a surgeon and *are* surgeons. In addition to being *seen* as surgeons, women in surgery want to be treated equitably, respected, and included in the surgical fraternity to which they belong, a much more challenging proposition.

There is clear evidence across careers that women think, interact, and learn differently. While it may be easier for women to adapt and attempt to fit in, they are perceived as outsiders on the basis of gender alone, and acknowledging and understanding such gender differences allows women to better cope with the stressors related to training and practice. There is a well-documented confidence gap between genders across occupations in which women project less confidence for the same level of skill as men (Kay & Shipman, 2014; Estes & Felker, 2012). Such a confidence gap can put women at a significant disadvantage in a profession like surgery that rewards confidence. Imposter syndrome refers to a syndrome in which one doubts her abilities and accomplishments and is fearful she will be exposed as a fraud (Koven, 2017). Imposter syndrome is more common among women (Botkus, Serchen, Moyer, Bornstein, & Hingle, 2018) and is itself associated with denigration of one's strengths and confidence.

Stereotype threat is another challenge that may impact women surgeons navigating their professional identity. Stereotype threat refers to individuals conforming to a socially accepted stereotype, which has been shown to impact performance (Salles, Mueller, & Cohen, 2016). For women working in environments that do not respect women as surgeons, it would be expected that their work performance suffers. Studies have shown that the mere presence of other people can evoke performance change, i.e., females taking math exams do worse in the presence of men (Inzlicht & Ben-Zeev, 2000).

Unconscious gender bias significantly affects women in surgery at every stage of career development. From training through practice, a woman surgeon's ability to garner respect in the workplace and establish credible relationships with her patients and their families is often challenged in ways that are different than for her male colleagues. Research on unconscious bias demonstrates that something as seemingly insignificant as word choice reveals and propagates unconscious bias. The website #BiasCorrect helps uncover unconscious gender bias (#BiasCorrect, 2019). For example, a female surgeon who is speaking up in a group setting may be described as pushy while the same behavior by a male surgeon is described as persuasive. Figure 1 demonstrates how a negative connotation is assigned to a word when used to describe a woman due to unconscious gender bias.

Women face additional challenges when demonstrating leadership skills. Leadership characteristics are typically equated to male qualities - decisive, tough, direct. When women lead, they are perceived to behave in a way that challenges gender-normative schemas. This causes a negative perception of a woman's authority and results in unfavorable relationship with both men and women on the team. Consequently, a woman is more likely to be unjustly criticized and rejected. By contrast, the more successful a man is, the more likable he is by both genders (Katsarou, 2019; O'Neill, 2019). At a fundamental level, women surgeons are challenging long held gender schemas (Greenberg, 2017).

Gender Bias, Discrimination, Harassment

The Accreditation Council for Graduate Medical Education (ACGME) upholds professionalism as one of six core competencies. Professionalism is defined by "compassion, integrity and respect for others", as well as "accountability to patients, society and the profession" (ACGME Common Program Requirements (Residency), 2019; "#BeEthical: A call to healthcare leaders", 2018). The medical profession embraces "a set of values, behaviors, and relationships that underpins the trust the public has in its doctors" (Smith, 2006). These principles embody the professional code of conduct of physician behavior. Unfortunately, there is mounting evidence that bias impacts women in the workplace and undermines the very foundation of professionalism espoused by our professional organizations, societies, and institutions.

Bias can be explicit or implicit. Explicit bias is defined as discrimination based on an individual's personal characteristics. Title VII of the Civil Rights Act of 1964 prohibits discrimination based on 5 protected classes, including race, color, sex, religion and national origin (Title VII, 2019). Title XI of the Education Amendments Act of 1972 states "no person in the United States shall, on the basis of sex, be excluded from participation in, be denied the benefits of, or be subjected to discrimination under any education program or activity receiving Federal financial assistance" (Title IX, 2019). Violations of these laws may be easier to identify than implicit bias, which is the tendency to be more comfortable with those who resemble us and reflect our values.

Implicit bias is ingrained in the subconscious, based on prior social and psychological interactions and experiences. The effects on the victim may be more draining on cognitive and emotional resources (King & Jones, 2016) as time and energy are spent trying to analyze, decipher, and plan responses to vague mistreatment. Files and colleagues (2017) compared the use of a professional title during introduction of Internal Medicine Grand Rounds speakers based on gender of the introducer and the speaker. Female introducers used the professional title ("Dr. Full Name" or "Dr. Last Name only") for female and male speakers 97.8% and 95% of the time, respectively. By contrast, male introducers used the full professional title 72.4% and 49.2% of the time for male versus female speakers, respectively. This public dismissal of a woman speaker's expertise might be viewed as disparaging. Introducing a woman speaker for grand rounds without her professional title undermines her authority as a content expert. These experiences of "un-titling" or "de-professionalism" in aggregate and in different professional environments can affect a woman's ability to gain respect and are interpreted as a form of microaggression (Devon, 2019), or daily slights or insults based on societal stereotypes that convey belittling or disparaging messages about a person ("Diversity in the Classroom", 2014).

Gender disparity is pervasive across surgical specialties and encompasses a range of inappropriate behaviors such as: microaggression, bullying, discrimination and harassment (including sexual harassment) ("ASA Task Force on Equity, Diversion, and Inclusion", 2018; Dossa & Baxter, 2018). Harassment starts in medical training and continues through one's professional career. More than 50% of medical students and 2/3 of residents experience at least one form of harassment, with sexual harassment commonly experienced by women and those in surgical programs (Fnais et al., 2014; Huang, Chua, Saw, & Young, 2018; Dzau & Johnson, 2018; Brown et al., 2019). While the main source of abuse was usually the consultant surgeon (31-34%), additional forms of abuse were perpetrated on behalf of administrators (28%), nurses (11%), and patients/families (21%) (Fnais et al., 2014; Huang, Chua, Saw, & Young, 2018). In a survey of early-career surgical faculty across eight academic institutions, 50% of women respondents experienced sexual discrimination, and 38.5% reported gender was a barrier to career advancement (Cochran et al., 2013). In another study of medical school faculty, female faculty were 2.5 times more likely than male faculty to perceive gender-based discrimination in the academic environment, with rates of discrimination increasing from early- to mid-career faculty (47% to 70%, respectively) (Carr et al., 2000).

Workplace bullying is categorized as "sabotage, verbal abuse, or conduct that is threatening, intimidating or humiliating" (Halverson, Neumayer, & Dagl, 2012). Bullying may include a threat to professional or personal standing, isolation, overwork or destabilization (Rayner & Hoel, 1997). A United States Workplace Bullying Survey revealed that 49% of workers from all industries are victims of bullying and a significant number of victims suffer from post-traumatic stress disorder (Pei & Cochran, 2019). A recent meta-analysis of discrimination, bullying, and harassment in surgery found incidences of 22.4%, 37.7%, and 31.2%, respectively, with recognition that these events are very likely underreported (Huang, Chua, Saw, & Young, 2018). The repercussions of bullying impair patient care, as bullying and other disruptive behaviors have been linked to intimidation, reduced interpersonal communication, and loss of teamwork (Dossa & Baxter, 2018). In addition, bullying has negative effects on the victim with documented reduction in self-esteem and resilience (Pei & Cochran, 2019). Women who report bullying have higher rates of depression, anxiety, and stress, which increases the risk of burnout and suicide (Dzau & Johnson, 2018).

Although there is not complete overlap, an environment that allows gender bias, microaggression, and bullying is one where sexual harassment may be tolerated. Sexual harassment encompasses a range of behaviors, including gender-based harassment (subtle sexual innuendo or sexist statements), unwanted sexual attention, and sexual coercion (sexual advances or threats) (Dzau & Johnson, 2018; Carr et al., 2000). The National Academies of Science, Engineering and Medicine (NASEM) issued a report on sexual harassment of women after evidence that more than 40% of students reported sexual harassment at multiple academic centers ("Sexual Harassment of Women: Climate, Culture and Consequences in Academic Sciences, Engineering, and Medicine", 2018). This report identified five factors that increase the likelihood of sexual harassment of women in medicine: (1) perceived tolerance for sexual harassment, (2) male-dominated work settings, (3) a hierarchical power structure, (4) symbolic compliance policies and procedures, and (5) uninformed leadership. Sexual harassment is associated with reduction in job satisfaction, disinvestment with the organization, a change in career and early retirement, and therefore negatively impacts women in the workplace.

Pay Inequity

The Equal Pay Act of 1963 prohibits unequal pay for equal work performed by men and women, despite this the gender wage gap in surgery persists. Although Doximity reported an annual narrowing of the gender pay gap in a recent article ("Doximity 2019 Physician Compensation Report", 2019), this was due to a relative plateau of male physician salaries not an increase in salaries for women. In 2018, full-time female surgeons earned approximately $75,000 less than male surgeons ("Medscape physician compensation report 2018", 2018). Women in surgery and surgical subspecialties experience the largest difference in adjusted salary ($32,000 and $44,000, respectively), with male surgeons earning 36% more than female surgeons (Jena, Olenski, & Blumenthal, 2016; Jagsi et al., 2012; Warner & Lehmann, 2019).

Pay discrepancy begins with career entry and continues through promotion. Early career female faculty with mentored career development (K23, K08) awards were found to make more than $30,000 less than male investigators (Jagsi et al., 2013). Among mid-career faculty researchers, male gender was an independent predictor of salary, even after adjusting for specialty, academic rank, work hours, research time, and other factors. In fact, a male researcher would earn $12,000 more simply by being male (Sanfey et al., 2017).

Common metrics used by academic centers to calculate compensation – including number of years since first academic appointment, duration of academic career, academic rank, departmental affiliation, and percent effort do not adequately account for gender pay disparity (Freund et al., 2016). In a study of 10,241 academic faculty, almost 39% of the gender difference in salary remained after adjusting for age, experience, clinical productivity, research productivity, specialty, and faculty rank (Jena, Olenski, & Blumenthal, 2016). Evaluation of salary discrepancy based on partnership (i.e. whether faculty had a full-time working partner) explained 17% of the pay gap, supporting the bias that women who have a partner that contributes financially may not need to make as much money (Warner & Lehmann, 2019). Other factors that potentially contribute to a gender wage gap in surgery are less tangible. Women surgeons may receive less administrative or clinical support than their male counterparts making their practices less efficient. Women are more likely to be assigned unpaid work, such as tasks related to scheduling or organization of a practice that do not easily translate into traditional performance metrics (Sanfey et al., 2015). Finally, while the direct impact on pay has not been quantified, parenting is associated as a detriment to female surgical faculty and may perpetuate stereotypes of undependability and lack of commitment due to potential work absence, desire for part-time status, and disinterest in leadership positions.

The impact of pay inequity extends into future financial security. Additional research has shed light on the lost accumulated wealth that women surgeons experience over their careers and how that wealth gap has implications on lifestyle, investing and retirement. A woman hired in 2005 would have $210,829 less in salary and investment returns despite gender equity initiatives that narrowed the pay gap from 2.6 to 1.9 percent (Johns Hopkins Medicine, 2019).

Recent research that confirms the gender pay gap should now be translated into policy that prevents perpetuation of such practices. In 2015, Oregon Health & Sciences University implemented an institution-wide compensation plan aimed to improve transparency and equity among surgical faculty. Investigators in the Department of Surgery subsequently found salaries for male and female surgical faculty were at the Association of American Medical Colleges (AAMC) median, which also remedied the gender wage gap (Hoops et al., 2018). Similarly, an objective compensation plan implemented at the University of Alabama - Birmingham in 2017 increased the percentage women surgeons earned compared to male surgeons (46% vs. 72% of male salary) (Morris, Chen, Heslin, & Krontiras, 2018). One example of a highly successful organization that maintains pay equity is the Mayo Clinic. At Mayo, physicians are paid a set salary based on experience regardless of clinical time, productivity or gender (Berry & Seltman, 2014). Running counter to the typical productivity model, the organization notes long-term commitment, with rates of physician turnover at 2.2% in 2012, compared to 6.1% for US health care systems overall. Executive leadership must acknowledge gender pay disparity and commit to a culture of "equal pay for equal work". It is the responsibility of academic institutions and health care systems to achieve salary parity.

Research and Funding

"To publish or perish" is the precept of academic success and embedded within the foundational culture of academic promotion. Publications serve as an academician's footprint of research productivity, one that requires financial support through new investigator start-up funds, or institutional and federal grant dollars. However, support is not equally provided to men and women researchers, which may portend gender differences in productivity and career success.

Initially, there is a considerable gap between the start-up funds provided to men and women early-career researchers. Data from two New England biomedical-research programs found that the median start-up package for women scientists was $350,000 as compared to $889,000 for men (McIntire, 2015). This discrepancy reduces quantity of lab supplies, and limits availability to hire appropriate staff and fund post-doctoral students. The unintended consequences not only restrict the productivity of a woman principal investigator, but has been associated with early-career attrition rates and delays in promotion (Hoops et al., 2018).

Grant funding is a factor in academic promotion and during reviews by tenure committees. As such, the disparity in awarded grant funding is another example of gender inequity that impacts career success and related satisfaction. Women first-time NIH principal investigators received a median grant of $126,615 while their male counter parts received $165,721, a $40,000 difference that establishes financial inequity and can limit professional advancement (Oliveira, Ma, Woodruff, & Uzzi, 2019). A similar rate of funding disparity was noted at the top 50 NIH-funded institutions, at Big Ten and Ivy League universities.

The percentage of NIH grants awarded to women principal investigators has increased since 1994 (Zhuge, Kaufman, Simeone, Chen, & Velazquez, 2011), with first-time R01 grant awards $15,913 higher for women ($364,509 mean award) (Kaiser, 2019). Men continue to represent approximately two-thirds of NIH grant applicants, with equal rates of men and women who apply receiving funding (19-20%) (NIH Data Book, 2019). However, men consistently receive larger NIH awards $507,279 vs $421,385, (Oliveira, Ma, Woodruff, & Uzzi, 2019) and consistently receive more R01 awards at all career stages (Pohlhaus, Jiang, Wagner, Schaffer, & Pinn, 2011). In addition, R01 Type 2 (renewal) applications were scored lower for women PIs at a single university, posing a potential risk to one's research career, professional advancement and leadership opportunities (Kaatz et al., 2016). Despite having similar rates of publications (for academic rank), and competitive or superior credentials, women academicians are awarded fewer federal grants and receive less institutional financial support than men.

Women Surgeons in Leadership

Inequities in the promotion of women in academic ranks are pervasive, with women representing 29% of Assistant Professors, 21% of Associate Professors and 12% of Professors in 2018 ("https://www.aamc.org/download/495048/data/18table13.pdf.", 2019). This translates into women occupying fewer executive leadership positions, with 24 women appointed as Chair of a Surgery Department in 2018 ("https://www.aamc.org/download/495102/data/supplementaltablec.pdf.", 2019). The limitation of women in leadership positions also correlates to a trickle down effect of fewer leadership opportunities and positions in other professional areas. Within professional surgical societies, women have been appointed to only 4 presidential positions for the American College of Obstetricians and Gynecologists (ACOG) (of 70) ("72. The American College of Obstetricians and Gynecologists Presidential Addresses", 2019) and 4 presidential positions for the American College of Surgeons (ACS) (of 99) ("The American College of Surgeons Archives.", 2019). Positions within professional societies, on editorial boards, and other outside professional activities are considered strongly in most academic departments as a metric for promotion. These activities allow access to networks of thought leaders who may spark or support clinical or research interests. Limited access to these professional opportunities may impede the advancement of women in academia and augment academic achievement gaps.

Low percentages of women in professional leadership roles serve to strengthen the stereotype of the accomplished surgeon as an older male. Board examiners remain overwhelmingly male (80%) disproportionate to women examinees (39%) (Fingeret, 2019). Within the ranks of leadership in surgical professional societies women have been unable to break the glass ceiling. Women hold few council or other executive positions in most surgical professional organizations (Lyons et al., 2019). Despite a significant increase in the proportion of women speakers at annual meetings of surgical professional societies, women remain in the minority of panelists and moderators, and approximately one-in-five panels contain no women speakers prompting the term "manels" (Wilcox, Trooboff, Lai, Turner, & Wong, 2019). On June 12, 2019, Francis Collins, the director of the NIH, went on record announcing his plan to end the manel tradition. His plan includes a requirement that any panel he participates in must include women speakers (Park, 2019). This precedent sets a new expectation for a diversity of content experts at professional meetings.

Like positions within professional societies, positions on editorial boards for journals are prestigious. Editors act as gatekeepers for the presentation of not only research but guidelines, commentaries, and editorials – thereby controlling the intellectual dialogue within a medical specialty. From 1997 to 2017 the proportion of women serving on high-impact surgery journals increased from 5% to 19%; however, the total number of women serving on editorial boards for surgical journals remains far below that of men (Harris et al., 2019). This difference may not only be reflective of, but contribute to, a gender gap in publications which is more pronounced in surgical fields than non-surgical specialties. Within *Annals of Surgery* between 1970 and 2004 women first authors only increased from 2.3% to 16.7% and women senior authors from 0.7% to 6.7%. These rates were lower than all other measured subspecialties (Jagsi et al., 2006). The lack of institutional opportunities for women in surgery appears to create a vicious cycle of exclusion from other national professional opportunities thereby reinforcing gender bias experienced by women surgeons. The Committee on Publication Ethics (COPE) is a nonprofit organization whose mission is to define best practice in the ethics of scholarly publishing and to assist editors and publishers to achieve this. COPE provides leadership in publication ethics and should therefore lead the charge of insisting that there is gender equity in this arena. Surgical specialties have recognized the difficulties related to women developing as leaders and certain specialties have developed initiatives to combat this. For example, the American Association for Thoracic Surgeons devoted their leadership academy in 2019 to developing women leaders.

Mentorship/Sponsorship

A lack of mentorship has been suggested as a critical barrier impeding the advancement of professional women. Women face considerable barriers in partnering with strong mentors, and this is most pronounced in the sciences (Bates et al., 2016). A 2012 survey of women physicians in academic medicine demonstrated that only half of women faculty report having a mentor, a third had previously had a mentor, and 13% report never having had a mentor. Interestingly women also prefer a gender concordant mentorship relationship. Notably, this study also demonstrated that full professors were less likely to have a current mentor compared to lower ranked faculty, although mentorship remains important as women rise in rank (Carapinha, Ortiz-Walters, McCracken, Hill, & Reede, 2016). Specific efforts to target the mentoring needs of senior women faculty should be considered by organizations interested in retaining senior female faculty, such that mentors remain available for women earlier in their careers. Because women currently hold a minority of the high-ranking positions within surgical departments and communities, a well-developed network of women available to act as mentors is unfortunately dramatically exceeded by the number of potential women mentees. Women surgeons consistently report a lack of mentoring as an obstacle in academic surgery (Weber et al., 2005; Wise et al. 2004; Caniano, Sonnino, & Paolo, 2004).

Organizational programs can help to alleviate a perceived lack of mentors. A multifaceted intervention including mentoring was implemented in 1990 through 1995 within the Department of Medicine at Johns Hopkins School of Medicine to correct gender-based career obstacles reported by women faculty. This translated to an increase in the number of women promoted to the rank of associate professor, as well as the proportion of women expecting to stay in academic medicine. There was a downside of mentoring for women: 32% of women (compared to 10% of men, p = .004) reported that their mentor used their work to advance their own career rather than that of the mentee (Sambunjak, Straus, & Marušić, 2006).

Today, the paucity of same sex mentors remains a problem. Women junior faculty are often desperate for women mentors to guide professional development opportunities, facilitate networking opportunities and champion developmental experiences. The few women in leadership are left burdened with requests for mentorship adding to their other job responsibilities. Mentorship is difficult to measure and is rarely considered as a performance metric in academic medicine. Therefore, for the women who act as mentors, this effort is not compensated nor recognized as a factor that may detract from other measures used to support academic promotion.

Some have suggested that an inadvertent negative effect of the #MeToo movement is less enthusiasm by men in leadership to mentor women faculty amplifying the scarcity of available mentors for women surgeons (Soklaridis et al., 2018).

Without mentors who have both national and institutional power, women surgeons may be left without an advocate to assist with career development and when faced with gender bias, sexual harassment, or burnout, all of which are more frequent among women surgeons. Building a diverse mentoring network that includes same-sex gender preferences may require reaching outside one's specialty, department, or institution. Implicit bias training may increase all mentors' sensitivity to gender related issues and may allow mentors to meet the needs of diverse mentees.

When Worlds Collide: Seeking Balance Between Professional and Personal Life

Surgical culture and the rules of engagement evolved at a time when women were not as prevalent in the workforce. At this time in history, when women are increasingly choosing surgical careers, the provisions for personal and professional satisfaction, support to succeed at both, and optimization of work-life balance are lagging behind needs.

A recent Pew Research Center analysis of the United States Census Bureau data found that the majority of women in their forties are mothers (Livingston, 2019). If this is any reflection of a woman's desire to be a mother and motherhood being a consistent lifetime goal for women in our society, it is not surprising that women opt out of surgical careers and make up less than one-quarter of 10 surgical specialties. A recent article in AAMC NEWS entitled *"Where are all the women in Surgery?"* opens with the following statement "for decades women have been discouraged from entering the surgical subspecialties" (Haskins, 2019). As women continue to overcome structural barriers to entering and practicing surgery, it follows that women (and #heforshe advocates) must break down the gendered cultural norms that fail to align with the unique needs of women. The International Journal of Surgery Global Health article *"Women in Surgery: challenges and opportunities"* highlights social deterrents to surgical careers for women, namely work-life balance. Women are subjected to the gendered expectations previously set by a traditionally male-dominated profession, steering women away from a career that might pose irreconcilable demands on their personal and professional life (de Costa, 2018).

Women remain disproportionately responsible for and impacted by familial caregiving, not withstanding the implicit physical, psychological, and emotional demands of pregnancy, childbirth, and nursing (Henry, 2019). Surgical training and early career establishment, which are grueling, stressful and tedious, coincide with a woman's fertility and typical timing to create a family. Taking leave for pregnancy, postpartum bonding and nursing do not conform to traditional norms for surgeons.

Women confront inflexibility and other obstacles related to the requisite time off needed to carry healthy pregnancies, deliver, bond, and adequately nurse their children, assuming they can conceive at all (Rangel et al., 2018). In a heartfelt piece published in TIME magazine, Dr. Arghavan Salles (2019) eloquently lays out the default expectation of uninterrupted training and putting other personal priorities on hold for career ambition and the ease of assimilating into the current surgical culture that makes more sense for men. Until our surgical community evolves to embrace a new normal that surgeons are parents and parenting is an accepted priority, there will continue to be gender bias, discrimination, and unequal numbers of women in surgery. It is therefore incumbent upon our professional leaders to work with national boards, professional societies, and affiliated institutions to develop policies and accommodations that invite, engage, and allow women to flourish in the surgical workforce.

At present the American Board of Surgery (ABS) offers several options for extending residency by one year but all require ABS and training program advanced approval. Given that not all pregnancies conform to one's anticipated optimal timing, this provision may not always be possible for women opting to have children during residency. The current option to use four weeks of vacation for maternity leave with a provision to take an additional 2 weeks for a "documented medical condition" is a preposterous solution that warrants immediate attention (General Surgery Leave Policy, 2019). Women can save up and borrow vacation time from other residency years for maternity leave (AWS Maternity Leave policy for Surgical Residents, 2019), effectively denying much needed vacation time in other years. Furthermore, the strain of pregnancy, delivery and adjusting to a newborn is not restorative and should serve as a valid argument that maternity leave should not be equated with vacation. Requiring the use of vacation for maternity leave is discriminatory, as there is no biological equivalent for men. Partner parental leave would allow a second parent to be of assistance in the postpartum period, but it is infrequently available. In a recent study of women who were pregnant during surgical residency 39% of women surveyed

Figure 1. An illustration of a #BiasCorrect

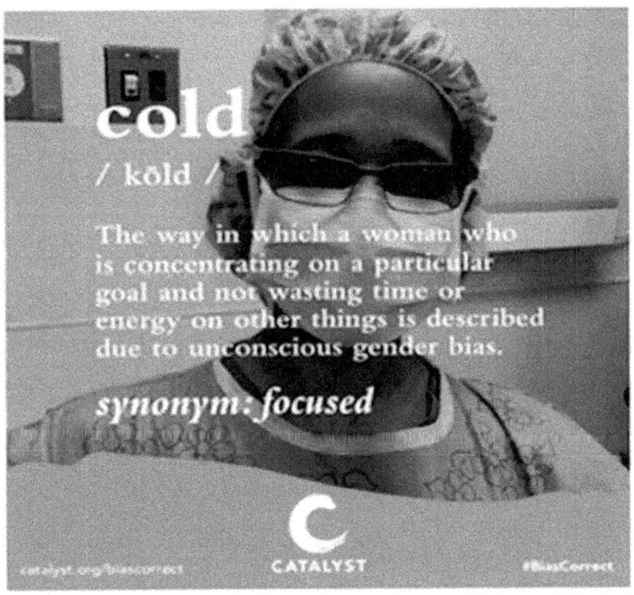

considered leaving residency and 30% would advise women medical students against pursuing a surgical career (Wall, 2019). Remarkably 40% of women surgeons are childless whereas 92% of male surgeons have children (Martinez, Daniels, & Chandra, 2012).

Other studies show that young physicians, both men and women, are searching for more balance between their personal and professional lives in the context of evolving life partnerships that do not conform to traditional heteronormative gender roles. There is an emerging movement to achieve balance in the medical profession as burn out and suicide reach epidemic proportions. This desire for a healthier more equitable work-life balance can only become realized by intentional culture change with compensatory action, part of which is happening by the presence of more women in leadership positions and the advocacy of men who support gender equity and equality.

CONCLUSION

It takes time to understand the benefits of change, diversity and inclusion, but research consistently supports the global benefits of a diverse workforce. The surgical workplace should be no different than any other industry workplace and yet the surgical workforce suffers from being one of the last bastions to preserve traditional male dominated hierarchical traditions and norms.

"We can make surgery a better profession: not just for women, but for everyone seeking to provide health care in an environment free from discrimination" (de Costa, 2018).

REFERENCES

AAMC Faculty Roster. (2018). U.S. Medical School Faculty by Sex, Rank, and Department, 2018. Retrieved from https://www.aamc.org/download/495048/data/18table13.pdf

AAMC Faculty Roster. (2018). Department Chairs by Department, Sex, and Race/Ethnicity, 2018. Retrieved from https://www.aamc.org/download/495102/data/supplementaltablec.pdf

ACGME Common Program Requirements (Residency), revised June 10, 2019. Retrieved from https://acgme.org/Portals/0/PFAssets/ProgramRequirements/CPRResidency2019.pdf

Ali, A. M., & McVay, C. L. (2016). Women in surgery: A history of adversity, resilience, and accomplishment. *Journal of the American College of Surgeons*, *223*(4), 670–673. doi:10.1016/j.jamcollsurg.2016.06.012 PMID:27374995

ASA Task Force on Equity, Diversity, and Inclusion 2018.

AWS Maternity Leave Policy for Surgical Residents. (2002). General format. Retrieved from https://cdn.ymaws.com/womensurgeons.site-ym.com/resource/resmgr/docs/Resource_Library/ResidentPolicy.pdf

Bates, C., Gordon, L., Travis, E., Chatterjee, A., Chaudron, L., Fivush, B., ... Moses, A. (2016). Striving for gender equity in academic medicine careers: A call to action. *Academic Medicine*, *91*(8), 1050–1052. doi:10.1097/ACM.0000000000001283 PMID:27332868

#BeEthical: A Call to Healthcare Leaders. Ending Gender Workforce Disparities is an Ethical Imperative. September 2018.

Berry, L. L., & Seltman, K. D. (2014). The enduring culture of Mayo Clinic. *Mayo Clinic Proceedings*, *89*(2), 144–147. doi:10.1016/j.mayocp.2013.10.025 PMID:24485127

#BiasCorrect.)(2019). Retrieved from https://www.catalyst.org/biascorrect/

Brown, J., Brury, L., Raub, K., Levy, B., Brantner, P., Krivak, T. C., … Naumann, R. W. (2019). Workplace harassment and discrimination in gynecology: results of the AAGL member survey. *JMIG*, published online March 4, 2019.

Brown, M. A., Erdman, M. K., Munger, A. M., & Miller, A. N. (2019). Despite growing number of women surgeons, authorship gender disparity in orthopaedic literature persists over 30 years. [Epub ahead of print]. *Clinical Orthopaedics and Related Research*, (Jun), 17. PMID:31283733

Butkus, R., Serchen, J., Moyer, D. V., Bornstein, S. S., & Hingle, S. T. (2018). Achieving gender equity in physician compensation and career advancement: A position paper of the American College of Physicians. *Annals of Internal Medicine*, *168*(10), 721–723. doi:10.7326/M17-3438 PMID:29710100

Caniano, D. A., Sonnino, R. E., & Paolo, A. M. (2004). Keys to career satisfaction: Insights from a survey of women pediatric surgeons. *J Ped Surg*, *39*(6), 984–990. doi:10.1016/j.jpedsurg.2004.02.039 PMID:15185240

Carapinha, R., Ortiz-Walters, R., McCracken, C. M., Hill, E. V., & Reede, J. Y. (2016). Variability in women faculty's preferences regarding mentor similarity: A multi-institution study in academic medicine. *Academic Medicine*, *91*(8), 1108–1118. doi:10.1097/ACM.0000000000001284 PMID:27332871

Carr, P. L., Ash, A. S., Friedman, R. H., Szalacha, L., Barnett, R. C., Palepu, A., & Moskowtiz, M. M. (2000). Faculty perceptions of gender discrimination and sexual harassment in academic medicine. *Annals of Internal Medicine*, *132*(11), 889–896. doi:10.7326/0003-4819-132-11-200006060-00007 PMID:10836916

Cochran, A., Elder, W. B., Crandall, M., Brasel, K., Hauschild, T., & Neumayer, L. (2013). Barriers to advancement in academic surgery: Views of senior residents and early career faculty. *American Journal of Surgery*, *206*(5), 661–666. doi:10.1016/j.amjsurg.2013.07.003 PMID:24011566

Davis, E. C., Risucci, D. A., Blair, P. G., & Sachdeva, A. K. (2011). Women in surgery residency programs: Evolving trends from a national perspective. *Journal of the American College of Surgeons*, *212*(3), 320–326. doi:10.1016/j.jamcollsurg.2010.11.008 PMID:21247778

de Costa, J., Chen-Xu, J., Bentounsi, Z., & Vervoort, D. (2018). Women in surgery: challenges and opportunities. *Inl J Surg Glob Health.*

Devon, K. M. (2019). Call Me by My Name: Doctor. *Annals of Surgery*, *270*(1), 29–30. doi:10.1097/SLA.0000000000003327 PMID:31021830

Diversity in the Classroom. UCLA Diversity & Faculty Development 2014.

Donington, J. S., Litle, V. R., Sesti, J., & Colson, Y. L. (2012). The WTS report on the current status of women in cardiothoracic surgery. *The Annals of Thoracic Surgery*, *94*(2), 452–458, discussion 458–459. doi:10.1016/j.athoracsur.2012.03.102 PMID:22698775

Dossa, F., & Baxter, N. N. (2018). Reducing gender bias in surgery. *BJS*, *105*(13), 1707–1709. doi:10.1002/bjs.11042 PMID:30462365

Doximity 2019 Physician Compensation Report. (2019, April 2). Retrieved from https://blog.doximity.com/articles/doximity-2019-physician-compensation-report-d0ca91d1-3cf1-4cbb-b403-a49b9ffa849f

Dzau, V. J., & Johnson, P. A. (2018). Ending sexual harassment in academic medicine. *The New England Journal of Medicine*, *379*(17), 1589–1591. doi:10.1056/NEJMp1809846 PMID:30207831

Elmore, L. C., Jeffe, D. B., Jin, L., Awad, M. M., & Turnbull, I. R. (2016). National Survey of Burnout among US General Surgery Residents. *Journal of the American College of Surgeons*, *223*(3), 440–451. doi:10.1016/j.jamcollsurg.2016.05.014 PMID:27238875

Estes, Z., & Felker, S. (2012). Confidence mediates the sex difference in mental rotation performance. *Archives of Sexual Behavior*, *41*(3), 557–570. doi:10.100710508-011-9875-5 PMID:22130691

Files, J. A., Mayer, A. P., Ko, M. G., Friedrich, P., Jenkins, M., Bryan, M. J., ... Hayes, S. N. (2017). Speaker. introductions at internal medicine grand rounds: Forms of address reveal gender bias J. *Women & Health*, *26*(5), 413–419. doi:10.1089/jwh.2016.6044 PMID:28437214

Fingeret, A. L. (2019). Room for improvement: Barriers and strategies to improve gender parity for American Board of Surgery certifying examiners. *The Journal of Surgical Research*, *237*, 136–137. doi:10.1016/j.jss.2018.06.009 PMID:30917896

Fnais, N., Soobiah, C., Chen, M. H., Lillie, E., Perrier, L., Tashkhandi, M., ... Tricco, A. C. (2014). Harassment and discrimination in medical training: A systematic review and meta-analysis. *Academic Medicine*, *89*, 817–827. doi:10.1097/ACM.0000000000000200 PMID:24667512

Frangou, C. (2018, Feb. 6). Surgeons (women and men) say it's time to close surgery's gender gap. *Gen Surg News*. Retrieved from https://www.generalsurgerynews.com/In-the-News/Article/02-18/Surgeons-Women-and-Men-Say-It-s-Time-to-Close-Surgery-s-Gender-Gap/46919?sub=2F10E432441735F412C78CC6CDB6D8ECDBE22B01D93E95F3569347DA5E5463C&enl=true

Freund, K. M., Raj, A., Kaplan, S. E., Terrin, N., Breeze, J. L., Urech, T. H., & Carr, P. L. (2016). Inequities in academic compensation by gender: A follow-up to the national faculty survey cohort study. *Academic Medicine*, *91*(8), 1068–1073. doi:10.1097/ACM.0000000000001250 PMID:27276007

General Surgery Leave Policy. (2017). General format. Retrieved from http://www.absurgery.org/default.jsp?policygsleave

Greenberg, C. C. (2017). Association for Academic Surgery presidential address: Sticky floors and glass ceilings. *The Journal of Surgical Research*, *219*, ix–xviii. doi:10.1016/j.jss.2017.09.006 PMID:29078918

Halverson, A. L., Neumayer, L., & Dagl, T. F. (2012). Leadership skills in the OR, part II: recognizing disruptive behavior. *ACS Bulletin*, 1-5.

Harris, C. A., Banerjee, T., Cramer, M., Manz, S., Ward, S. T., Dimick, J., & Telem, D. A. (2019). Editorial (spring) board? Gender composition in high-impact general surgery journals over 20 years. *Annals of Surgery*, *269*(3), 582–588. doi:10.1097/SLA.0000000000002667 PMID:29342020

Haskins, J. (2019, July 15). General format. Retrieved from https://news.aamc.org/diversity/article/where-are-all-the-women-in-surgery/

Henry, T. A. (2019, June 3). General format. Retrieved from https://www.ama-assn.org/practice-management/physician-health/higher-physician-burnout-risk-moms-sandwich-generation

Hoops, H. E., Brasel, K. J., Dewey, E., Rodgers, S., Merrill, J., Hunter, J. G., & Azarow, K. S. (2018). Analysis of gender-based differences in surgery faculty compensation, promotion, and retention: Establishing equity. *Annals of Surgery*, *268*(3), 479–487. doi:10.1097/SLA.0000000000002920 PMID:30063494

Huang, Y., Chua, T. C., Saw, R. P. M., & Young, C. J. (2018). Discrimination, bullying and harassment in surgery: A systematic review and meta-analysis. *World Journal of Surgery*, *42*(12), 3867–3873. doi:10.100700268-018-4716-5 PMID:29971462

Hughes, K. A. (2015). #ILookeLikeASurgeon goes viral: How it happened. *FACs Bulletin*, *100*, 10–16. PMID:26677529

Inzlicht, M., & Ben-Zeev, T. (2000). A threatening intellectual environment: Why females are susceptible to experiencing problem-solving deficits in the presence of males. *Psychological Science*, *11*(5), 365–371. doi:10.1111/1467-9280.00272 PMID:11228906

Jagsi, R., Griffith, K. A., Stewart, A., Sambuco, D., DeCastro, R., & Ubel, P. A. (2012). Gender differences in the salaries of physician researchers. *Journal of the American Medical Association*, *307*(22), 2410–2417. doi:10.1001/jama.2012.6183 PMID:22692173

Jagsi, R., Griffith, K. A., Stewart, A., Sambuco, D., DeCastro, R., & Ubel, P. A. (2013). Gender differences in salary in a recent cohort of early-career physician-researchers. *Academic Medicine*, *88*(11), 1689–1699. doi:10.1097/ACM.0b013e3182a71519 PMID:24072109

Jagsi, R., Guancial, E. A., Worobey, C. C., Henault, L. E., Chang, Y., Starr, R., ... Hylek, E. M. (2006). The "gender gap" in authorship of academic medical literature— A 35-year perspective. *The New England Journal of Medicine*, *355*(3), 281–287. doi:10.1056/NEJMsa053910 PMID:16855268

Jena, A. B., Olenski, A. R., & Blumenthal, D. M. (2016). Sex differences in physician salary in US public medical schools. *JAMA Internal Medicine*, *176*(9), 1294–1304. doi:10.1001/jamainternmed.2016.3284 PMID:27400435

Johns Hopkins Medicine. (2019, Jan. 29). How gender disparities in salary add up over a lifetime. *ScienceDaily*. Retrieved from https://www.sciencedaily.com/releases/2019/01/190128111728.htm

Kaatz, A., Lee, Y. G., Potvien, A., Magua, W., Filut, A., Bhattacharya, A., ... Carnes, M. (2016). Analysis of NIH R01 Application critiques, impact and criteria scores: Does the sex of the principal investigator make a difference. *Academic Medicine*, *91*, 1080–1088. doi:10.1097/ACM.0000000000001272 PMID:27276003

Kaiser, J. (2019, March 8). Men get larger first NIH grants, but is the news all bad for female scientists? Retrieved from https://www.sciencemag.org/news/2019/03/men-get-larger-first-nih-grants-news-all-bad-female-scientists

Katsarou, M. (2019). *Women and the Leadership Labyrinth Howard vs Heidi*. Leadership Psychol Inst.

Kay, K., & Shipman, C. (2014). The Confidence Gap. *Atlantic (Boston, Mass.)*.

King, E., & Jones, K. (2016). Why subtle bias is so often worse than blatant discrimination. *Harvard Business Review*.

Koven, S. (2017). Letter to a Young Female Physician. *The New England Journal of Medicine, 376*(20), 1907–1909. doi:10.1056/NEJMp1702010 PMID:28514609

Livingston, G. (2018, Jan. 18). General format. Retrieved from http://www.pewsocialtrends.org/2018/01/18/theyre-waiting-longer-but-u-s-women-today-more-likely-to-have-children-than-a-decade-ago

Lyons, N. B., Bernardi, K., Huang, L., Holihan, J. L., Cherla, D., Martin, A. C., ... Hydo, L. (2019). Gender. disparity in surgery: An evaluation of surgical societies. *Surgical Infections, 20*(5), 406–410. doi:10.1089ur.2018.220 PMID:30892131

Martinez, G., Daniels, K., & Chandra, A. (2012). Fertility of men and women aged 15-44 years in the United States: National survey of family growth, 2006-2010. *National Health Statistics Reports, 12*, 1–28. PMID:22803225

McIntire, M. E. (2015, Sept. 17). Another Research Gender Gap: Men get more start-up money. Retrieved from https://www.chronicle.com/article/Another-Research-Gender-Gap-/233177

Medscape. (2018). Medscape physician compensation report 2018. Retrieved from https://www.medscape.com/slideshow/2018-compensation-surgeon-6009657

Morris, M., Chen, H., Heslin, M. J., & Krontiras, H. (2018). A structured compensation plan improves but does not erase the sex pay gap in surgery. *Annals of Surgery, 268*(3), 442–448. doi:10.1097/SLA.0000000000002928 PMID:29979249

Mouly, F. & Bormes, G. (2017). The New Yorker Cover that's Being Replicated by Women Surgeons Around the World.

National Academies of Sciences, Engineering and Medicine. (2018). Sexual Harassment of Women: Climate, Culture and Consequences in Academic Sciences, Engineering, and Medicine.

NIH Data Book. (2019, April). [Graph illustration the Cumulative Investigator Rate: Research Project Grants, R21, P01, or R01-Equivalents] Retrieved from https://report.nih.gov/nihdatabook/index.aspx

O'Neill, T. (2019). *Success and Likability for Women in the Workplace, The Heidi-Howard Study*. Morgan McKinley Go Beyond.

Oliveira, D. F. M., Ma, Y., Woodruff, T. K., & Uzzi, B. (2019). Comparison of National Institutes of Health Grant Amounts to First-Time Male and Female Principal Investigators. *Journal of the American Medical Association, 321*(9), 898–900. doi:10.1001/jama.2018.21944 PMID:30835300

Park, A. (2019, June 25). NIH Director Francis Collins has a plan to help eliminate "manels". *Time*. Retrieved from https://time.com/5611142/manels-nih-director-francis-collins/?amp=true

Pei, K. Y., & Cochran, A. (2019). Workplace bullying among surgeons – the perfect crime. *Annals of Surgery*, *269*(1), 43–44. doi:10.1097/SLA.0000000000003018 PMID:30247324

Pohlhaus, J. R., Jiang, H., Wagner, R. M., Schaffer, W. T., & Pinn, V. W. (2011). Sex differences in application success, and funding rates for NIH extramural programs. *Academic Medicine*, *86*(6), 759–767. doi:10.1097/ACM.0b013e31821836ff PMID:21512358

Rangel, E. L., Smink, D. L., Castillo-Angeles, M., Kwakye, G., Changala, M., Haider, A. H., & Doherty, G. M. (2018). Pregnancy and motherhood during surgical training. *JAMA Surgery*, *153*(7), 644–652. doi:10.1001/jamasurg.2018.0153 PMID:29562068

Rayner, C., & Hoel, H. (1997). A summary review of literature relating to workplace bullying. *Journal of Community & Applied Social Psychology*, *7*(3), 181–191. doi:10.1002/(SICI)1099-1298(199706)7:3<181::AID-CASP416>3.0.CO;2-Y

Reed, C. E., Vaporciyan, A. A., Erikson, C., Dill, M. J., Carpenter, A. J., Guleserian, K. J., & Merrill, W. H. (2010). Factors dominating choice of surgical specialty. *Journal of the American College of Surgeons*, *210*(3), 319–324. doi:10.1016/j.jamcollsurg.2009.11.016 PMID:20193895

Rutkow, I. M. (2000). Mary Edwards Walker. *Archives of Surgery (Chicago, Ill.)*, *135*(4), 489–489. doi:10.1001/archsurg.135.4.489 PMID:10768718

Salles, A. (2019, Jan. 3). I spent my fertile years training to be a surgeon. Now, it might be too late for me to have a baby. *TIME*. Retrieved from https://time.com/5484506/fertility-egg-freezing/

Salles, A., Mueller, C. M., & Cohen, G. L. (2016). A values affirmation intervention to improve female residents' surgical performance. *Journal of Graduate Medical Education*, *8*(3), 378–383. doi:10.4300/JGME-D-15-00214.1 PMID:27413441

Sambunjak, D., Straus, S. E., & Marušić, A. (2006). Mentoring in academic medicine: A systematic review. *Journal of the American Medical Association*, *296*(9), 1103–1115. doi:10.1001/jama.296.9.1103 PMID:16954490

Sanfey, H., Crandall, M., Shaughnessy, E., Stein, S. L., Cochran, A., Parangi, S., & Laronga, C. (2017). Strategies for identifying and closing the gender salary gap in surgery. *Journal of the American College of Surgeons*, *225*(2), 333–338. doi:10.1016/j.jamcollsurg.2017.03.018 PMID:28400299

Sanfey, H., Fromson, J., Mellinger, J., Rakinic, J., Williams, M., & Williams, B. (2015). Surgeons in difficulty: An exploration of differences in assistance between male and female surgeons. *Journal of the American College of Surgeons*, *221*, 621–627. doi:10.1016/j.jamcollsurg.2015.02.015 PMID:25872689

Schmidt, L. E., Cooper, C. A., & Guo, W. A. (2016). Factors influencing US medical students' decision to pursue surgery. *The Journal of Surgical Research*, *203*(1), 64–74. doi:10.1016/j.jss.2016.03.054 PMID:27338536

Sexton, K. W., Hocking, K. M., Wise, E., Osgood, M. J., Cheung-Flynn, J., Komalavilas, P., ... Brophy, C. M. (2012). Women in academic surgery: The pipeline is busted. *Journal of Surgical Education, 69*(1), 84–90. doi:10.1016/j.jsurg.2011.07.008 PMID:22208838

Smith, R. (2006). Medical professionalism: Out with the old and in with the new. *Journal of the Royal Society of Medicine, 99*(2), 48–50. doi:10.1177/014107680609900202 PMID:16449765

Soklaridis, S., Zahn, C., Kuper, A., Gillis, D., Taylor, V. H., & Whitehead, C. (2018). Men's fear of mentoring in the #MeToo era— What's at stake for academic medicine? *The New England Journal of Medicine, 379*(23), 2270–2274. doi:10.1056/NEJMms1805743 PMID:30281387

Spetzler, R. F. (2011). Progress of women in neurosurgery. *Asian Journal of Neurosurgery, 6*(1), 6–12. doi:10.4103/1793-5482.85627 PMID:22059098

Stephens, E. H., Robich, M. P., Walters, D. M., DeNino, W. F., Aftab, M., Tchantchaleishvili, V., ... Shah, A. A. (2016). Gender and Cardiothoracic Surgery Training: Specialty Interests, Satisfaction, and Career Pathways. *The Annals of Thoracic Surgery, 102*(1), 200–206. doi:10.1016/j.athoracsur.2016.03.043 PMID:27157051

The American College of Obstetricians and Gynecologists Presidential Addresses. (2019, April 15). General format. Retrieved from https://www.acog.org/About-ACOG/ACOG-Departments/Resource-Center/Presidents-and-Their-Inaugural-Addresses?IsMobileSet=false

The American College of Surgeons Archives. (2019). General format. Retrieved from https://www.facs.org/about-acs/archives/acshistory/presidentslist

Title VII of the Civil Rights Act of 1964. Retrieved from www.eeoc.gov/laws/statutes/titlevii.cfm

Title XI of the Education Ammendments Act of 1972. Retrieved from http://www.ncaa.org/about/resources/inclusion/title-ix-frequently-asked-questions

Valsangkar, N., Fecher, A. M., Rozycki, G. S., Blanton, C., Bell, T. M., Freischlag, J., ... Koniaris, L. G. (2016). Understanding the barriers to hiring and promoting women in surgical subspecialties. *Journal of the American College of Surgeons, 223*(2), 387–398. doi:10.1016/j.jamcollsurg.2016.03.042 PMID:27109779

Vaporciyan, A. A., Reed, C. E., Erikson, C., Dill, M. J., Carpenter, A. J., Guleserian, K. J., & Merrill, W. (2009). Factors affecting interest in cardiothoracic surgery: Survey of North American general surgery residents. *The Annals of Thoracic Surgery, 87*(5), 1351–1359. doi:10.1016/j.athoracsur.2009.02.096 PMID:19379863

Wall, A. (2018, March 30). Pregnancy, new moms, and surgical residency. Association of Academic Surgery. Retrieved from http://www.aasurg.org/blog/pregnancy-new-moms-surgical-residency/

Warner, A. S., & Lehmann, L. S. (2019). Gender wage disparities in medicine: Time to close the gap. *Journal of General Internal Medicine, 34*(7), 1334–1336. doi:10.100711606-019-04940-9 PMID:30963441

Weber, T., Reidel, M., Graf, S., Hinz, U., Keller, M., & Büchler, M. (2005). Careers of women in academic surgery. *Chirurg, 76*(7), 703–711, discussion 11. doi:10.100700104-005-1017-y PMID:15770490

Wilcox, A. R., Trooboff, S. W., Lai, C. S., Turner, P. L., & Wong, S. L. (2019). Trends in gender representation at the American College of Surgeons Clinical Congress and the Academic Surgical Congress: a mixed picture of progress. *J Am Coll Surg*.

Wise, M. R., Shapiro, H., Bodley, J., Pittini, R., McKay, D., Willan, A., & Hannah, M. E. (2004). Factors affecting academic promotion in obstetrics and gynaecology in Canada. *Journal of Obstetrics and Gynaecology Canada*, *26*(2), 127–136. doi:10.1016/S1701-2163(16)30488-1 PMID:14965478

Yeo, H. L., Abelson, J. S., Symer, M. M., Mao, J., Michelassi, F., Bell, R., ... Sosa, J. A. (2018). Association of time to attrition in surgical residency with individual resident and programmatic factors. *JAMA Surgery*, *153*(6), 511–517. doi:10.1001/jamasurg.2017.6202 PMID:29466536

Zhuge, Y., Kaufman, J., Simeone, D. M., Chen, H., & Velazquez, O. C. (2011). Is there still a glass ceiling for women in academic surgery? *Annals of Surgery*, *253*(4), 637–643. doi:10.1097/SLA.0b013e3182111120 PMID:21475000

Chapter 19
Prophylaxis in Action:
#MeToo for Women of Medical and Surgical Disciplines

Catherine Hayes
Faculty of Health Sciences and Wellbeing, University of Sunderland, Sunderland, UK

Yitka N. H. Graham
Faculty of Health Sciences and Wellbeing, University of Sunderland, Sunderland, UK

ABSTRACT

The empowerment of women as a consequence of the #MeToo initiative has undoubtedly impacted perpetrators, who are now at risk. It has also enabled an agenda for change that has visibly impacted the global workforce and placed a spotlight on the concept of authentic womanhood and the need for its protection. This is a prophylactic measure for the future, so other women who dedicate their lives to the service of others might not be subject to the violation and indignity in 21st Century workforces that has characterised generations of misogyny before them This chapter seeks to illuminate the contexts, settings, and experiences of women working at the front line of medical care and their interactions with colleagues, and is balanced by an illumination of their male counterparts and their reactions to these reported perceptions.

INTRODUCTION

Where transcendence between the lines of human attraction to a colleague in the context of the workplace descends into the liminal shift towards sexual harassment, recent evidence of global contemporary debate prevails in modern societies (Barlow, 2018). Where people are physically assaulted or people are positively stereotyped and favoured in the workplace because of their willingness to undertake intimate relations with those in power, cultures are irrevocably damaged. The empowerment of women as a consequence of the #MeToo initiative, has undoubtedly impacted on the increasing level of vulnerability to exposure that these perpetrators are now at risk of (Ford, 2018). It has also enabled this to drive an agenda for change that has visibly impacted on the global workforce and placed a spotlight on the con-

DOI: 10.4018/978-1-5225-9599-1.ch019

cept of authentic womanhood and the need for protection of it. This is a prophylactic measure for the future, so that other women who dedicate their lives to the service of others might not be subject to the violation and indignity in 21st Century workforces that has characterised generations of misogyny before them (Lovell, 2018). This chapter, which focuses on European and United Kingdom perspectives, seeks to illuminate the contexts, settings and experiences of women working at the front line of medical care, their interactions with colleagues and is balanced by an illumination of their male counterparts and their reactions to these reported perceptions.

Context and Intentionality in Workplace Sexism

It is the ambiguity or nuanced nature of sexual harassment that moves discussion away from binary thinking around whether an act of predatory sexual nature has occurred to one of a much more nebulous dialogue around the appropriateness of human interaction, the context of it but more importantly the intentionality belying it, bearing in mind that flirtatious behaviour and even romantic and emotional attachment are very much equal realities of all global workplaces where men and women, work alongside one another (Bareket et al., 2018; Campbell et al., 2018).

Each presenting case of discrimination has its own particular set of variables, all of which are open to interpretation through lenses of scrutiny by people with differing sets of values, beliefs and ethical principles (Zarkov and Davis, 2018). If healthcare institutions are to protect their staff against extraneous variables such as these then there must be a zero tolerance of the acceptability of harassment in the workplace and all concerns regarding the possibility of this occurring there, must be forcefully addressed from the outset (Bates et al., 2018).

The systemic prevention of women ensuring their rights in the workplace is socially constructed around the concept of 'girliness'. It is the bureaucratic approaches which have ensured the normalisation of deviance with male peers, resulting in a raft of sexism in the workplace that is avoided by little more than tokenism in practice. This has originated from a wider positional stance of sexism at an ontological level, which consequently became epistemologically aligned with exploitation, unwitting oppression and integration into societal expectation. The need for a systematic overhaul in the positionality of womanhood across global communities has never been more apparent (Supriya, 2018; Huff et al., 2018).

Parameters of the Spectrum of Sexual Misconduct in the Workplace

Defining and classifying behaviours that constitute sexual misconduct in the workplace Decisions about which category a behaviour falls into depend on the situation, the context and the overall tone of communication, delivery and nonverbal behaviours (McClure, 2019; Gertner, 2018). One of the greatest issues is that organisationally institutions fail to define exactly what these parameters ought to constitute in the workplace. In terms of classifying what is 'non-offensive' there are generally comments about personal appearance or clothing that ought not to enter the workplace but when they do not generally cause offence. Those comments that are cringe worthy or awkward in nature usually pertain directly to gender – for example 'that's a typical woman comment' or 'ladies before gentlemen, when inviting open discussion'. Those things which are offensive, but which may not necessarily have a sexual intentionality are things such as hugging people with complete disregard as to whether this is appropriate, referring to the physical attributes of women (for example dumb blonde jokes). Implying family issues are the only priority women have. The liminal threshold between being offensive and sexual misconduct lies with a move towards intimate contact such as kissing, which is not invited and is unwelcome, physical grabbing and overt sexual intentionality. Using derogatory terms regarding a woman's career progression in relation to her sexuality and her capacity to gain promotion on the basis of this. Serious sexual misconduct implies physical assertion of sexuality, uninvited with a women, exposure of the genitals or inappropriately suggestive bodily contact, which is again uninvited. Coercion of the use of physical force to engage women in sexual activity.

Initiating and Sustaining Change in the Context of the Workplace and Professional Practice

Establishing exactly why boundaries have not yet been established/maintained in the workplace in relation to sexual harassment and liminal thresholds of behaviour is multi-faceted and at times an ambiguous issue in relation to the acceptability of human interrelationships in practice. As a consequence addressing and making sustainable workplace changes, can become an ambiguous task, which tend to be locally implemented approaches rather than recognised national initiatives or guidelines. Considering this also provides an opportunity to address whether something is a Human Resource issue or whether it is a legal matter for the police authorities (Spraitz, 2018). Organisational infrastructure can often be a barrier to change in circumstances which would protect women against unwanted sexual attention, with a cultural normalisation of deviance in relation to professional practice levels of acceptable behaviour (Sundaram and Jackson, 2018).

Delineating Sexism and Misogyny

Manne posits misogyny as being better understood as a moral manifestation of sexist ideology and provides an operational definition as 'a social sciences or environment where when women face hostility and hatred because they are women in a man's world, from which historical patriarchy originates (Manne, 2016). The very means by which men have been nurtured by since birth, in most instances is subsequently weaponised in advocating that women adhere to stereotypical perceptions of the female role so that they can continue to benefit from a relationship, which is no longer appropriate. Misogyny this serves to reinforce sexist perspectives or the patriarchal social relations underpinning (Manne, 2017). Cohn and Blumberg (2019) rightly denounce the bureaucracy underpinning the active subordination of women in the 21st Century workforce, this appears to transcend universal perspectives of fairness and equity for all women, not just those in the UK or Europe.

Economic Implications of the Subordination of Women

The subordination of women in the workplace has stemmed from a lack of commitment by progressive generations to close the divisions of labour which has ensured women experience insufficient support in the social infrastructure within which they live and work (Pateman, 2018). Undoubtedly this links heavily to the concept of physiological and social evolution in relation to the reproductive capacity of women. The language and discourse surrounding the holistic progression of women away from population demands. Perhaps the reality of words such as oppression, exploitation and denigration, which lie at the heart of organisational infrastructures led predominantly by white middle class men, in the context of labour force norms ought to be the first issue for address. The transectionality of this with other social issues is clear – white supremacy and racial prejudice being the obvious counterparts of a society now led by politicians whose mantra is to control rather than empower and whose coarse intentionality belies their societal position. Where bureaucratic change focuses predominantly on weaponising policy to serve a greater misogyny and the divisive intentionality of global governments, in reality what hope for society can there be unless women use a collective voice to challenge it?

Re-Framing a New Lens for Historical Contexts and Cultures

In instances where harassment has occurred at differing levels of an organisational hierarchy then, historically, all evidence pointed to the member lowest in the hierarchy being asked to prove their credibility beyond the context of professionalism. It is this historical approach to the perceived legitimacy of positional power which is fundamentally wrong. The assumption of innocence which has been attributed to positionality has now been removed. Men and women are fundamentally equal but different and their relative positions in organisational hierarchies around the world's workplaces cannot skew their capacity to be assumed innocent because of their academic and professional achievements or the consequent perceived respectability based on them (Healy and Kirton, 2000). It is also at this point when the boundaries between criminality and inappropriateness are drawn, however discernment by an astute Human Resources department ought first to establish core facts and the testable consistency of potential witnesses. Institutionally organisations are now ethically and morally expected to protect staff against unwanted sexual protection and their staff can regard this with a degree of entitlement (Cater et al., 2018).

The provision of a safe environment in which all people feel free to go about their daily work without the need for undue concern about unwarranted attention is one which in certain contexts, has not been possible, for an array of differing cultural norms, the normalisation of deviance and the imbalance between genders, which has fuelled and demeaned both professional men and women. As such this predicament necessitates a collective sense of responsibility to not only verbalise and raise awareness of the need for change but perhaps more importantly to ensure that change is sustained, fair and transparent for every member of every workforce. Whilst a panacea for change at present, it is this vision, which will contribute to better working conditions in the future and an active recognition of the difference between acceptability and cultural normalisation of deviant behaviour, regardless of age, gender, race, faith or sexual orientation.

Medicine is just one context where this vision must be phronetically applied and adhered to (Han et al., 2018). The relative and evident lack of women in leadership roles in the context of medicine has ensured action to redress the balance in gender representations across the majority of healthcare hierarchies and to a certain extent this has been achieved. It is evident that more women than ever are occupying executive positions, leadership roles and professorial positions, however evidence reveals that the perceived realities of these women in relation to sexist remarks, inappropriate sexually suggestive behaviour and coercion to sexual activity for reward in the form of promotion still represent a need for wholesale address across our societies.

The historically male constructed narrative accounts of the contribution of women to the progression and development of democratic freedom, often fail to acknowledge just how significant these contributions are and continue to be. We often fail to remember, for example that Nancy, Viscountess Astor, became the first Member of Parliament (MP) but not until 1919, only a century ago. Whilst this represented a landmark progression at the time, one hundred years later it also represents a benchmark of just how far we have left to go to ensure equity and parity of dignity and respect for all in public service, of which medical practice is a typical example (Quinn, 2017). What is ironical is that the suffrage that women died to gain, has also engendered subsequent generations of both women and men to support feminism and to see the evolution of Fourth Wave Feminism. This Fourth Wave Feminism arrived as a consequence of change in our technological societies and ironically this change was borne out of a trajectory of protest against containment, limitation and silencing of speaking out against the 21st Century workplace contexts of sexual harassment, rape and oppression, where education and relative privilege have served only to protect those at the helm of these acts (Fullagar and Pavlidis, 2018).

Socially constructed, gender is largely determined by the societies and communities to whom people belong (Mihaila and Botezat, 2016). It is largely characterised by our human perception of whether physical characteristics express femininity or masculinity in relation to mannerisms and observable actions and which are enhanced by clothing and the way we choose to dress and present ourselves in public. These fuel the perceptions and value judgements we all resonate, but more significantly highlight that dominance and submission can become issues for people whose assumptions of outward appearance are then translated to attitudes, then a degree of proactive behavioural expression, which is at best offensive and degrading and at worst potentially harmful to those in enforced submissive roles, either through clear evidence of wrongful gender stereotyping or willful disregard for the mutual respect of colleagues.

Perceived vs. Actual Reality: What is the State of Play in Medicine and Surgery Today?

Our recent qualitative research into the context of women in surgery highlighted the complexity of working in the context of an inherently male-dominated profession (Bellini et al., 2018). The aim of this research was to survey women working within a surgical discipline, to understand their current perceptions, providing insight into their practical day-to-day lives and unashamedly supporting the potential for an action-oriented change within the profession. The study provided surgeons with link to a confidential, online survey was distributed through the Association of Surgeons of Great Britain and Ireland (ASGBI) social media platforms on Facebook and Twitter over a 2-week period in October 2017. We ensured that participants were those women working in surgical specialties and actively responding to the link shared through the ASGBI social media platforms. The data sets we collated were analysed through a mixed-methods approach which made it possible to identify the most salient themes that these women in surgery identified and articulated. The findings of this research bore testimony to the sexism women in surgery experienced with a total of 81 female participants replying and eighty eight percent of these women also reporting that they perceived surgery as a male-dominated field of practice. Over half of these women had personally experienced sexual discrimination in their surgical roles where they also reported experiencing a ‘glass ceiling’ in the facilitation of their surgical training. Orthopaedics was reported as the most sexist surgical specialty by over half of women. Reports of bias in gendered language in the workplace were reported by fifty nine percent of women, where a lack of formal mentorship, inflexibility towards part-time careers, gender stereotypes and poor work–life balance were the main perceived barriers for women in surgical careers. Perhaps most significantly, this research highlighted the implicit nature of the perceived discrimination that women report in their surgical careers. In essence this points to the need to create an action-oriented change of cultures and subcultures in surgical disciplines by allowing all staff, regardless of gender, to reflect on their own behaviour, perceptions and the culture in which they work. Our work is consolidated by the findings of a raft of other researchers who have reported similar recent outcomes to their own explorations of women in health and medicine (Smith, Bethune and Hurley, 2018; Hughes and Bernstein, 2018;

Lighting Fires Not Filling Buckets: Role Modelling for a More Positive Future

Education is not the filling of a bucket but the lighting of a fire. ~W.B.Yeats

At the heart of transformative education lies the internalisation of meaning making that can affect people to the point their attitudes and behaviours change (Reimann and Alfermann, 2018). This change must begin with the awareness raising, re-education and facilitation of reflection that leads to behavioural change and thinking in action in everyday practice (Magee, 2017; Taylor, 2017). This change necessitates a wholesale change to undergraduate curricula, where early professional identities are framed and consolidated by intergenerational transmission and the enculturation into a professional identity (Morgan et al., 2018; Liston and Rahimi, 2017).

In an age where the now historical philosophies of Nietzche and Mailer remain widely taught, often by women to women as a means of underpinning scholarly activity, ought we really to be surprised at the perpetuation of a subculture of misogyny? This question is now at the fore of change initiatives (Reid-Pharr, 2019). The obvious response is that the #MeToo movement needs to penetrate more deeply than the hymen of media publicity, the casting couch and Hollywood red carpets to operationalise any potential for real life impact. Real women work in all contexts and settings of society; the awareness we seek to raise for women in medicine and surgery via a collective voice is merely a middle-class megaphone for women who have become little more regarded than a social underclass and deviants of physiologically based destiny.

Both the pedagogical opportunity and challenge this provides, needs little indication. As numbers of women entering these professions increase, it is disheartening to see the ongoing wide scale evidence of a two-tier society, where woman still traditionally occupy positions of subservience (Bucknor et al., 2018; Hughes and Bernstein, 2018; Fee, 2019).

Horton and Freire's (1990) now seminal debate on the power of pedagogy in practice, resonates across the tympanic membrane of those people for whom hope of change resonates. Whether transformational solidarity for women was even possible was the debate that characterised 1980's feminist writing. The small differences that exist between women across global societies were identified as a source of unjust domination and oppressive relationships. Political solidarity has never been the preserve of the woman yet thankfully it now serves and characterises the currency of debate around the #MeToo movement by women who are now instead making it work for women instead of just being by women.

Whatever their nature, current ontological and consequently epistemological paradigm shifts bode well for intergenerational focus on operational change for women and girls contemplating careers in medicine and surgery. However, this must be tempered by the ethos of critical postmodern educational praxes which maintain a scope for ethical imagination and progression. The situated nature of this in medicine and surgery contexts is not unique but using the female workforce in these settings to illustrate the need for change can be highlighted. Accompanying it though, needs to be a complementary raft of liberating pedagogy that strikes at the minds and conscience of all those working in situations and contexts that have to date proven themselves impenetrable and remain largely untouched by the concept of social justice.

In the context of pedagogic practice, what Freire postulated as the only mechanism of transformative change is active dialogue – dialogue beyond that of the declarative but that which represents a real prospect of proactive intervention for the benefit of future generations of women (Horton and Freire, 1990). This is potentially one of few transferrable directives for mediation in the reclamation of women's voices both on an individual and collective basis, stating,

Dialogue is the encounter between men, mediated by the world, in order to move the world.... Those who have been denied their primordial potential right to speak their word must first reclaim and prevent the continuation of this dehumanising aggression (Freire, 1990)

Igniting a Spark for Structure and Agency in Medicine and Surgery

The structural power relationships identified in the work of Cohen, deal with the taxonomies and classifications of power that exist within and between genders in society. The fact that these structural power relationships also determine the degree of accessibility that people have to the specific resources that fuel the potential of professional identity for millions worldwide (Coyle, 2010). The epistemic injustice of context and situational circumstance for women necessitates a consideration of the fluidity of representation and how this has been impacted upon by different historical eras, all of which can be mapped back to the characteristically recognisable feminist waves. The capacity of women to engage, achieve and progress within the context of medicine and surgery will ultimately be determined by whether a commitment to change. The #MeToo initiative will potentially do much to raise awareness and further concern for such a fundamental societal issue. Coyle's concept of passion or dedication and intrinsic motivation to achieve a goal is something he termed 'ignition', where he posits that the identity that has the potential to inspire others comes from having an origin that is ultimately recognisable, where it is possible to see how familiar boundaries and challenges can be overcome, to remain authentic and accessible (ibid, 2010). In the context of a global sisterhood these features are something all women can aspire to and ones which we all ought to remember, will enhance not only our own lives, but which extends reach to a level of intergenerational solidarity, in the true essence of suffrage.

Beyond Blaming and Framing: Reclaiming Dignity Through Authentic Womanhood

As people in support of the reclamation of dignity for women in all professions, the recognition of the contribution of our own grandmothers, mothers, sisters and best friends has to pervade our intrinsic motivation and our passion to drive tangible social change. These women provided our own aspirational identities, in many instances gave selflessly to our accomplishments and remained steadfast in the belief of our potential success in the contributions we could make professionally and to the concept of womanhood. Let us honour great women, not just of this generation but those who made what we do today possible. Let us honour their memories with a legacy of positive change for the future women of medicine and surgery today. We are womanhood, sisterhood and stand together for this future positive change. A century on from suffrage, let us continue to advocate true acceptance of our gender and intellectual endeavours so that we might remain clearly both identifiable and imminently aspirational to a whole new generation of medics and surgeons who remember this legacy with pride.

CONCLUSION

The active momentum that has driven the #MeToo movement for the last five years has provided a platform for the address of the need for ongoing dialogue and advocacy for women in the workplace generally and for women in the medical and surgical sphere, specifically. This paper heightens debate of whether it is for the individual/organisations/professional societies or the wider community to address all of these issues. This will undoubtedly involve corrective measures being adopted and maintained. Importantly this will require ongoing advocacy on the part of women, as we have indicated in this chapter. This means that change must occur but it is more than just the bureaucratic structures that are impeding the progress of women, there is also the enabling role of patriarchy which is a direct driver of misogyny and consequently sexism. Identifying corrective and sustainable measures which need to be adopted and applied in practice, is the next major challenge for global societies in which women occupy an ever-increasing number of roles in the workplace

REFERENCES

Bareket, O., Shnabel, N., Abeles, D., Gervais, S., & Yuval-Greenberg, S. (2018). Evidence for an Association between Men's Spontaneous Objectifying Gazing Behavior and their Endorsement of Objectifying Attitudes toward Women. *Sex Roles*, 1–12.

Barlow, A. (2018). "Can I take out my penis?" Navigating Sex and Intimacy in the Workplace: An Empirical Test of Black's Theory of Conflict. *Deviant Behavior*, 1–14.

Bates, C. K., Jagsi, R., Gordon, L. K., Travis, E., Chatterjee, A., Gillis, M., ... Fivush, B. (2018). It is time for zero tolerance for sexual harassment in academic medicine. *Academic Medicine*, *93*(2), 163–165. doi:10.1097/ACM.0000000000002050 PMID:29116986

Bellini, M. I., Graham, Y., Hayes, C., Zakeri, R., Parks, R., & Papalois, V. (2019). A woman's place is in theatre: Women's perceptions and experiences of working in surgery from the Association of Surgeons of Great Britain and Ireland women in surgery working group. *BMJ Open*, *9*(1). doi:10.1136/bmjopen-2018-024349 PMID:30617103

Bucknor, A., Kamali, P., Phillips, N., Mathijssen, I., Rakhorst, H., Lin, S. J., & Furnas, H. (2018). Gender Inequality for Women in Plastic Surgery: A Systematic Scoping Review. *Plastic and Reconstructive Surgery*, *141*(6), 1561–1577. doi:10.1097/PRS.0000000000004375 PMID:29794715

Campbell, K., Nelson, J., Parker, M. L., & Johnston, S. (2018). Interpersonal Chemistry in Friendships and Romantic Relationships. *Interpersona: An International Journal on Personal Relationships*, *12*(1), 34–50. doi:10.5964/ijpr.v12i1.289

Cater, S. W., Yoon, S. C., Lowell, D. A., Campbell, J. C., Sulioti, G., Qin, R., ... Grimm, L. J. (2018). Bridging the gap: Identifying global trends in gender disparity among the radiology physician workforce. *Academic Radiology*, *25*(8), 1052–1061. doi:10.1016/j.acra.2017.12.021 PMID:29398433

Cohn, S., & Blumberg, R. L. (Eds.). (2019). *Gender and Development: The Economic Basis of Women's Power*. Sage.

Coyle, D. (2010). *The Talent Code: Greatness isn't born, it's grown*. Random House.

Fee, E. (2019). *Women and health: The politics of sex in medicine*. Routledge. doi:10.4324/9781315223346

Ford, C. (2018). The turning point: One man's downfall,# MeToo, and the rising up. *Meanjin*, *77*(2), 40.

Freire, P. (2018). *Pedagogy of the oppressed.* USA: Bloomsbury Publishing.

Fullagar, S., & Pavlidis, A. (2018). Feminist theories after the poststructuralist turn. In *Feminisms in Leisure Studies* (pp. 48–71). Routledge. doi:10.4324/9781315108476-3

Gertner, N. (2018). Sexual Harassment and the Bench. *Stan. L. Rev. Online*, *71*, 86.

Han, H., Kim, Y., Kim, S., Cho, Y., & Chae, C. (2018). Looking into the labyrinth of gender inequality: Women physicians in academic medicine. *Medical Education*, *52*(10), 1083–1095. doi:10.1111/medu.13682 PMID:30255527

Healy, G., & Kirton, G. (2000). Women, power and trade union government in the UK. *British Journal of Industrial Relations*, *38*(3), 343–360. doi:10.1111/1467-8543.00168

Horton, M., & Freire, P. (1990). *We make the road by walking: Conversations on education and social change*. Temple University Press.

Huff, S., Rudman, D. L., Magalhães, L., & Lawson, E. (2018). 'Africana womanism': Implications for transformative scholarship in occupational science. *Journal of Occupational Science*, *25*(4), 554–565. doi:10.1080/14427591.2018.1493614

Hughes, F., & Bernstein, P. S. (2018). Sexism in obstetrics and gynecology: Not just a "women's issue". *American Journal of Obstetrics and Gynecology*, *219*(4), 364–e1. doi:10.1016/j.ajog.2018.07.006 PMID:30017680

Liston, D. D., & Rahimi, R. (Eds.). (2017). *Promoting Social Justice Through the Scholarship of Teaching and Learning*. Indiana University Press. doi:10.2307/j.ctt2005zc2

Lovell, K. N. (2018). "Everyone Gets a Blister": Sexism, Gender Empowerment, and Race in the People's Park Movement. *Women's Studies Quarterly*, *46*(3), 103–119. doi:10.1353/wsq.2018.0034

Magee, R. V. (2017). One Field, Different Doors In: Contemplative Higher Education, Transformative Education, and Education for Social Justice. Social Justice, Inner Work & Contemplative Practice, 119.

Manne, K. (2016). The logic of misogyny. *Boston Review*, *41*(4), 8–23.

Manne, K. (2017). Down girl: The logic of misogyny. Oxford, UK: Oxford University Press. doi:10.1093/oso/9780190604981.001.0001

McClure, E. (2019). Theorizing a Spectrum of Aggression: Microaggressions, Creepiness, and Sexual Assault. *the pluralist, 14*(1), 91-101.

Mihaila, R., & Botezat, O. (2016). The Gender Construction of Society. *Journal of Research in Gender Studies*, *6*(2), 187.

Morgan, A. U., Chaiyachati, K. H., Weissman, G. E., & Liao, J. M. (2018). Eliminating Gender-Based Bias in Academic Medicine: More than Naming the "Elephant in the Room". *Journal of General Internal Medicine*, 1–3. PMID:29564608

Nietsche, F. (1911). Beyond good and evil (vol. 12 of The complete works. Ed.: O. Levy) Foulis.

Pateman, C. (2018). *The disorder of women: Democracy, feminism and political theory*. John Wiley & Sons.

Quinn, T. A. (2017). Opening the Doors of Medicine to Women. *The Journal of the American Osteopathic Association, 117*(3), 149–149. doi:10.7556/jaoa.2017.028 PMID:28241325

Reid-Pharr, R. F. (2019). The Disappearance of Great Men: Or, If You Want to Understand the Wounded Celebrity of Donald Trump, Just Ask Norman Mailer. *Minnesota Review, 2019*(92), 58-72.

Reimann, S., & Alfermann, D. (2018). Female Doctors in Conflict: How Gendering Processes in German Hospitals Influence Female Physicians' Careers. *Gender Issues*, *35*(1), 52–70. doi:10.100712147-017-9186-9

Smith, V., Bethune, C., & Hurley, K. F. (2018). Examining medical student specialty choice through a gender lens: An orientational qualitative study. *Teaching and Learning in Medicine*, *30*(1), 33–44. doi: 10.1080/10401334.2017.1306447 PMID:28497985

Spraitz, J. (2018). Institutional Sexual Abuse. *Contemporary Issues in Victimology: Identifying Patterns and Trends*, 225.

Sundaram, V., & Jackson, C. (2018). 'Monstrous men' and 'sex scandals': The myth of exceptional deviance in sexual harassment and violence in education. *Palgrave Communications*, *4*(1), 147. doi:10.105741599-018-0202-9

Supriya, K. E. (2018). Judgment and the Problem of Agency/Accountability: A Postcolonial Critique of Poststructuralist Theory. In Judgment Calls (pp. 42-62). Routledge.

Taylor, E. W. (2017). Transformative learning theory. In *Transformative Learning Meets Bildung* (pp. 17–29). Rotterdam, The Netherlands: SensePublishers. doi:10.1007/978-94-6300-797-9_2

Zarkov, D. & Davis, K. (2018). Ambiguities and dilemmas around# MeToo:# ForHow Long and# WhereTo?

Compilation of References

2018 . Global mobile consumer trends. Deloitte. (2018). Retrieved from https://www2.deloitte.com/global/en/pages/technology-media-and-telecommunications/articles/gx-global-mobile-consumer-trends.html

AAMC (2014). The State of Women in Academic Medicine: The Pipeline and Pathways to Leadership.

AAMC Faculty Roster. (2018). Department Chairs by Department, Sex, and Race/Ethnicity, 2018. Retrieved from https://www.aamc.org/download/495102/data/supplementaltablec.pdf

AAMC Faculty Roster. (2018). U.S. Medical School Faculty by Sex, Rank, and Department, 2018. Retrieved from https://www.aamc.org/download/495048/data/18table13.pdf

AAMC. (2005). *Women in U.S. academic medicine statistics and medical school benchmarking, 2004–2005*. Washington, DC: Association of American Medical Colleges.

Abrantes, A., & Simões,, J. (2017). Thinking Ahead: Portugal's Health in 2027. Port. *J Public Health*, *35*, 141–144. doi:10.1159/000488336

Academy of Medical Royal Colleges. (2015). Exercise the miracle cure and the role of the doctor in promoting it. Retrieved from http://www.aomrc.org.uk/publications/reports-guidance/exercise-the-miracle-cure-0215/

ACGME Common Program Requirements (Residency), revised June 10, 2019. Retrieved from https://acgme.org/Portals/0/PFAssets/ProgramRequirements/CPRResidency2019.pdf

ACOG (The American College of Obstetricians and Gynaecologists). (2015). Early pregnancy loss. Available at https://www.acog.org/Patients/FAQs/Early-Pregnancy-Loss?IsMobileSet=false

ACSS. (2005-2007). Relatório Social do Ministério da Saúde e do Serviço Nacional de Saúde, 2005-2007. Retrieved from http://www.acss.min-saude.pt

ACSS. (2017). *Relatório Social do Ministério da Saúde e do Serviço Nacional de Saúde*. Retrieved from http://www.acss.min-saude.pt

ACSS. (2017). Relatório Social do Ministério da Saúde e do Serviço Nacional de Saúde. Retrieved from http://www.acss.min-saude.pt/

Adams, R. B., & Ferreira, D. (2009). Women in the Boardroom and Their Impact on Governance and Performance. *Journal of Financial Economics*, *94*(2), 291–309. doi:10.1016/j.jfineco.2008.10.007Catalyst Report. (1999). Catalyst Report: 1999 Catalyst Census of Women Corporate Officers and Top Earners. Retrieved from https://www.catalyst.org/

Aditi Ramakrishnan, M. A., Dana Sambuco, M. P. P. A., Reshma Jagsi, M. D., & Phil, D. (2014). Women's Participation in the Medical Profession: Insights from Experiences in Japan, Scandinavia, Russia, and Eastern Europe. *Journal of Women's Health*, *23*(11), 927–934. doi:10.1089/jwh.2014.4736 PMID:25320867

Agostoni, C., Braegger, C., Decsi, T., Kolacek, S., Koletzko, B., Michaelsen, K. F., ... van Goudoever, J. (2009). Breastfeeding: A commentary by the ESPGHAN Committee on Nutrition. *Journal of Pediatric Gastroenterology and Nutrition*, *49*(1), 112–125. doi:10.1097/MPG.0b013e31819f1e05 PMID:19502997

Al-Awami, S. M. (2000). Surgery in Saudi Arabia. *Archives of Surgery (Chicago, Ill.)*, *135*(3), 354–357. doi:10.1001/archsurg.135.3.354 PMID:10722041

Albakr, F., Bruce, E., Davidson, P., Schlaffer, E., & Kropiunigg, U. (2017). Empowered but not equal: Challenging the traditional gender roles as seen by university students in Saudi Arabia. *Forum for International Research in Education*, *4*(1), 52-66.

Alghamdi, T. (2014). Balance between career and family among female doctors at KAMC, Riyadh, Saudi Arabia. *International Journal of Medical Science and Public Health*, *3*(2), 203–211. doi:10.5455/ijmsph.2013.021220133

Ali, A. M., & McVay, C. L. (2016). Women in surgery: A history of adversity, resilience, and accomplishment. *Journal of the American College of Surgeons*, *223*(4), 670–673. doi:10.1016/j.jamcollsurg.2016.06.012 PMID:27374995

Amanatullah, E. T., & Morris, M. W. (2010). Negotiating gender roles: Gender differences in assertive negotiating are mediated by women's fear of backlash and attenuated when negotiating on behalf of others. *Journal of Personality and Social Psychology*, *98*(2), 256–267. doi:10.1037/a0017094 PMID:20085399

Amanatullah, E. T., & Tinsley, C. H. (2013). Punishing female negotiators for asserting too much…or not enough: Exploring why advocacy moderates backlash against assertive female negotiators. *Organizational Behavior and Human Decision Processes*, *120*(1), 110–122. doi:10.1016/j.obhdp.2012.03.006

Andreen, A. (1988). *Karolina Widerström, En levnadsteckning*. Norstedts.

Angier, M., & Axelrod, B. (2014). Realizing the power of talented women. *The McKinsey Quarterly*.

Annan, K. (2005). Empowerment of Women is the Most Effective Development Tool.

Antoniadis, S., Passauer-Baierl, S., Baschnegger, H., & Weigl, M. (2014). Identification and interference of intraoperative distractions and interruptions in operating rooms. *The Journal of Surgical Research*, *188*(1), 21–29. doi:10.1016/j.jss.2013.12.002 PMID:24405613

AoMRC (The Academy of Medical Royal Colleges). (2016). Maternity/Paternity Survey Results. Available from http://aomrc.org.uk/wp-content/uploads/2016/06/Maternity_paternity_survey_200416-1.pdf

Appleby, J. (2018, April 5). The gender pay gap in the NHS: the story so far. Retrieved from https://www.nuffieldtrust.org.uk/news-item/the-gender-pay-gap-in-the-nhs-the-story-so-far

Arab board web. *About the Board.* Available at http://arab board.org/en/content/about-board

Arabian Gulf University. *Homepage*. Available at http://www.agu.edu.bh/english/university/uni_facts.aspx

Arabian Gulf University. *University Facts*. Available at http://www.agu.edu.bh/english/university/uni_facts.aspx

Arbetsdepartementet/Swedish government. (1977). Retrieved from www.riksdagen.se/sv/dokument-lagar/dokument/svensk-forfattningssamling/semesterlag-1977480_sfs-1977-480

Arrizabalaga, P., Abellana, R., Viñas, O., Merino, A., & Ascaso, C. (2014). Gender inequalities in the medical profession: Are there still barriers to women physicians in the 21st century? *Gaceta Sanitaria*, *28*(5), 351–438. doi:10.1016/j.gaceta.2014.03.014 PMID:24889702

Artz, B., Goodall, A. H., & Oswald, A. J. (2018). Do Women Ask? *Industrial Relations*, *57*(4), 611–636. doi:10.1111/irel.12214

ASA Task Force on Equity, Diversity, and Inclusion 2018.

Association of American Medical College. (2018). Retrieved from www.aamc.org

Association of American Medical Colleges (AAMC). (2016). The state of women in academic medicine: the pipeline and pathways to leadership, 2015-2016. Retrieved from (https:// www.aamc.org/members/gwims/statistics/)

Association of American Medical Colleges, Annual Report 2014.

Association of American Medical Colleges. (2013-2014). The State of Women in Academic Medicine. The Pipeline and Pathways to Leadership. Retrieved from https://members.aamc.org/eweb/upload/The%20State%20of%20Women%20in%20Academic%20Medicine%202013-2014%20FINAL.pdf

Association of American Medical Colleges. (2017). *More Women Than Men Enrolled in U.S. Medical Schools in 2017.* Retrieved from https://news.aamc.org/content/downloadable/117/

Author's note (Machado MC): Many years later, he was my role model to enter the medical school and he was the most supportive within my family

AWS Maternity Leave Policy for Surgical Residents. (2002). General format. Retrieved from https://cdn.ymaws.com/womensurgeons.site-ym.com/resource/resmgr/docs/Resource_Library/ResidentPolicy.pdf

Babcock, L., & Laschever, S. (2008). *Why Women Don't Ask: The high cost of avoiding negotiation - and positive strategies for change*. Princeton, NJ: Princeton University Press.

Babcock, L., & Laschever, S. (2009). *Women don't ask: Negotiation and the gender divide*. Princeton, NJ: Princeton University Press.

Badawy, R. L., Gazdag, B. A., Bentley, J. R., & Brouer, R. L. (2018). Are all impostors created equal? Exploring gender differences in the impostor phenomenon-performance link. *Personality and Individual Differences*, *131*, 156–163. doi:10.1016/j.paid.2018.04.044

Badham, V. (2018). Think sexism in medicine is unique to Japan? Think again. *The Guardian.* Retrieved from https://www.theguardian.com/commentisfree/2018/aug/13/think-sexism-in-medicine-is-unique-to-japan-think-again

Bagheritari, M. & David, M. (2013). Legislation and Policy – GEA – Gender and Education Association. Retrieved from http://www.genderandeducation.com/resources-2/legislative-frameworks/

Baird, J. (2018). Women, Own Your 'Dr' Titles. The New York Times. Retrieved from https://www.nytimes.com/2018/06/28/opinion/women-dont-back-down-online.html

Baird, M., Daugherty, L., Kumar, K. B., & Arifkhanova, A. (2015). Regional and gender differences and trends in the anesthesiologist workforce. *Anesthesiology*, *123*(5), 997–1012. doi:10.1097/ALN.0000000000000834 PMID:26291778

Bala, N. (2014). The 3 Biggest Reasons that India's Girls Drop Out of School.

Baqi, S., Albalbeesi, A., Iftikhar, S., Baig-Ansari, N., Alanazi, M., & Alanazi, A. (2017, October). Perceptions of gender equality, work environment, support and social issues for women doctors at a university hospital in Riyadh, Kingdom of Saudi Arabia. *PLoS One*, *12*(10). doi:10.1371/journal.pone.0186896 PMID:29073172

Bareket, O., Shnabel, N., Abeles, D., Gervais, S., & Yuval-Greenberg, S. (2018). Evidence for an Association between Men's Spontaneous Objectifying Gazing Behavior and their Endorsement of Objectifying Attitudes toward Women. *Sex Roles*, 1–12.

Barlow, A. (2018). "Can I take out my penis?" Navigating Sex and Intimacy in the Workplace: An Empirical Test of Black's Theory of Conflict. *Deviant Behavior*, 1–14.

Baron-Cohen, S. (2012). *The Essential Difference: men, women and extreme male brain*. London, UK: Penguin.

Bass, B. L., & Napolitano, L. M. (2004). Gender and diversity considerations in surgical training. *The Surgical Clinics of North America, 84*(6), 1537–1555. doi:10.1016/j.suc.2004.06.008 PMID:15501274

Bass, B. M., Bass, R., & Bass, B. M. (2009). *The Bass handbook of leadership: theory, research, and managerial applications*. Simon and Schuster.

Bates, C. K., Jagsi, R., Gordon, L. K., Travis, E., Chatterjee, A., Gillis, M., ... Fivush, B. (2018). It is time for zero tolerance for sexual harassment in academic medicine. *Academic Medicine, 93*(2), 163–165. doi:10.1097/ACM.0000000000002050 PMID:29116986

Bates, C., Gordon, L., Travis, E., Chatterjee, A., Chaudron, L., Fivush, B., ... Moses, A. (2016). Striving for gender equity in academic medicine careers: A call for action. *Academic Medicine, 91*(8), 1050–1052. doi:10.1097/ACM.0000000000001283 PMID:27332868

Baumhäkel, M., Müller, U., & Böhm, M. (2009). Influence of gender of physicians and patients on guidelinerecommended treatment of chronic heart failure in a cross-sectional study. *European Journal of Heart Failure, 11*(3), 299–303. doi:10.1093/eurjhf/hfn041 PMID:19158153

Baxter, A. D., Boet, S., Reid, D., & Skidmore, G. (2014). The aging anesthesiologist: a narrative review and suggested strategies. *Canadian Journal of Anaesthesia = Journal Canadien d'anesthesie, 61*(9), 865–875. doi:10.100712630-014-0194-x

Baxter, A., Thompson, C., & McCartney, C. (2016, October). "Winding down" guidelines for anesthesiologists: The Ottawa Hospital plan. *Canadian Journal of Anaesthesia = Journal Canadien d'anesthesie*. United States. doi:10.100712630-016-0692-0

Baxter, J. (2014). *Double-voicing at work. Power, gender and linguistic expertise*. Basingstoke, UK: Palgrave Macmillan. doi:10.1057/9781137348531

Beagan, B. L. (2000). Neutralizing differences: Producing neutral doctors for (almost) neutral patients. *Social Science & Medicine, 51*(8), 1253–1265. doi:10.1016/S0277-9536(00)00043-5 PMID:11037215

Beard, M. (2017). *Women and Power*. London, UK: Profile Books.

Bellini, M. I., Graham, Y., Hayes, C., Zakeri, R., Parks, R., & Papalois, V. (2019). A Woman´s place in theatre: women´s perceptions and experiences of working in surgery from the Association of Surgeons of Great Britain and Ireland. Women in Surgery working group. *BJM Open. 7;9*(1). doi:10.1136/bmjopen-2018-024349

Beltaib, M. (n.d.). *Tunisia's First Female Doctor: The Life of Tawhida Belsheikh*. Available at https://raseef22.com/article/1068287-tunisias-first-female-doctor-life-tawhida-belsheikh

Benziger, C. P., Roth, G. A., & Moran, A. E. (2016). The Global Burden of Disease Study and the Preventable Burden of NCD. *Global Heart, 11*(4), 393–397. doi:10.1016/j.gheart.2016.10.024 PMID:27938824

Berger, A., Giacalone, J., Barlow, P., Kapadia, M., & Keith, J. (2017). Choosing surgery as a career: Early results of a longitudinal study of medical students. *Surgery, 161*(6), 1683–1689. doi:10.1016/j.surg.2016.12.016 PMID:28161006

Bernard, D. L., Hoggard, L. S., & Neblett, E. W. (2018). Racial discrimination, racial identity, and impostor phenomenon: A profile approach. *Cultural Diversity & Ethnic Minority Psychology, 24*(1), 51–61. doi:10.1037/cdp0000161 PMID:28414495

Bernard, N. S., Dollinger, S. J., & Ramaniah, N. V. (2002). Applying the Big Five personality factors to the impostor phenomenon. *Journal of Personality Assessment*, *78*(2), 321–333. doi:10.1207/S15327752JPA7802_07 PMID:12067196

Berry, C. A. (2014). They Call Me Dr. Berry. *New York Times.* Retrieved from https://www.nytimes.com/2014/11/02/opinion/sunday/they-call-me-doctor-berry.html

Berry, L. L., & Seltman, K. D. (2014). The enduring culture of Mayo Clinic. *Mayo Clinic Proceedings*, *89*(2), 144–147. doi:10.1016/j.mayocp.2013.10.025 PMID:24485127

Besley, T., Folke, O., Persson, T., & Rickne, J. (2017). Gender Quotas and the Crisis of the Mediocre Man: Theory and Evidence from Sweden. *The American Economic Review*, *107*(8), 2204–2242. doi:10.1257/aer.20160080

Bhadra, M. (2011, January). Indian women in medicine: An enquiry since 1880. *Indian Anthropologist*, *1*, 17.

Bickel, J., Wara, D., Atkinson, B., Cohen, L., Dunn, M., Hostler, S., & Stokes, E. (2002). Increasing Women's Leadership in Academic Medicine: Report of the AAMC Project Implementation Committee. *Academic Medicine*, *77*(10), 1043–1061. doi:10.1097/00001888-200210000-00023 PMID:12377686

Binder, R., Garcia, P., Johnson, B., & Fuentes-Afflick, E. (2018). Sexual Harassment in Medical Schools. *Academic Medicine*, *93*(12), 1770–1773. doi:10.1097/ACM.0000000000002302 PMID:29794528

Bismark, M., Morris, J., Thomas, L., Loh, E., Phelps, G., & Dickinson, H. (2015). Reasons And Remedies For Under-Representation Of Women In Medical Leadership Roles: A Qualitative Study From Australia. *BMJ Open*, *5*(11). doi:10.1136/bmjopen-2015-009384 PMID:26576814

Bjurman, A. & Paul, U. (1988). I Karolina Widerströms Fotspår. 100 år med kvinnliga läkare i Sverige, särtryck av föreläsningar.

Blackmore, S. (2013). *Elizabeth Blackwell: the first woman to qualify as a doctor in America*. University of Bristol. The Wellcome Trust 2013. Retrieved from http://blog.wellcome.ac.uk/2013/07/22/elizabeth-blackwell/

Blair, J. E., Mayer, A. P., Caubet, S. L., Norby, S. M., O'Connor, M. I., & Hayes, S. N. (2015). Pregnancy and Parental Leave During Graduate Medical Education. *Academic Medicine*, *1*(November). doi:10.1097/ACM.0000000000001006 PMID:26606722

Blau, F. D. & Kahn, L. M. (2017). The Gender Wage Gap: Extent, Trends, and Explanations. *The New York Times, 55*(3), 789–865. doi:10.1257/jel.20160995

Blik op nieuws. (2018). Subsidie zorgt voor toename vrouwelijke hoogleraren. Retrieved from https://www.blikopnieuws.nl/nieuws/269428/subsidie-zorgt-voor-toename-vrouwelijke-hoogleraren.html

BMA (British Medical Association). (2015a). Less-than-full-time training guidance update. Available from https://www.bma.org.uk/news/2015/august/less-than-full-time-training-guidance-update

BMA (British Medical Association). (2015b). Less than full time guidance. Available at https://www.bma.org.uk/-/media/files/pdfs/developing%20your%20career/bma%20less%20than%20full%20time%20guidance.pdf

BMA, British Medical Association Equal Opportunities Committee. (2009). Equality and diversity in UK medical schools. BMA.

Bohnet, I. (2016). *What works: Gender equality by design*. Cambridge, MA: Belknap Press of Harvard University Press. doi:10.4159/9780674545991

Boiko, J. R., Anderson, A. J. M., & Gordon, R. A. (2017). Representation of women among academic grand rounds speaker. *JAMA Internal Medicine*, *177*(5), 722–724. doi:10.1001/jamainternmed.2016.9646 PMID:28264094

Bongiovanni, T., Yeo, H., Sosa, J. A., Yoo, P. S., Long, T., Rosenthal, M., ... Nunez-Smith, M. (2015). Attrition from surgical residency training: Perspectives from those who left. *American Journal of Surgery, 210*(4), 648–654. doi:10.1016/j.amjsurg.2015.05.014 PMID:26238074

Bonilla, G. (2010). Teoría feminista, ilustración y modernidad: Notas para un debate. *Cuadrenos de literatura del Caribe e Hispanoamericana*. Enero-junio 2010.

Borges, N., Navarro, A., & Grover, A. (2012). Women Physicians: Choosing a Career in Academic Medicine. *Academic Medicine, 87*(1), 105–114. doi:10.1097/ACM.0b013e31823ab4a8 PMID:22104052

BOTA (British Orthopaedic Trainees Association). (2017). Cut it out/ Hammer it out. http://www.bota.org.uk/hammer-it-out/

Boulouta, I. (2013). Hidden Connections: The Link Between Board Gender Diversity and Corporate Social Performance. *Journal of Business Ethics. Springer Netherlands, 113*(2), 185–197. doi:10.100710551-012-1293-7

Bowles, H. R., Babcock, L., & Lai, L. (2007). Social incentives for gender differences in the propensity to initiate negotiations: Sometimes it does hurt to ask. *Organizational Behavior and Human Decision Processes, 103*(1), 84–103. doi:10.1016/j.obhdp.2006.09.001

Braun, D. L., & Susman, V. L. (1992). Pregnancy during psychiatry residency: A study of attitudes. *Academic Psychiatry, 16*(4), 178–185. doi:10.1007/BF03341390 PMID:24435425

Briggs Myers, I., & Myers, P. B. (1995). *Gifts Differing: Understanding Personality Type*. Palo Alto, CA: Davies-Black Publishing.

British Broadcasting Corporation. (2017). *Do you have a gender-bias?* [Video]. Retrieved from https://www.youtube.com/watch?v=J69HkKz9g4A

Brottsförebyggande rådet, BRÅ. (2019). Statistics March 2019. Retrieved from https://www.bra.se/om-bra/nytt-fran-bra/arkiv/press/2019-03-28-slutlig-brottsstatistik-2018

Brown, A. & Ruzycki, S. (2018). The idea that medicine is above sexism is false – and destructive. Healthy Debate. Retrieved from https://healthydebate.ca/opinions/sexism-in-medicine

Brown, J., Brury, L., Raub, K., Levy, B., Brantner, P., Krivak, T. C., … Naumann, R. W. (2019). Workplace harassment and discrimination in gynecology: results of the AAGL member survey. *JMIG*, published online March 4, 2019.

Brown, C., Harries, R. L., Abdelrahman, T., Thomas, C., Pollitt, M. J., & Lewis, W. G. (2018). Surgical gender gap: A curriculum concordance and career vector perspective. *Postgraduate Medical Journal, 94*(1115), 483–488. doi:10.1136/postgradmedj-2017-135437 PMID:30355590

Brown, E. G., Galante, J. M., Keller, B. A., Braxton, J., & Farmer, D. L. (2014). Pregnancy-Related Attrition in General Surgery. *JAMA Surgery, 149*(9), 893. doi:10.1001/jamasurg.2014.1227 PMID:25029501

Brown, M. A., Erdman, M. K., Munger, A. M., & Miller, A. N. (2019). Despite growing number of women surgeons, authorship gender disparity in orthopaedic literature persists over 30 years. [Epub ahead of print]. *Clinical Orthopaedics and Related Research*, (Jun), 17. PMID:31283733

Bruce, A., Battista, A., Plankey, M., Johnson, L., & Marshall, M. (2015). Perceptions of gender-based discrimination during surgical training and practice. *Medical Education Online, 20*(1), 25923. doi:10.3402/meo.v20.25923 PMID:25652117

Bryan, P. [petrajbryan]. (2018, March 28). @MandipRandhawa7 @ChrisOliverNHS @hcwomenleaders Agree may not be talked about widely - but I've found it to be a common subject when I'm coaching others. Particularly with women leaders #NHSwomen [Tweet]. Retrieved from https://twitter.com/petrajbryan/status/979073494922211328

Buckley, L., Sanders, K., & Hampton, C. (2000). Obstacles to promotion? Values of women faculty about career success and recognition. *Academic Medicine, 75*(3), 283–288. doi:10.1097/00001888-200003000-00021 PMID:10724319

Bucknor, A., Kamali, P., Phillips, N., Mathijssen, I., Rakhorst, H., Lin, S. J., & Furnas, H. (2018). Gender Inequality for Women in Plastic Surgery: A Systematic Scoping Review. *Plastic and Reconstructive Surgery, 141*(6), 1561–1577. doi:10.1097/PRS.0000000000004375 PMID:29794715

Burkhart, S. (1987). Sexism in medical writing. *British Medical Journal, 295,* 19-26. Retrieved from https://www.ncbi.nlm.nih.gov/pmc/articles/PMC1257479/

Butkus, R., Serchen, J., Moyer, D. V., Bornstein, S. S., & Hingle, S. T. (2018). Achieving gender equity in physician compensation and career advancement: A position paper of the American College of Physicians. *Annals of Internal Medicine, 168*(10), 721–723. doi:10.7326/M17-3438 PMID:29710100

Butler, J. (2006). *Gender Trouble*. London, UK: Routledge.

Byrnes, K. D., & Lester, D. (2016). The imposter phenomenon in teachers and accountants. *Psychological Reports, 77*(1), 350–350. doi:10.2466/pr0.1995.77.1.350 PMID:7501775

Cameron, D. (2007) What language barrier? *The Guardian.* Retrieved from https://www.theguardian.com/world/2007/oct/01/gender.books

Cameron, D. (1985). *Feminism and linguistic theory*. London, UK: Macmillan. doi:10.1007/978-1-349-17727-1

Cameron, D. (1995). *Verbal Hygiene*. London, UK: Routledge.

Cammarata, B. & Thomas, B. (2014). Technology's Escalating Impact on Perioperative Care: Clinical, Compliance, and Medicolegal Considerations - Anesthesia Patient Safety Foundation. *APFS Newsletter, 29*(1). Retrieved from https://www.apsf.org/article/technologys-escalating-impact-on-perioperative-care-clinical-compliance-and-medicolegal-considerations/

Campbell, D. (2019, March 29). Male NHS doctors earn 17% more than their female peers. *The Guardian.*

Campbell, K., Nelson, J., Parker, M. L., & Johnston, S. (2018). Interpersonal Chemistry in Friendships and Romantic Relationships. *Interpersona: An International Journal on Personal Relationships, 12*(1), 34–50. doi:10.5964/ijpr.v12i1.289

Caniano, D. A., Sonnino, R. E., & Paolo, A. M. (2004). Keys to career satisfaction: Insights from a survey of women pediatric surgeons. *J Ped Surg, 39*(6), 984–990. doi:10.1016/j.jpedsurg.2004.02.039 PMID:15185240

Capaciteitsorgaan. (2016). Capaciteitsplan 2016. Retrieved from (https://capaciteitsorgaan.nl/app/uploads/2016/10/2016_10_21-Capaciteitsplan-2016-Deelrapport-4-SG-DEFINITIEF.pdf)

Carapinha, R., Ortiz-Walters, R., McCracken, C. M., Hill, E. V., & Reede, J. Y. (2016). Variability in women faculty's preferences regarding mentor similarity: A multi-institution study in academic medicine. *Academic Medicine, 91*(8), 1108–1118. doi:10.1097/ACM.0000000000001284 PMID:27332871

Cardoso, S., Carvalho, T., & Videira, P. (2018). Is It Still Worth Working In Academia? The Views from Portuguese Academics. *Higher Education Policy*. doi:10.105741307-018-0123-7

Carling, P. C., Hayward, K., Coakley, E. H., & Wolf, A. M. (1999). Part-time residency training in internal medicine: Analysis of a ten-year experience. *Academic Medicine, 74*(3), 282–284. doi:10.1097/00001888-199903000-00020 PMID:10099652

Carnes, M., & Bland, C. (2007). Viewpoint: A challenge to academic health centers and the National Institutes of Health to prevent unintended gender bias in the selection of clinical and translational science award leaders. *Academic Medicine*, *82*(2), 202–206. doi:10.1097/ACM.0b013e31802d939f PMID:17264704

Carnes, M., Morrissey, C., & Geller, S. E. (2008). Women's health and women's leadership in academic medicine: Hitting the same glass ceiling? *Journal of Women's Health*, *17*(9), 1453–1462. doi:10.1089/jwh.2007.0688 PMID:18954235

Carpenter, A. M., Tan, S. A., Costopoulos, K., Cooper, L. A., Sarosi, G. A., & Shaw, C. M. (2018). Gender Diversity in General Surgery Residency Leadership. *Journal of Surgical Education*, *75*(6), e68–e71. doi:10.1016/j.jsurg.2018.07.021 PMID:30177356

Carr, P. L., Ash, A. S., Friedman, R. H., Szalacha, L., Barnett, R. C., Palepu, A., & Moskowtiz, M. M. (2000). Faculty perceptions of gender discrimination and sexual harassment in academic medicine. *Annals of Internal Medicine*, *132*(11), 889–896. doi:10.7326/0003-4819-132-11-200006060-00007 PMID:10836916

Carr, P., Raj, A., Kaplan, S., Md, M. P. H., Terrin, N., Breeze, J., ... Md, M. P. H. (2018). Gender Differences in Academic Medicine: Retention, Rank, and Leadership Comparisons from the National Faculty Survey. *Academic Medicine*, *93*(11), 1694–1699. doi:10.1097/ACM.0000000000002146 PMID:29384751

Catalyst Report. (2003). Catalyst Report: 2003 Catalyst Census of Women Board Directors of the Fortune 500. Retrieved from https://www.catalyst.org/

Cater, S. W., Yoon, S. C., Lowell, D. A., Campbell, J. C., Sulioti, G., Qin, R., ... Grimm, L. J. (2018). Bridging the gap: Identifying global trends in gender disparity among the radiology physician workforce. *Academic Radiology*, *25*(8), 1052–1061. doi:10.1016/j.acra.2017.12.021 PMID:29398433

Central Bureau of Statistics Sweden. (2018). Women and men in Sweden. Facts and figures.

Ceu Machado, M. (2003). A feminização da Medicina. *Analise Social*, *166*, 127–7.

Chadda, R., & Sood, M. (2010, June). Women in medicine: A perspective. *Indian Journal of Gender Studies*, *17*(2), 277–285. doi:10.1177/097152151001700204

Chae, J.-H., Piedmont, R. L., Estadt, B. K., & Wicks, R. J. (1995). Personological evaluation of Clance's Imposter Phenomenon Scale in a Korean sample. *Journal of Personality Assessment*, *65*(3), 468–485. doi:10.120715327752jpa6503_7 PMID:16367710

Chakelian, A. (2018, April 4). What to say when someone tries to mansplain away the gender pay gap. *New Statesman (London, England)*.

Chandramouli, C., & General, R. (2011). *Census of India 2011*. Provisional Population Totals.

Chapman, B. (2017, June 19). Workplace gender quotas weed out incompetent men and make businesses more efficient, study finds. *The Independent*.

Cheng, L., & Yang, H. (2015). Learning about gender on campus: An analysis of the hidden curriculum for medical students. *Medical Education*, *49*(3), 321–331. doi:10.1111/medu.12628 PMID:25693991

Chen, M. M., Yeo, H. L., Roman, S. A., Bell, R. H. Jr, & Sosa, J. A. (2013). Life events during surgical residency have different effects on women and men over time. *Surgery*, *154*(2), 162–170. doi:10.1016/j.surg.2013.03.014 PMID:23889946

Chen, S., Huang, P., Shih, Y., & Chang, L. (2016). Investigation of multiple human factors in personalized learning. *Interactive Learning Environments*, *24*(1), 119–141. doi:10.1080/10494820.2013.825809

Chinchilla, N. (2018). *Integrar la vida. "Integrate life*. Barcelona, Spain: Ariel.

Choo, E. K., Kass, D., Westergaard, M., Watts, S. H., Berwald, N., Regan, L., ... Nobay, F. (2016). The Development of Best Practice Recommendations to Support the Hiring, Recruitment, and Advancement of Women Physicians in Emergency Medicine. *Academic Emergency Medicine, 23*(11), 1203–1209. doi:10.1111/acem.13028 PMID:27286760

Choudhry, N. K., Fletcher, R. H., & Soumerai, S. B. (2005). Systematic Review: The Relationship between Clinical Experience and Quality of Health Care. *Annals of Internal Medicine, 142*(4), 260. doi:10.7326/0003-4819-142-4-200502150-00008 PMID:15710959

Chrisman, S. M., Pieper, W. A., Clance, P. R., Holland, C. L., & Glickauf-Hughes, C. (1995). Validation of the Clance Impostor Phenomenon Scale. *Journal of Personality Assessment, 65*(3), 456–467. doi:10.120715327752jpa6503_6 PMID:16367709

ChrissieMoz. (2018, March 28). My imposter syndrome was fuelled by a male boss who once told me that I needed to learn "the power of silence," that fuelled my self doubt on the validity of my opinions. Speak up! #NHSwomen [Tweet]. Retrieved from https://twitter.com/ChrissieMoz/status/979084803336232962

Christensen, M., Aubeeluck, A., Fergusson, D., Craft, J., Knight, J., Wirihana, L., & Stupple, E. (2016). Do student nurses experience imposter phenomenon? An international comparison of final year undergraduate nursing students readiness for registration. *Journal of Advanced Nursing, 72*(11), 2784–2793. doi:10.1111/jan.13034 PMID:27240171

Chuchu, N., Takwoingi, Y., Dinnes, J., Matin, R. N., Bassett, O., & Moreau, J. F., … Group, C. S. C. D. T. A. (2018). Smartphone applications for triaging adults with skin lesions that are suspicious for melanoma. *Cochrane Database of Systematic Reviews*, (12). doi:10.1002/14651858.CD013192 PMID:30521685

Chung, M., Raman, G., Chew, P., Magula, N., Trikalinos, T., & Lau, J. (2007). Breastfeeding and maternal and infant health outcomes in developed countries. *Evidence Report/Technol Assessment., 153*, 1–186. PMID:17764214

CIG. (2017). Comissão para a Cidadania e Igualdade de Género (2017). Igualdade de Género em Portugal, Indicadores-Chave 2017. Retrieved from https://www.cig.gov.pt/2017/07/igualdade-de-genero-em-portugal-indicadores-chave-2017/

CIG. (2017). Comissão para a Cidadania e Igualdade de Género. Boletim estatístico 2017. Retrieved from https://www.cig.gov.pt/2018/02/igualdade-genero-portugal-boletim-estatistico-2017/

Cislak, A., Formanowicz, M., & Saguy, T. (2018). Bias against research on gender bias. *Scientometrics, 115*(1), 189–200. doi:10.100711192-018-2667-0 PMID:29527071

Clance, P. R. (n.d.). Clance Impostor Phenomenon Test. Retrieved from https://paulineroseclance.com/pdf/IPTestandscoring.pdf

Clance, P. & O`Toole, M. A. (1998). The impostor phenomenon: an internal barrier to empowerment and achievement. Special issue: Treating women's fear of failure. *Women & Therapy, 6*, 51–64.

Clance, P. R. (1985). *The Impostor Phenomenon: When Success Makes You Feel Like A Fake* (pp. 20–22). Toronto, Canada: Bantam Books.

Clance, P. R. , & O'Toole, M. A. (1988). *The Imposter Phenomenon: An Internal Barrier To Empowerment and Achievement*. Philadelphia, PA: Haworth Press.

Clance, P. R., & Imes, S. (1978). The imposter phenomenon in high achieving women: Dynamics and therapeutic intervention. *Psychotherapy (Chicago, Ill.), 15*.

Clark, N. F. (2014). Act now to shrink the confidence gap. *Forbes*.

Clemente, P. (2018). *El poder de flexibilizar dinámicas*. El mundo. Retrieved from http://www.elmundo.es/economia/innovadores/2018/12/20/5c17e4e721efa0e31d8b461e.html

Cochran, A., Elder, W. B., Crandall, M., Brasel, K., Hauschild, T., & Neumayer, L. (2013). Barriers to advancement in academic surgery: Views of senior residents and early career faculty. *American Journal of Surgery*, *206*(5), 661–666. doi:10.1016/j.amjsurg.2013.07.003 PMID:24011566

Codd, E. (2016). *Women in STEM. Technology, career pathways and the gender pay gap* (pp. 1–24). Deloitte. Retrieved from https://www2.deloitte.com/uk/en/pages/growth/articles/technology-career-pathways-gender-pay-gap.html

Cohen, D. (2015). Facebook Offers All Employees 4 Months' Parental Leave. AdWeek. Retrieved from http://www.adweek.com/digital/four-months-parental-leave/

Cohen, M. J. M., Kay, A., Youakim, J. M., & Balaicuis, J. M. (2009). Identity transformation in medical students. *American Journal of Psychoanalysis*, *69*(1), 43–52. doi:10.1057/ajp.2008.38 PMID:19295620

Cohen, R. (2016, Sept. 7). What Programming's Past Reveals About Today's Gender-Pay Gap. *Atlantic (Boston, Mass.)*.

Cohn, S., & Blumberg, R. L. (Eds.). (2019). *Gender and Development: The Economic Basis of Women's Power*. Sage.

Cokley, K., Stone, S., Krueger, N., Bailey, M., Garba, R., & Hurst, A. (2018). Self-esteem as a mediator of the link between perfectionism and the impostor phenomenon. *Personality and Individual Differences*, *135*, 292–297. doi:10.1016/j.paid.2018.07.032

Comissão para a Cidadania e Igualdade de Género. Presidência do Conselho de Ministros. *Igualdade de Género em Portugal*. Boletim Estatístico, 2017

Compton, M., Frank, E., Elon, L., & Carrera, J. (2008). Changes in U. S. Medical Students' Specialty Interests Over the Course of Medical School. *J Gen Intern Med Jul; 23*(7), 1095–1100. doi:10.100711606-008-0579-z

Contessa, J., Suarez, L., Kyruakides, T., & Nadzam, G. (2013). The Influence of Surgeon Personality Factors on Risk Tolerance: A Pilot Study. *Journal of Surgical Education*, *70*(6), 806–812. doi:10.1016/j.jsurg.2013.07.014 PMID:24209660

Cook, A. & Glass, C. (2014) Women and Top Leadership Positions: Towards an Institutional Analysis. *Gender, Work & Organization*. Hoboken, NJ: John Wiley & Sons. 21(1), pp. 91–103. doi:10.1111/gwao.12018

Cookman, L. (n.d.). *UAE ranks highest for gender equality in GCC, says Human Development Report*. Available at https://www.thenational.ae/uae/uae-ranks-highest-for-gender-equality-in-gcc-says-human-development-report-1.737261

Cooper, W. O., Spain, D. A., Guillamondegui, O., Kelz, R. R., Domenico, H. J., Hopkins, J., ... & Webb, L. E. (2019). Association of coworker reports about unprofessional behavior by surgeons with surgical complications in their patients. *JAMA surgery*. doi:10.1001/jamasurg.2019.1738

Cooper-Patrick, L., Gallo, J. J., Gonzales, J. J., Vu, H. T., Powe, N. R., Nelson, C., & Ford, D. E. (1999). Race, gender, and partnership in the patient-physician relationship. *Journal of the American Medical Association*, *282*(6), 583–589. doi:10.1001/jama.282.6.583 PMID:10450723

Coptic Medical Society UK. (n.d.). *Dr. Helena Sidarous*. Available at http://copticmedical.com/dr-helena-sidarous/

Cowman, S. E., & Ferrari, J. R. (2002). "Am I for real?" Predicting impostor tendencies from self-handicapping and affective components. *Social Behavior and Personality*, *30*(2), 119–125. doi:10.2224bp.2002.30.2.119

Coyle, D. (2010). *The Talent Code: Greatness isn't born, it's grown*. Random House.

Cozzarelli, C., & Major, B. (1990). Exploring the validity of the impostor phenomenon. *Journal of Social and Clinical Psychology*, *9*(4), 401–417. doi:10.1521/jscp.1990.9.4.401

CRESAP. (2017). Comissão de Recrutamento e Seleção para a Administração Pública, "Relatório de Atividades 2017". Retrieved from http://www.cresap.pt/

Crown Copyright. (2019). Unpaid parental leave. UK Government. Available at https://www.gov.uk/parental-leave/print

Cujec, B., Oancia, T., Bohm, C., & Johnson, D. (2000). Career and parenting satisfaction among medical students, residents and physician teachers at a Canadian medical school. *Canadian Medical Association Journal*, *162*(5), 637–640. PMID:10738448

Danell, R., & Hjerm, M. (2013). Career prospects for female university researchers have not improved. *Scientometrics*, *94*(3), 999–1006. doi:10.100711192-012-0840-4

Darzi, A. (2008). *A high quality workforce: NHS Next Stage Review*. London, UK: Department of Health.

Davis, E. C., Risucci, D. A., Blair, P. G., & Sachdeva, A. K. (2011). Women in surgery residency programs: Evolving trends from a national perspective. *Journal of the American College of Surgeons*, *212*(3), 320–326. doi:10.1016/j.jamcollsurg.2010.11.008 PMID:21247778

Dawson, J. (2018). *Links between NHS staff experience and patient satisfaction: Analysis of surveys from 2014 and 2015.* nhsstaffsurveys.com.

de Costa, J., Chen-Xu, J., Bentounsi, Z., & Vervoort, D. (2018). Women in surgery: challenges and opportunities. *Inl J Surg Glob Health.*

De Hert, S. & Honorato-Cia, C. (2018). Gender and leadership positions in Anaesthesiology: take on the challenge. *ESA Newsletter*, Issue 75. Retrieved from http://newsletter.esahq.org/gender-leadership-positions-anaesthesiology-take-challenge/

De Hert, S. (2018). Burnout Among Anesthesiologists: It's Time for Action! *Journal of Cardiothoracic and Vascular Anesthesia*, *32*(6), 2467–2468. doi:10.1053/j.jvca.2018.06.010 PMID:30093191

De Jonckheere, J., Jeanne, M., Keribedj, A., Delecroix, M., & Logier., R. (2018). Closed-loop administration of analgesic drugs based on heart rate variability analysis*. In *2018 40th Annual International Conference of the IEEE Engineering in Medicine and Biology Society (EMBC)* (Vol. 2018, pp. 506–509). IEEE. doi:10.1109/EMBC.2018.8512330

De Oliveira, G. S. J. (2017, September). Biological evidence of the impact of burnout on the health of anesthesiologists. *Journal of Clinical Anesthesia*. United States. doi:10.1016/j.jclinane.2017.06.011

Dean, E. (2017) The gender pay gap in surgery. *Bulletin Royal College of Surgeons of England* *99*(1), 12-14. Retrieved from https://publishing.rcseng.ac.uk/doi/full/10.1308/rcsbull.2017.12

Dean, E. (2017). The Gender Pay Gap in Surgery. *Royal College of Surgeons Bulletin*, *99*(1), 12–14. doi:10.1308/rcsbull.2017.12

Decree Law N° 485/77, Diário da República n.° 266/1977, Série I, 1977-11-17.

Decree-Law n° 202/2006 of 27 October, Diário da República, 1ª série—N° 208— 27 October 2006.

Deech, R. (2009). *Women doctors: making a difference. Report of the Chair of the National Working Group on Women in Medicine*. London, UK: Department of Health.

Delisle, M. & Wirtzfeld, D. (n.d.). Why do we lack gender diversity in academic medical leadership. *Are we there yet?*

Department of Health and Social Care UK. (2016). New £816 million investment in health research. Retrieved from https://www.gov.uk/government/news/new-816-million-investment-in-health-research on 22/07/2019

Department of Health and Social Care. (2019, March 29). New data on gender pay gap in medicine. Retrieved from https://www.gov.uk/government/news/new-data-on-gender-pay-gap-in-medicine

Devillard, S., Sancier, S., Werner, C., Maller, I., & Kossoff, C. (2013). Gender diversity in top management: Moving corporate culture, moving boundaries. Women Matter.

Devon, K. M. (2019). Call Me by My Name: Doctor. *Annals of Surgery*, *270*(1), 29–30. doi:10.1097/SLA.0000000000003327 PMID:31021830

DGEEC. (2015). *Portuguese scientific production: Statistics series 2005-2015*. General Direction of Statistics in Education and Science. Retrieved from http://www.dgeec.mec.pt/

DGEEC. (2016). Direção Geral de Estatísticas da Educação e Ciência. InCitesTM, Clarivate Analytics. Data updated in November 2016. Retrieved from http://www.dgeec.mec.pt/

Diamond, S., Thomas, C. Jr, Desai, S., Holliday, E., Jagsi, R., Schmitt, C., & Enestvedt, B. K. (2016). Gender Differences in Publication Productivity, Academic Rank, and Career Duration Among U.S. Academic Gastroenterology Faculty. *Academic Medicine*, *91*(8), 1158–1163. doi:10.1097/ACM.0000000000001219 PMID:27144993

Diderichsen, S. (2017). *It's just a job, a new generation of physicians dealing with career and work ideals.* (Dissertation, Umeå University).

Digman, J. M. (1990). Personality structure: Emergence of the Five-Factor Model. *Annual Review of Psychology*, *41*(1), 417–440. doi:10.1146/annurev.ps.41.020190.002221

Diversity in the Classroom. UCLA Diversity & Faculty Development 2014.

Dixit, A., Feldman-Winter, L., & Szucs, K. (2015). Parental leave policies and pediatric trainees in the United States. *Journal of Human Lactation, 31*(3), 434–439.

Domino, K. B., & Sessler, D. I. (2012). Internet Use during Anesthesia Care. *Anesthesiology*, *117*(6), 1156–1158. doi:10.1097/ALN.0b013e31827515fb PMID:23099739

Donington, J. S., Litle, V. R., Sesti, J., & Colson, Y. L. (2012). The WTS report on the current status of women in cardiothoracic surgery. *The Annals of Thoracic Surgery*, *94*(2), 452–458, discussion 458–459. doi:10.1016/j.athoracsur.2012.03.102 PMID:22698775

Donnelly, L. (2017, July 29). Hospital consultants gender pay gap revealed: Four times as many men get bonuses than women. *The Telegraph.*

Dossa, F., & Baxter, N. N. (2018). Reducing gender bias in surgery. *British Journal of Surgery*, *105*(13), 1707–1709. doi:10.1002/bjs.11042 PMID:30462365

Dowd, S. B., & Davidhizar, R. (1997). Do you feel like an impostor? *The Health Care Supervisor*, *15*(3), 51–56. PMID:10165429

Downs, J., Reif, L., Hokororo, A., & Fitzgerald, D. (2014). Increasing Women in Leadership in Global Health. *Academic Medicine*, *89*(8), 1103–1107. doi:10.1097/ACM.0000000000000369 PMID:24918761

Doximity 2018 Physician Compensation Report. (2018). Doximity 2018 Physician Compensation Report. Retrieved from https://blog.doximity.com/articles/doximity-2018-physician-compensation-report

Doximity 2019 Physician Compensation Report. (2019, April 2). Retrieved from https://blog.doximity.com/articles/doximity-2019-physician-compensation-report-d0ca91d1-3cf1-4cbb-b403-a49b9ffa849f

DuBrin, A. J. (2016). *Leadership: research findings, practice, and skills. Eighth*. Boston, MA: Cengage Learning.

Dudău, D. P. (2014). The relation between perfectionism and impostor phenomenon. *Procedia: Social and Behavioral Sciences*, *127*, 129–133. doi:10.1016/j.sbspro.2014.03.226

Dutch Association of Medical Specialists. (2017). Medical Specialist 2025. Retrieved from https://www.demedischspecialist.nl/sites/default/files/FMS_visiedoc_MS2025%28eng%29_2017_PL_v02%28lr%29.pdf)

Dyrbye, L. N., Shanafelt, T. D., Balch, C. M., Satele, D., Sloan, J., & Freischlag, J. (2011). Relationship between work-home conflicts and burnout among American surgeons: a comparison by sex. *Archives of surgery. American Medical Association, 146*(2), pp. 211–217.

Dzau, V. J., & Johnson, P. A. (2018). Ending Sexual Harassment in Academic Medicine. *The New England Journal of Medicine*, *379*(17), 17. doi:10.1056/NEJMp1809846 PMID:30207831

Eagly, A. H., Johannesen-Schmidt, M. C., & Van Engen, M. L. (2003) Transformational, transactional, and laissez-faire leadership styles: a meta-analysis comparing women and men. *Psychological bulletin. American Psychological Association, 129*(4), p. 569.

Eagly, A. (1987). *Sex differences in social behaviour: A social-role interpretation*. Hillsdale, NJ: Lawrence Erlbaum.

Eagly, A., & Mladinic, A. (1994). Are people prejudiced against women? Some answers from research on attitudes, gender stereotypes, and judgments of competence. *European Review of Social Psychology*, *5*(1), 1–35. doi:10.1080/14792779543000002

Eagly, A., Wood, W., & Diekman, A. B. (2000). Social role theory of sex differences and similarities: A current appraisal. In T. Eckes & H. M. Traunter (Eds.), *The developmental social psychology of gender*. Mahwah, NJ: Lawrence Erlbaum.

Eaton, E. & Jackson, C. (2018). Want to improve gender equality at work? Help men take parental leave. *Mercer*. Available at https://www.mercer.com/our-thinking/want-to-improve-gender-equality-at-work-help-men-take-parental-leave.html

Eckert, P. & McConnell-Ginet, S. (1992). Communities of practice: where language, gender and power all live. In K. Hall, M. Bucholtz, & B. Moonwoman (Eds.), *Locating Power, Proceedings of the 1992 Berkeley Women and Language Conference*. Berkeley, CA: Berkeley Woman and Language Group. Retrieved from https://web.stanford.edu/~eckert/PDF/Communitiesof.pdf

Edmunds, L., Ovseiko, P., Shepperd, S., Greenhalgh, T., Frith, P., Roberts, N., & Buchan, A. M. (2016). Why do Women Choose or Reject Careers in Academic Medicine? A Narrative Review of Empirical Evidence. *Lancet*, *388*(10062), 2948–2958. doi:10.1016/S0140-6736(15)01091-0 PMID:27105721

Egger Halbeis, C. B., Cvachovec, K., Scherpereel, P., Mellin-Olsen, J., Drobnik, L., & Sondore, A. (2007). Anaesthesia workforce in Europe. *European Journal of Anaesthesiology*, *24*(12), 991–1007. doi:10.1017/S0265021507000762 PMID:17608964

Egwurugwu, J., Ugwuezumba, P., Ohamaeme, M., Dike, E., Eberendu, I., & Egwurugwu, E. (2018). Relationship between self-esteem and impostor syndrome among undergraduate medical students in a Nigerian university. *International Journal of Brain and Cognitive Sciences*, *7*(1), 9–16. doi:10.5923/j.ijbcs.20180701.02

EIGE. (2015). European Institute for Gender Equality, about Portugal. Retrieved from https://eige.europa.eu/

Ellwood, S., & Garcia-Lacalle, J. (2015). The Influence of Presence and Position of Women on the Boards of Directors: The Case of NHS Foundation Trusts. *Journal of Business Ethics. Springer Netherlands, 130*(1), 69–84. doi:10.100710551-014-2206-8

Elmore, L. C., Jeffe, D. B., Jin, L., Awad, M. M., & Turnbull, I. R. (2016). National Survey of Burnout among US General Surgery Residents. *Journal of the American College of Surgeons, 223*(3), 440–451. doi:10.1016/j.jamcollsurg.2016.05.014 PMID:27238875

Elsevier. (2017). *Gender in the Global Research Landscape.* Available at Elsevier.com/ research-intelligence/resource-library/gender-report

Elston, M. A. (2009). *Women and medicine: the future.* London, UK: Royal College of Physicians. Retrieved from www.rcplondon.ac.uk/pubs/brochure.aspx?e=277

Epstein, R. M. & Privitera, M. R. (2016). *Doing something about physician burnout, 388*(10057), 2216–2217. doi:10.1016/S0140-6736(16)31332-0

Estatísticas - Direção-Geral de Estatísticas da Educação e Ciência. Retrieved from www.dgeec.mec.pt/np4/estatisticas

Estes, Z., & Felker, S. (2012). Confidence mediates the sex difference in mental rotation performance. *Archives of Sexual Behavior, 41*(3), 557–570. doi:10.100710508-011-9875-5 PMID:22130691

Faculdade de Medicina de Lisboa (Lisbon Medical School) – Relatório. (2017). Retrieved from www.medicina.ulisboa.pt/wp-content

Fee, E. (2019). *Women and health: The politics of sex in medicine.* Routledge. doi:10.4324/9781315223346

Fernández, Evaristo, & Bermúdez, José. (2000). El pesimismo defensivo y el síndrome del impostor:análisis de sus componentes afectivos y cognitivos. *Revista de Psicopatología y Psicología Clínica, 5*(2), 115–130.

Ferrari, J. R., & Olivette, M. J. (2000). Parental authority influences on the development females dysfunctional procrastination. *Journal of Research in Personality, 7*, 495–502.

Files, J. A., Mayer, A. P., Ko, M. G., Friedrich, P., Jenkins, M., Bryan, M. J., ... Hayes, S. N. (2017). Speaker introductions at internal medicine grand rounds: Forms of address reveal gender bias. *Journal of Women's Health, 26*(5), 413–419. doi:10.1089/jwh.2016.6044 PMID:28437214

Finch, G. & Hellier, D. (2018, March 16). Goldman Sachs Pays Females in U.K. 56% Less Than Male Colleagues. Retrieved from https://www.bloomberg.com/news/articles/2018-03-16/goldman-sachs-pays-female-staff-56-less-than-male-colleagues

Fingeret, A. L. (2019). Room for improvement: Barriers and strategies to improve gender parity for American Board of Surgery certifying examiners. *The Journal of Surgical Research, 237*, 136–137. doi:10.1016/j.jss.2018.06.009 PMID:30917896

Fisher, D. (2018). Want men to share parental leave? Just give them equality. The Guardian. Available at https://www.theguardian.com/commentisfree/2018/feb/15/men-share-parental-leave-entitlement-women-equality-fathers

Fitzpatrick, T. A., & Curran, C. R. (2014). Waiting for your coronation: A career-limiting trap. *Nursing Economics, 32*(3), 162–165. PMID:25137816

Flacking, R., Dykes, F., & Ewald, U. (2010). The influence of fathers' socio- economic status and paternity leave on breastfeeding duration: A population-based cohort study. *Scandinavian Journal of Public Health, 38*(4), 337–343. doi:10.1177/1403494810362002 PMID:20147577

Fleming, N. (2018, Feb. 28). How the gender pay gap permeates science and engineering. *New Scientist, 237*(3167), 22–23. doi:10.1016/S0262-4079(18)30389-0

Fnais, N., Soobiah, C., Chen, M. H., Lillie, E., Perrier, L., Tashkhandi, M., ... Tricco, A. C. (2014). Harassment and discrimination in medical training: A systematic review and meta-analysis. *Academic Medicine, 89*, 817–827. doi:10.1097/ACM.0000000000000200 PMID:24667512

Forcing employers to reveal their gender pay gaps is making them think. (2018, April 5). Forcing employers to reveal their gender pay gaps is making them think. *The Economist.*

Ford, C. (2018). The turning point: One man's downfall,# MeToo, and the rising up. *Meanjin, 77*(2), 40.

Foundation Programme. (2017). *UK Foundation Programme Career Destinations Report 2017.* Retrieved from http://www.foundationprogramme.nhs.uk/sites/default/files/2018-07/2017%20F2%20Career%20Destinations%20Report_0.pdf

Francis, R. (2013) Report of the Mid Staffordshire NHS foundation trust public inquiry: executive summary. The Stationery Office, 947.

Franco, K., Evans, C. L., Best, A. P., Zrull, J. P., & Pizza, G. A. (1983). Conflicts associated with physicians' pregnancies. *The American Journal of Psychiatry, 140*(7), 902–904. doi:10.1176/ajp.140.7.902 PMID:6859310

Frangou, C. (2018, Feb. 6). Surgeons (women and men) say it's time to close surgery's gender gap. *Gen Surg News.* Retrieved from https://www.generalsurgerynews.com/In-the-News/Article/02-18/Surgeons-Women-and-Men-Say-It-s-Time-to-Close-Surgery-s-Gender-Gap/46919?sub=2F10E432441735F412C78CC6CDB6D8ECDBE22B01D93E95F3569347DA5E5463C&enl=true

Freire, P. (2018). *Pedagogy of the oppressed.* USA: Bloomsbury Publishing.

Freund, K. M., Raj, A., Kaplan, S. E., Terrin, N., Breeze, J. L., Urech, T. H., & Carr, P. L. (2016). Inequities in academic compensation by gender: A follow-up to the national faculty survey cohort study. *Academic Medicine, 91*(8), 1068–1073. doi:10.1097/ACM.0000000000001250 PMID:27276007

Fried-Buchalter, S. (1992). Fear of success, fear of failure, and the imposter phenomenon: A factor analytic approach to convergent and discriminant validity. *Journal of Personality Assessment, 58*(2), 368–379. doi:10.120715327752jpa5802_13 PMID:16370869

Fullagar, S., & Pavlidis, A. (2018). Feminist theories after the poststructuralist turn. In *Feminisms in Leisure Studies* (pp. 48–71). Routledge. doi:10.4324/9781315108476-3

G. M. C. (Great Britain). (2017) *The State of Medical Education and Practice in the UK: 2017.* General Medical Council.

Gaio Alves, M. & Lopes, P. (2012). Ensino Superior em Portugal: retrato sociográfico. Gabinete de Estudos da SNESUP, Dezembro 2012. Retrieved from www.snesup.pt/htmls/_dlds/relatorio-retrato-sociografico-af.pdf

Gallagher, P. (2017, June 28). Stop the increasing gender pay gap, doctors tell BMA conference. *I News.*

Gardner, S. V., James, M. F., & Evans, N. R. (2002). Gender issues among South African anaesthetists. *South African Medical Journal, 92*(9), 732–736. PMID:12382361

Gargiulo, D. A., Hyman, N. H., & Hebert, J. C. (2006). Women in surgery: Do we really understand the deterrents? *Archives of Surgery, 141*(4), 405–408. doi:10.1001/archsurg.141.4.405 PMID:16618901

Garrett, J. [JenniferGarrett]. (2018a, March 28). Good point Chris, it's about being a minority: gender, nationality, race, social class, sexuality all feed #ImposterSyndrome Also environments where there's lots of critical peer review #nhswomen https://t.co/1POhv8ETEQ [Tweet]. Retrieved from https://twitter.com/JenniferGarrett/status/979074080010899457

Garrett, J. [JenniferGarrett]. (2018b, March 28). I agree @ana_brankovic organisations that allow staff to show doubt, make mistakes and be vulnerable are less likely to have staff who suffer from #ImposterSyndrome #NHSwomen https://t.co/WHScauj0jV [Tweet]. Retrieved from https://twitter.com/JenniferGarrett/status/979074514788212736

Garrett, J. [JenniferGarrett]. (2018c, March 28). This is an important point, the only person I now compare myself to is me. Am I better than I was a week, a month, a year ago? If there's growth, I am happy #impostersyndrome #nhswomen #ditchcomparison https://t.co/zS0kxKrbGH [Tweet]. Retrieved from https://twitter.com/JenniferGarrett/status/979078285199015936

Garza, R. M., Weston, J. S., & Furnas, H. J. (2017). Pregnancy and the Plastic Surgery Resident. *Plastic and Reconstructive Surgery*, *139*(1), 245–252. doi:10.1097/PRS.0000000000002861 PMID:28027263

GBD. (2017). A fragile world. (2018). *Lancet*, *329*, 1683. doi:10.1016/S0140-6736(18)32858-7

GCC. (n.d.). *GCC Charter*. Available at http://www.gcc-sg.org/en-us/Pages/default.aspx

GCC. (n.d.). *Population-STAT*. [Online].

General Medical Council. (2018). *Factsheet Dr Bawa-Garba* [Ebook]. Retrieved from https://www.gmc-uk.org/-/media/documents/20180419-factsheet---dr-bawa-garba-case-final_pdf-74385491.pdf

General Surgery Leave Policy. (2017). General format. Retrieved from http://www.absurgery.org/default.jsp?policygsleave

Gertner, N. (2018). Sexual Harassment and the Bench. *Stan. L. Rev. Online*, *71*, 86.

Ghatan, C. E., Fassiotto, M., Jacobsen, J. P., Sze, D. Y., & Kothary, N. (2016). Occupational Radiation Exposure during Pregnancy: A Survey of Attitudes and Practices among Interventional Radiologists. *Journal of Vascular and Interventional Radiology*, *27*(7), 1013–20.e3. doi:10.1016/j.jvir.2016.03.040 PMID:27236211

Ghosh, K. (2018, August). Violence against doctors: A wake-up call. *The Indian Journal of Medical Research*, *148*(2), 130. doi:10.4103/ijmr.IJMR_1299_17 PMID:30381535

Ghossain, A., Freiha, F., & Geahchan, N. (2003). Surgery in Lebanon. *Archives of Surgery (Chicago, Ill.)*, *138*(2), 215–219. doi:10.1001/archsurg.138.2.215 PMID:12578423

Giacalone, M., Zaouter, C., Mion, S., & Hemmerling, T. M. (2016). Impact of age on anaesthesiologists' competence: A narrative review. *European Journal of Anaesthesiology*, *33*(11), 787–793. doi:10.1097/EJA.0000000000000534 PMID:27635955

Gjerberg, E. (2003). Women doctors in Norway: The challenging balance between career and family life. *Social Science & Medicine*, *57*(7), 1327–1341. doi:10.1016/S0277-9536(02)00513-0 PMID:12899913

GlaxoSmithKline. (2019) *Inclusion and diversity*. Retrieved from https://www.gsk.com/cn-gb/responsibility/our-people/inclusion-and-diversity/

Glick, P. & Fiske, S. T. (1996). The ambivalent sexism inventory: differentiating hostile and benevolent sexism. *Personality and social psychology, 70*(3), 491-512. doi:10.1037/0022-3514.70.3.491

GMC (General Medical Council). (2017). Training Environments 2017. Key findings from the national training survey. Available at https://www.gmc-uk.org/about/what-we-do-and-why/data-and-research/-/media/documents/nts-report-20173_pdf-72689147.pdf

GMC (The General Medical Council). (2016). The State of Medical Education and Practice in the UK 2016. Executive Summary. Available at http://www.gmcuk.org/GMC_SOMEP_2016___Executive_summary.pdf_68137466.pdf

Goldacre, M., Laxton, L., & Lambert, T. (2010). Medical graduates' early career choices of specialty and their eventual specialty destinations: UK prospective cohort studies. *BMJ, 341*(jul06 1). doi:10.1136/bmj.c3199

Goldhill, O. (2016, Feb. 1). Is imposter syndrome a sign of greatness? *Quartz.*

Gomes, A. (2004). (in press). O primeiro congresso feminista em Portugal realizou-se há 80 anos. O Público 4 May 2004. Retrieved from https://www publico.pt/2004/05/04/sociedade/noticia/

Gonzales, K. L., Noonan, C., Goins, R. T., Henderson, W. G., Beals, J., Manson, S. M., ... Roubideaux, Y. (2016). Assessing the everyday discrimination scale among American Indians and Alaska Natives. *Psychological Assessment, 28*(1), 51–58. doi:10.1037/a0039337 PMID:26146948

Gordon, M. B., McGuinness, G. A., Stanton, B. F., Brooks, S., Chiang, V. W., Vinci, R., & Sectish, T. C. (2008). Part-time training in pediatric residency programs: Principles and practices. *Pediatrics, 122*(4), e938–e944. doi:10.1542/peds.2008-0719 PMID:18809596

Goveas, S. (2012, August). Growth in the Number of Female Medical Doctors in Oman. What are the reasons? *Sultan Qaboos University Medical Journal, 12*(3), 380–381. doi:10.12816/0003159 PMID:23269954

Government Equalities Office. (n.d.). *Reducing the gender pay gap and improving gender equality in organisations: Evidence-based actions for employers.* Retrieved from gender-pay-gap.service.gov.uk

Government of India . (n.d.). 9th Five Year Plan (Vol-2).

GPEARI. (2011). *Fluxos e situação profissional dos doutorados em Portugal – 2009.* Ministério da Ciência e Ensino Superior, Estatísticas Oficiais. Junho 2011. Retrieved from http://www.dgeec.mec.pt/np4/208

Grady, D. (2014). Carolyn Kaelin, Breast Cancer Surgeon Patient Advocate and Patient, Dies at 54. *New York Times.* Retrieved from https://www.nytimes.com/2015/08/10/us/carolyn-kaelin-breast-cancer-surgeon-dies-at-54.html

Gratton, L., & Scott, A. (2016). *The 100-year life Living and Working in an Age of Longevity.* London, UK: Bloomsbury Information Ltd.

Gravett, G. (2013). Tell Me Something I Don't Know About Women in the Workplace. *Harvard Business Review*, (August). Retrieved from https://hbr.org/2013/08/tell-me-something-i-dont-know

Gray, S. F., Goodyear, H. M., & Jones, M. J. T. (2005). Outcomes of flexible training compared to full time training during the Specialist Registrar Grade in the UK. *Med Educ Online.* Retrieved from www.med-ed-online.org/pdf/10000007.pdf

Gray, J. (1992). *Men are from Mars, Women are from Venus.* London, UK: HarperCollins.

Gray, S., Alexander, K., & Eaton, J. (2004). Equal opportunity for all? Trends in flexible training 1995-2001. *Medical Teacher, 26*(3), 256–259. doi:10.1080/0142159042000191993 PMID:15203504

Greenberg, C. C. (2017). Association for Academic Surgery presidential address: Sticky floors and glass ceilings. *Journal of Surgical Research. Elsevier, 219*, ix–xviii. doi:10.1016/j.jss.2017.09.006 PMID:29078918

Greenhill, J., McKimm, J., Da Silva, A. S., Taylor, C., & Edwards, S. (2015). Women and Leadership in Medicine and Medical Education: International Perspectives. In Gender, Careers and Inequalities in Medicine and Medical Education: International Perspectives (pp. 69-98).

Griffin, E. (2018, March 12). What's to blame for the gender pay gap? The housework myth. *The Guardian.*

Gross, G. (2014). *Men are from Mars, women are from Venus... or are they? Are the differences between boys and girls really that great? Or is our biological determinism more of a self-fulfilled prophecy?* Human Behaviour, Parenting, and Education.

Grossman, R. (2018, Nov. 1). Gender parity and diversity are being used in the private sector by investors as a quality marker. - @RuthSealy #LiftAsYouClimb @hcwomenleaders [Tweet]. Retrieved from https://twitter.com/rebgross/status/1057949609027399680

Grossman, R. (2018). The surgical personality: Does it matter? *The Bulletin of the Royal College of Surgeons of England, 100*(3), 130–132. doi:10.1308/rcsbull.2018.130

Guille, C., Frank, E., Zhao, Z., Kalmbach, D. A., Nietert, P. J., Mata, D. A., & Sen, S. (2017). Work- family conflict and the sex difference in depression among training physicians. *JAMA Internal Medicine, 177*(12), 1766–1772. doi:10.1001/jamainternmed.2017.5138 PMID:29084311

Gulf Business. (n.d.). *UAE, Bahrain, Saudi rise, Kuwait, Qatar fall in gender equality ranking*. Available at https://gulfbusiness.com/uae-bahrain-saudi-climb-kuwait-qatar-fall-gender-equality-ranking/

Gupta, A., Meriwether, K., & Hewlett, G. (2019). Impact of training specialty on breastfeeding among resident physicians: A National Survey. *Breastfeeding Medicine, 14*(1), 46–56. doi:10.1089/bfm.2018.0140 PMID:30346796

Gustavson-Kaddaka, E. (2010). Om kvinnliga medicine vid Karolinska Institutet i slutet av 1800-talet. Retrieved from https://issuu.com/ki200/docs/evi_g_kadaka_om_karolina_widerstrom

Hafsi, T., & Turgut, G. (2013). Boardroom Diversity and its Effect on Social Performance: Conceptualization and Empirical Evidence. *Journal of Business Ethics. Springer Netherlands, 112*(3), 463–479. doi:10.100710551-012-1272-z

Häggström, S. (2016). Shadow's Law. Bullet point publishing.

Hall, J. A., Irish, J. T., Roter, D. L., Ehrlich, C. M., & Miller, L. H. (1994). Gender in medical encounters: an analysis of physician and patient communication in a primary care setting. *Health Psychology,* 13, 384-293. Retrieved from https://www.ncbi.nlm.nih.gov/pubmed/7805632

Haller, G., Delhumeau, C., Mamie, C., Zoccatelli, D., & Clergue, F. (2016, August). Gender difference in career advancement and job satisfaction in anaesthesia: A cross-sectional study. *European Journal of Anaesthesiology*. England. doi:10.1097/EJA.0000000000000471

Hall, S. J., & Williams, S. T. (2017). The pregnant urologist. *BJU International, 120*(5), 731–734. doi:10.1111/bju.13927 PMID:28581066

Halverson, A. L., Neumayer, L., & Dagl, T. F. (2012). Leadership skills in the OR, part II: recognizing disruptive behavior. *ACS Bulletin*, 1-5.

Hamberg, K. (2008). Gender Bias in Medicine. *Women's Health (London, England), 4*(3), 237–243. doi:10.2217/17455057.4.3.237 PMID:19072473

Hamilton LC. The lesser-spotted pregnant surgeon. *RCS Bull., 100*(4), 172-175.

Hampton, T., Greenhalgh, R., Ryan, D., & Das-Purkayastha, P. (2016) Female surgical trainee attrition. *Bulletin of Royal College of Surgeons, 98*(3), 134-137. doi:10.1308/rcsbull.2016.134

Hancock, M. (2019, April 25). The NHS is a huge employer of women – I want it to be one of the best as well. *The Guardian.*

Han, H., Kim, Y., Kim, S., Cho, Y., & Chae, C. (2018). Looking into the labyrinth of gender inequality: Women physicians in academic medicine. *Medical Education, 52*(10), 1083–1095. doi:10.1111/medu.13682 PMID:30255527

Harries, R. L., Gokani, V. J., & Smitham, P. F. (2016). JEF on behalf of the councils of the Association of Surgeons in Training and the British Orthopaedic Trainees Association. Less than full-time training in surgery: a cross-sectional study evaluating the accessibility and experiences of flexible training in the surgical trainee workforce. *BMJ Open 4*(6), 1-7. Retrieved from https://bmjopen.bmj.com/content/bmjopen/6/4/e010136.full.pdf

Harries, R. L., Gokani, V. J., Smitham, P., & Fitzgerald, J. E. F. (2016). Less than full-time training in surgery: A cross-sectional study evaluating the accessibility and experiences of flexible training in the surgical trainee workforce. *BMJ Open, 6*(4), e010136. doi:10.1136/bmjopen-2015-010136 PMID:27091819

Harris, B. (2017, Nov. 6). *What the pay gap between men and women really looks like.* Retrieved from https://www.weforum.org/agenda/2017/11/pay-equality-men-women-gender-gap-report-2017/

Harris, C. A., Banerjee, T., Cramer, M., Manz, S., Ward, S. T., Dimick, J., & Telem, D. A. (2019). Editorial (spring) board? Gender composition in high-impact general surgery journals over 20 years. *Annals of Surgery, 269*(3), 582–588. doi:10.1097/SLA.0000000000002667 PMID:29342020

Harris, C. A., Blencowe, N., & Telem, D. A. (2017). What is in a pronoun?: Why Gender-Fair Language Matters. *Annals of Surgery, 266*(6), 932–933. doi:10.1097/SLA.0000000000002505 PMID:28902666

Harvey, J. C. (1981). The impostor phenomenon and achievements: A failure to internalize success (Doctoral thesis: Temple University, 1981). *Dissertation Abstracts International, 42*, 4969B.

Harvey, J. C., & Katz, C. (1985). *If I'm So Successful, Why Do I Feel Like a Fake: The Impostor Phenomenon.* New York, NY: Random House.

Hasebrook, J., Hahnenkamp, K., Buhre, W., de Korte-de Boer, D., Hamaekers, A., Metelmann, B., & Pfleiderer, B. (2017). Medicine Goes Female: Protocol for Improving Career Options of Females and Working Conditions for Researching Physicians in Clinical Medical Research by Organizational Transformation and Participatory Design. *JMIR Research Protocols, 6*(8), e152. doi:10.2196/resprot.7632 PMID:28768613

Haskins, J. (2019, July 15). General format. Retrieved from https://news.aamc.org/diversity/article/where-are-all-the-women-in-surgery/

he_reeves. (2018, March 1). I have often felt that some success has been down to luck (right place/right time) it's difficult to shake, however, luck only gets you so far the rest is down to you. The gremlins push me to be better, learn [Tweet]. Retrieved from https://twitter.com/he_reeves/status/969245903956660226

HE-Advance. (2018). *Athena SWAN Charter, Equality Charters.* Available at https://www.ecu.ac.uk/equality-charters/athena-swan/

Health & Care Women Leaders Network [hcwomenleaders]. (2018, March 27). Some have never heard of it. Some know it only too well. That confidence-sapping feeling that it's luck rather than ability that lies behind your success. Share your thoughts, experiences and coping strategies in our tweet chat, tomorrow from 8pm [Tweet]. Retrieved from https://twitter.com/hcwomenleaders/status/978646347082616839

Health at a Glance: Europe 2018. (2018). OECD. doi:10.1787/health_glance_eur-2018-en

Healy, G., & Kirton, G. (2000). Women, power and trade union government in the UK. *British Journal of Industrial Relations, 38*(3), 343–360. doi:10.1111/1467-8543.00168

Healy, N., Cantillon, P., Malone, C., & Kerin, M. (2012). Role models and mentors in surgery. *American Journal of Surgery, 204*(2), 256–261. doi:10.1016/j.amjsurg.2011.09.031 PMID:22621833

Hedvall, G. (1974). *Särtryck ur Nordisk Medicinhistorisk årsbok*. Fingraf Tryckeri.

HEE (Health Education England). (2017). Supported Return to Training. Available at https://www.hee.nhs.uk/sites/default/files/documents/Supported%20Return%20to%20Training.pdf

Heiligers, P. (2012). Gender differences in medical students' motives and career choice. *BMC Medical Education, 12*(1), 82. doi:10.1186/1472-6920-12-82 PMID:22913471

Helitzer, D., Newbill, S., Morahan, P., Magrane, D., Cardinali, G., Wu, C.-C., & Chang, S. (2014). Perceptions of Skill Development of Participants in Three National Career Development Programs for Women Faculty in Academic Medicine. *Academic Medicine, 89*(6), 896–903. doi:10.1097/ACM.0000000000000251 PMID:24871241

Hellman, C. M., & Caselman, T. D. (2004). A psychometric evaluation of the Harvey Imposter Phenomenon Scale. *Journal of Personality Assessment, 83*(2), 161–166. doi:10.120715327752jpa8302_10 PMID:15456652

Henderson, J. T. & Weisman, C. S. (2001). Physician gender effects on preventive screening and counseling: an analysis of male and female patients' health care experience. *Medical Care, 39,* 1281-1292. Retrieved from https://www.ncbi.nlm.nih.gov/pubmed/11717570

Henning, K., Ey, S., & Shaw, D. (1998). Perfectionism, the impostor phenomenon and psychological adjustment in medical, dental, nursing and pharmacy students. *Medical Education, 32*(5), 456–464. doi:10.1046/j.1365-2923.1998.00234.x PMID:10211285

Henry, T. A. (2019, June 3). General format. Retrieved from https://www.ama-assn.org/practice-management/physician-health/higher-physician-burnout-risk-moms-sandwich-generation

Henry, A., Clements, S., Kingston, A., & Abbott, J. (2012). In search of work/life balance: Trainee perspectives on part-time obstetrics and gynaecology specialist training. *BMC Research Notes, 5*(1), 19. doi:10.1186/1756-0500-5-19 PMID:22233566

Heuss, L. T., & Haenggeli, C. (2003). Open access to part-time specialist training- the Swiss experience. *Swiss Medical Weekly, 133*(17-18), 263–266. PMID:12833197

Hicks, J. (2018, April 11). Women and Black Doctors Still Make Far Less Than White Male Doctors. Retrieved from https://tonic.vice.com/en_us/article/bjp595/women-and-black-doctors-still-make-far-less-than-white-male-doctors

Hijabs & Bare Below the Elbows Toolkits. (2017). [Society Guidance] Retrieved from http://www.britishima.org/hbbe-toolkits/

Hill, E., Bowman, K., Stalmeijer, R., & Hart, J. (2014). You've got to know the rules to play the game: How medical students negotiate the hidden curriculum of surgical careers. *Medical Education, 48*(9), 884–894. doi:10.1111/medu.12488 PMID:25113115

Holliday, E. B., Ahmed, A. A., Jagsi, R., Stentz, N. C., Woodward, W. A., Fuller, C. D., & Thomas, C. R. Jr. (2015). Pregnancy and Parenthood in Radiation Oncology, Views and Experiences Survey (PROVES): Results of a Blinded Prospective Trainee Parenting and Career Development Assessment. *Radiation Oncology Biology, 92*(3), 516–524. doi:10.1016/j.ijrobp.2015.02.024 PMID:25892584

Holliday, E., Jagsi, R., Wilson, L. D., Choi, M., Thomas, C. R. Jr, & Fuller, C. D. (2014). Gender Differences in Publication Productivity, Academic Position, Career Duration, and Funding Among U.S. Academic Radiation Oncology Faculty. *Academic Medicine, 89*(5), 767–773. doi:10.1097/ACM.0000000000000229 PMID:24667510

Holmberg, K. (2017). Statistics from SLF and AFA, lecture April 22, 2017.

Holmes, S. W., Kertay, L., Adamson, L. B., Holland, C. L., & Clance, P. R. (1993). Measuring the impostor phenomenon: A comparison of Clance's IPScale and Harvey's IPScale. *Journal of Personality Assessment, 60*(1), 48–59. doi:10.120715327752jpa6001_3 PMID:8433268

Hoops, H. E., Brasel, K. J., Dewey, E., Rodgers, S., Merrill, J., Hunter, J. G., & Azarow, K. S. (2018). Analysis of Gender-based Differences in Surgery Faculty Compensation, Promotion, and Retention. *Annals of Surgery, 268*(3), 479–487. doi:10.1097/SLA.0000000000002920 PMID:30063494

Hopkins, C. (2018). Confronting unconscious bias. *Royal College of Surgeons Bulletin, 100*(8), 321–323. doi:10.1308/rcsbull.2018.321

Horton, M., & Freire, P. (1990). *We make the road by walking: Conversations on education and social change*. Temple University Press.

HSE (Health and Safety Executive). (2015). Working safely with ionising radiation: Guidance for expectant and breast-feeding mothers. Available at http://www.hse.gov.uk/pubns/indg334.pdf

Huang, Y., Chua, T. C., Saw, R. P. M., & Young, C. J. (2018). Discrimination, bullying and harassment in surgery: A systematic review and meta-analysis. *World Journal of Surgery, 42*(12), 3867–3873. doi:10.100700268-018-4716-5 PMID:29971462

Huff, S., Rudman, D. L., Magalhães, L., & Lawson, E. (2018). 'Africana womanism': Implications for transformative scholarship in occupational science. *Journal of Occupational Science, 25*(4), 554–565. doi:10.1080/14427591.2018.1493614

Hughes, F., & Bernstein, P. S. (2018). Sexism in obstetrics and gynecology: Not just a "women's issue". *American Journal of Obstetrics and Gynecology, 219*(4), 364–e1. doi:10.1016/j.ajog.2018.07.006 PMID:30017680

Hughes, K. A. (2015). #ILookeLikeASurgeon goes viral: How it happened. *FACs Bulletin, 100*, 10–16. PMID:26677529

Hultcrantz, E., & … . (1998). *Läkare doktor kvinna*. Studentlitteratur.

Humphreys, H., Russell, A., Marshall, R., Ricketts, V., & Reeves, D. (1991). The effect of surgical theatre head-gear on air bacterial counts. *The Journal of Hospital Infection, 19*(3), 175–180. doi:10.1016/0195-6701(91)90221-S PMID:1685505

Humphries, L., Lyon, S., Garza, R., Butz, D., Lemelman, B., & Park, J. (2017). Parental leave policies in graduate medical education: A systematic review. *The American college of surgeons.*

Hunt, V., Layton, D., & Prince, S. (2015, February). Why diversity matters. Retrieved from https://www.mckinsey.com/business-functions/organization/our-insights/why-diversity-matters

Ibarra, H., Ely, R., & Kolb, D. (2013). Women rising: the unseen barriers. *Harvard Business Review*, (September). Retrieved from https://hbr.org/2013/09/women-rising-the-unseen-barriers

Ibarra, H., Ely, R., & Kolb, D. (2013). Women rising: The unseen barriers. *Harvard Business Review, 91*(9), 60–66. PMID:23593768

Ilkhchi, S. V., Poursharifi, H., & Alilo, M. M. (2011). The effectiveness of Cognitive-Behavioral Group Therapy on self-efficacy and assertiveness among anxious female students of high schools. *Procedia: Social and Behavioral Sciences, 30*, 2586–2591. doi:10.1016/j.sbspro.2011.10.506

IMO (Irish Medical Organisation). (2017). IMO Position Paper on Women in Medicine. Available at https://www.imo.ie/policy-international-affair/documents/IMO-Position-Paper-on-Women-in-Medicine-Final.pdf

INE. (2018). Health personnel statistics. Source: Pordata. Last update: Aug. 8, 2018. Retrieved from https://www.pordata.pt/

INE. (2019). *População*. Instituto Nacional de Estatística. Retrieved from https://www.ine.pt/

Ingelman-Sundberg, C. (2009). *Boken om vikingarna*. Norstedts.

Instituto de la Mujer y para la Igualdad de Oportunidades. (n.d.). Retrieved from http://www.inmujer.gob.es/MujerCifras/PoderDecisiones/RealesAcademias.htmhttp://www.ine.es/jaxi/Datos.htm?path=/t15/p416/serie/l0/&file=s01001.px

integrativpsych. (2018, March 28). @hcwomenleaders I lost out on lots of early opportunities in life (e.g., work placements) due to #impostersyndrome because I had the mentality of "I don't know enough yet (to do this)". Thankfully, I have now developed a growth mindset. And [Tweet]. Retrieved from https://twitter.com/integrativpsych/status/979075774044045313

International Labour Organization (ILO). (2016). Women at work. Retrieved from https://www.ilo.org/wcmsp5/groups/public/- --dgreports/---dcomm/---publ/documents/publication/wcms_457317.pdf

Inzlicht, M., & Ben-Zeev, T. (2000). A threatening intellectual environment: Why females are susceptible to experiencing problem-solving deficits in the presence of males. *Psychological Science*, *11*(5), 365–371. doi:10.1111/1467-9280.00272 PMID:11228906

Isaac, C., Chertoff, J., Lee, B., & Carnes, M. (2011). Do Students' and Authors' Genders Affect Evaluations? A Linguistic Analysis of Medical Student Performance Evaluations. *Academic Medicine*, *86*(1), 59–66. doi:10.1097/ACM.0b013e318200561d PMID:21099389

Isabel, L. (2010). *Adelaide Cabete (1867 - 1935). Comissão para a Cidadania e a Igualdade de Género*. Lisbon, Portugal: Presidência do Conselho de Ministros.

Jagsi, R. (2018). Sexual harassment in medicine - #MeToo. *The New England Journal of Medicine*, *378*(3), 209–211. doi:10.1056/NEJMp1715962 PMID:29236567

Jagsi, R., Griffith, K. A., Stewart, A., Sambuco, D., DeCastro, R., & Ubel, P. A. (2012). Gender differences in the salaries of physician researchers. *Journal of the American Medical Association*, *307*(22), 2410–2417. doi:10.1001/jama.2012.6183 PMID:22692173

Jagsi, R., Griffith, K. A., Stewart, A., Sambuco, D., DeCastro, R., & Ubel, P. A. (2013). Gender differences in salary in a recent cohort of earlycareer physician-researchers. *Academic Medicine*, *88*(11), 1689–1699. doi:10.1097/ACM.0b013e3182a71519 PMID:24072109

Jagsi, R., Guancial, E. A., Worobey, C. C., Henault, L. E., Chang, Y., Starr, R., ... Hylek, E. M. (2006). The "gender gap" in authorship of academic medical literature— A 35-year perspective. *The New England Journal of Medicine*, *355*(3), 281–287. doi:10.1056/NEJMsa053910 PMID:16855268

Janz, O. & Schonpflug, D. (Eds.). (2014). Gender History in a Transnational Perspective: Networks, Biographies, Gender Orders, (pp. 53, 61–62). New York, NY: Berghahn Books. doi:10.2307/j.ctt9qcxnt

Jena, A. B., Olenski, A. R., & Blumenthal, D. M. (2016). Differences in Physician Salary in US Public Medical Schools. *Journal of the American Medical Association Internal Medicine*, *176*, 1294–1304. doi:10.1001/jamainternmed.2016.3284 PMID:27400435

Jenkins, M., Herrmann, A., Tashjian, A., Ramineni, T., Ramakrishnan, R., Raef, D., ... Shatzer, J. (2016). Sex and gender in medical education: A national student survey. *Biology of Sex Differences*, *7*(S1), 45. doi:10.118613293-016-0094-6 PMID:27785347

Jerg-Bretzke, L., & Limbrecht, K. (2012). Where have they gone?- a discussion on the balancing act of female doctors between work and family. *GMS Zeitschrift für Medizinische*, *29*(2), 19. PMID:22558025

Jindal, R., Ryan, J., Sajjad, I., Murthy, M., & Baines, L. (2005). Kidney Transplantation and Gender Disparity. *American Journal of Nephrology*, *25*(5), 474–483. doi:10.1159/000087920 PMID:16127268

Joffe, M., MacLeod, S., Kedziora, M., & Main, P. (2016). GP trainers and trainees – trait and gender differences in personality: Implications for GP training. *Education for Primary Care*, *27*(3), 205–213. doi:10.1080/14739879.2016.1147135 PMID:27059247

Johns Hopkins Medicine. (2019, Jan. 29). How gender disparities in salary add up over a lifetime. *ScienceDaily*. Retrieved from https://www.sciencedaily.com/releases/2019/01/190128111728.htm

Johnson, S. K., Hekman, D. R., & Chan, E. T. (2016, April 26). If There's Only One Woman in Your Candidate Pool, There's Statistically No Chance She'll Be Hired. *Harvard Business Review*.

Joint Committee on Surgical Training. (2017). *Guidance on the management of surgical trainees returning to clinical training after extended leave*. Retrieved from https://www.jcst.org/-/media/files/jcst/key-documents/return-to-work-guidance-final.pdf

Joosten, A., Delaporte, A., Cannesson, M., Rinehart, J., Dewilde, J. P., Van Obbergh, L., & Barvais, L. (2016). Fully Automated Anesthesia and Fluid Management Using Multiple Physiologic Closed-Loop Systems in a Patient Undergoing High-Risk Surgery. *A & A Case Reports*, *7*(12), 260–265. doi:10.1213/XAA.0000000000000405 PMID:27669030

Jung, C. G. (1971). Psychological types. In *Collected works of C* (Vol. 6). G. Jung.

Kaatz, A., Lee, Y. G., Potvien, A., Magua, W., Filut, A., Bhattacharya, A., ... Carnes, M. (2016). Analysis of NIH R01 Application critiques, impact and criteria scores: Does the sex of the principal investigator make a difference. *Academic Medicine*, *91*, 1080–1088. doi:10.1097/ACM.0000000000001272 PMID:27276003

Kaatz, A., Magua, W., Zimmerman, D. R., & Carnes, M. (2015). A quantitative linguistic analysis of National Institutes of Health R01 application critiques from investigators at one institution. *Academic Medicine*, *90*(1), 69–75. doi:10.1097/ACM.0000000000000442 PMID:25140529

Kabat-Zinn, J. (1994). *Wherever you go, there you are*. New York, NY: Hyperion.

Kaderli, R., Guller, U., Muff, B., Stefenelli, U., & Businger, A. (2010). Women in surgery: A survey in Switzerland. *Archives of Surgery*, *145*(11), 1119–1121. doi:10.1001/archsurg.2010.245 PMID:21079102

Kaiser, H. J. (2018). *Professionally active physicians by Gender*. Retrieved from https://www.kff.org/other/state-indicator/physicians-by-gender

Kaiser, J. (2019, March 8). Men get larger first NIH grants, but is the news all bad for female scientists? Retrieved from https://www.sciencemag.org/news/2019/03/men-get-larger-first-nih-grants-news-all-bad-female-scientists

Kaiser, R. B., Hogan, R., & Craig, S. B. (2008). Leadership and the fate of organizations. *The American Psychologist*, *63*(2), 96–110. doi:10.1037/0003-066X.63.2.96 PMID:18284278

Kaplan, S. H., Greenfield, S., Gandek, B., Rogers, W. H., & Ware, J. E. (1996). Characteristics of Physicians with Participatory Decision-Making Styles. *Annals of Internal Medicine*, *124*(5), 497–504. doi:10.7326/0003-4819-124-5-199603010-00007 PMID:8602709

Kass, R. B., Souba, W. W., & Thorndyke, L. E. (2006). Challenges Confronting Female Surgical Leaders: Overcoming the Barriers. *The Journal of Surgical Research*, *132*(2), 179–187. doi:10.1016/j.jss.2006.02.009 PMID:16564542

Katsarou, M. (2019). *Women and the Leadership Labyrinth Howard vs Heidi.* Leadership Psychol Inst.

Katz, J. D. (2016). The aging anesthesiologist. *Current Opinion in Anaesthesiology, 29*(2), 206–211. doi:10.1097/ACO.0000000000000299 PMID:26705128

Kausz, A. T., Obrador, G. T., Arora, P., Ruthazer, R., Levey, A. S., & Pereira, B. J. (2000). Late initiation of dialysis among women and ethnic minorities in the United States. *Journal of the American Society of Nephrology, 11*, 2351–2357. PMID:11095658

Kautzky-Willer, A. (2012). Sex and gender differences in endocrinology. In S. Oertelt-Prigione & V. Regitz-Zagrosek (Eds.), *Sex and Gender Aspects in Clinical Medicine* (pp. 125–149). London, UK: Springer. doi:10.1007/978-0-85729-832-4_9

Kavilanz, P. (2018, March 14). The gender pay gap for women doctors is big -- and getting worse. Retrieved from https://money.cnn.com/2018/03/14/news/economy/gender-pay-gap-doctors/index.html

Kay, K., & Shipman, C. (2014). The Confidence Gap. *Atlantic (Boston, Mass.).*

Kets de Vries, M. F. R. (2005). The dangers of feeling like a fake. *Harvard Business Review, 83*(9), 108–16–159.

Kim, C., McEwen, L. N., Gerzoff, R. B., Merrero, D. G., Mangione, C. M., Selby, J. V., & Herman, W. H. (2005). Is physician gender associated with the quality of diabetes care? *Diabetes Care, 28*(7), 1594–1598. doi:10.2337/diacare.28.7.1594 PMID:15983306

King, E., & Jones, K. (2016). Why subtle bias is so often worse than blatant discrimination. *Harvard Business Review.*

Klebanoff, M. A., Shiono, P., & Rhoads, G. (1990). Outcomes of pregnancy in a national sample of resident physicians. *The New England Journal of Medicine, 323*(15), 1040–1045. doi:10.1056/NEJM199010113231506 PMID:2215563

Klingensmith, M., & Anderson, K. (2006). Educational scholarship as a route to academic promotion: A depiction of surgical education scholars. *American Journal of Surgery, 191*(4), 533–537. doi:10.1016/j.amjsurg.2006.01.007</jrn>

Kolb, D. A., Boyatzis, R. E., & Mainemelis, C. (1999) *Experiential learning theory: previous research and new directions.* Working Paper 99-98. Cleveland, OH: Case Western Reserve University Hippocrates of Cos, (1923) The Oath [Internet]. Loeb Classical Library. 1923; 147, 298–299. doi:10.4159/DLCL.hippocrates_cos-oath

-Koligian, J. & Sternberg, R. J. (2000). Perceived fraudulence in young adults: Is there an imposter syndrome? *Journal of personality assessment, 56*(2), 308-326.

Kosny, A. & MacEachen, E. (2009). Gendered, invisible work in non-profit social service organizations: Implications for worker health and safety. *Gender, Work & Organization, 17*(4), 359-380.

Koven, S. (2017). Letter to a young female physician. *The New England Journal of Medicine, 376*(20), 1907–1909. doi:10.1056/NEJMp1702010 PMID:28514609

Krawczyk, M. (2017). Are all researchers male? Gender misattributions in citations. *Scientometrics, 110*(3), 1397–1402. doi:10.100711192-016-2192-y PMID:28255187

Krivkovich, A., Robinson, K., Starikova, I., Valentino, R., & Yee, L. (2017). Women in the workplace 2017. McKinsey Report.

Kruger, J., & Dunning, D. (1999). Unskilled and unaware of it: How difficulties in recognizing one's own incompetence lead to inflated self-assessments. *Journal of Personality and Social Psychology, 77*(6), 1121–1134. doi:10.1037/0022-3514.77.6.1121 PMID:10626367

Krupat, E., Rosenkranz, S. L., Yeager, C. M., Barnard, K., Putnam, S. M., & Inui, T. S. (2000). The practice orientations of physicians and patients: The effect of doctor-patient congruence on satisfaction. *Patient Education and Counseling*, *39*(1), 49–59. doi:10.1016/S0738-3991(99)00090-7 PMID:11013547

Kuwait Institute for Medical Specialties. (2016-2017). Manual of Policies for postgraduate. *Medical Education.*

Kuwait Institute for Medical Specialties. About KIMS. Available at https://www.kims.org.kw

Kuwait University Health Sciences Center. *Undergraduate Handbook.* 2018-2019.

Kuwait University. *Faculty of Medicine Homepage.* Available at http://www.hsc.edu.kw/FOM/

Kuwick, L. (2018, March 7). Commit to a conversation about the gender pay gap. Retrieved from https://www.kevinmd.com/blog/2018/03/commit-conversation-gender-pay-gap.html

Kvaerner, K. J., Aasland, O. G., & Botten, G. S. (1999). Female medical leadership: Cross sectional study. *BMJ (Clinical Research Ed.)*, *318*(7176), 91–94. doi:10.1136/bmj.318.7176.91 PMID:9880281

Kvinnsam- National Library for Gender Research. (2019). Notable years, Gothenburg university library. Retrieved from http://www.ub.gu.se/kvinn/artal

LaDonna, K. A., Ginsburg, S., & Watling, C. (2018). Rising to the level of your incompetence. *Academic Medicine*, *93*(5), 763–768. doi:10.1097/ACM.0000000000002046 PMID:29116983

Läkarförbund, S. (2016). Läkarfakta, statistik över medlemmar, Sveriges läkarförbund. Retrieved from https://slf.se/app/uploads/2018/04/laxxkarfakta-2016.pdf

Lakoff, R. (1963). Language and Woman's Place. *Language in Society*, *2*(1), 45–80. doi:10.1017/S0047404500000051

Lam, B. (2016, July 27). What Gender Pay-Gap Statistics Aren't Capturing. *Atlantic (Boston, Mass.).*

Lam, B. (2017, March 28). Education Doesn't Solve the Gender Pay Gap. *Atlantic (Boston, Mass.).*

Lashbrook, D. L., Frazier, L. M., Horbelt, D. V., Stembridge, T. W., & Rall, M. J. (2003). Pregnancy during obstetrics and gynecology residency: Effect on surgical experience. *American Journal of Obstetrics and Gynecology*, *189*(3), 662–665. doi:10.1067/S0002-9378(03)00877-9 PMID:14526288

Laurance, J. (2004) The medical timebomb: too many women doctors. Retrieved from http://www.independent.co.uk/life-style/health-and-families/health-news/the-medicaltimebomb-too- many-women-doctors-6260011.html

Lave, J., & Wenger, E. (1991). *Situated learning legitimate peripheral participation.* Cambridge, UK: Cambridge University Press. doi:10.1017/CBO9780511815355

Law n.º 64/2011 22 December, Diário da República, 1ª série-N°244- Dec. 22, 2011.

Laws, P., Rosborough, P., & Poodry, F. (1999). Women's responses to an activity-based introductory physics program. *American Journal of Physics*, *67*(S1), S32–S37. doi:10.1119/1.19077

Leach, P. K., Nygaard, R. M., Chipman, J. G., Brunsvold, M. E., & Marek, A. P. (2018). Impostor phenomenon and burnout in general surgeons and general surgery residents. *Journal of Surgical Education*, 1–8. doi:10.1016/j.jsurg.2018.06.025 PMID:30122638

Leary, M. R., Patton, K. M., Orlando, A. E., & Wagoner Funk, W. (2000). The impostor phenomenon: Self-perceptions, reflected appraisals, and interpersonal strategies. *Journal of Personality*, *68*(4), 725–756. doi:10.1111/1467-6494.00114 PMID:10934688

Lefebvre, L. G. & Kaufmann, I. M. (2017). The identification and management of substance use disorders in anesthesiologists. *Canadian Journal of Anaesthesia = Journal Canadien d'anesthesie, 64*(2), 211–218. doi:10.100712630-016-0775-y

Legassie, J., Zibrowski, E. M., & Goldszmidt, M. A. (2008). Measuring Resident Well-Being: Impostorism and Burnout Syndrome in Residency. *Journal of General Internal Medicine, 23*(7), 1090–1094. doi:10.100711606-008-0536-x PMID:18612750

Legewie, J., & DiPrete, T. (2014). The High School Environment and the Gender Gap in Science and Engineering. *Sociology of Education, 87*(4), 259–280. doi:10.1177/0038040714547770 PMID:27857451

Leonhardt, M., Bechtoldt, M. N., & Rohrmann, S. (2017). All impostors aren't alike – differentiating the impostor phenomenon. *Frontiers in Psychology, 8*, 424. doi:10.3389/fpsyg.2017.01505 PMID:28936188

Leslie, K., Hopf, H. W., Houston, P., & O'Sullivan, E. (2017). Women, minorities, and leadership in anesthesiology: Take the pledge. *Anesthesia and Analgesia, 124*(5), 1394–1396. doi:10.1213/ANE.0000000000001967 PMID:28426582

Le, T. A. N., Lo Sasso, A. T., & Vujicic, M. (2017). Trends in the earnings gender gap among dentists, physicians, and lawyers. *The Journal of the American Dental Association, 148*(4), 257–262.e2. doi:10.1016/j.adaj.2017.01.005 PMID:28238360

Leung, L. Y. (2018). Encouraging female undergraduate student to consider a surgical career [Abstract]. *Association of Surgeons of Great Britain and Ireland, 53*(Winter), 88-89. Retrieved from http://asgbi.org/Journals/Winter%202018%20 JASGBI.pdf

Leung, P. W. L., & Kwan, K. S. F. (1998). Parenting style, motivational orientation and self-perceived academic competence: A meditational model. *Merrill-Palmer Quarterly, 44*, 1–19.

Levanon, A., England, P., & Allison, P. (2009). Occupational Feminization and Pay: Assessing Causal Dynamics Using 1950-2000 U.S. Census Data. *Social Forces, 88*(2), 865–891. doi:10.1353of.0.0264

Liang, R., Dornan, T., & Nestel, D. (2019) Why do women leave surgical training? A qualitative and feminist study. *Lancet 393*(10171), 541-549. doi:10.1016/S0140-6736(18)32612-6

Lindsay, E. K., & Creswell, J. D. (2017). Mechanisms of mindfulness training: Monitor and Acceptance Theory (MAT). *Clinical Psychology Review, 51*, 48–59. doi:10.1016/j.cpr.2016.10.011 PMID:27835764

Lis, L. D., Wood, W. C., Petkova, E., & Shatkin, J. (2009). Mentoring in psychiatric residency programs: A survey of chief residents. *Academic Psychiatry, 33*(4), 307–312. doi:10.1176/appi.ap.33.4.307 PMID:19690111

Liston, D. D., & Rahimi, R. (Eds.). (2017). *Promoting Social Justice Through the Scholarship of Teaching and Learning*. Indiana University Press. doi:10.2307/j.ctt2005zc2

Livingston, G. (2015, July 6). For most highly educated women, motherhood doesn't start until the 30s. Washington, DC. Retrieved from http://www.pewresearch.org/fact-tank/2015/01/15/for-most- highly-educated-women-motherhood-doesnt-start-until-the-30s/

Livingston, G. (2018, Jan. 18). General format. Retrieved from http://www.pewsocialtrends.org/2018/01/18/theyre-waiting-longer-but-u-s-women-today-more-likely-to-have-children-than-a-decade-ago

Logghe, H., Jones, C., McCoubrey, A., & Fitzgerald, E. (2017). #ILookLikeASurgeon: Embracing diversity to improve patient outcomes. *BMJ (Clinical Research Ed.), j4653*. doi:10.1136/bmj.j4653 PMID:29018031

Lord, A. (2019, April 15). Also perhaps women tend to choose other things (e.g. teaching) over research? Which is fine as long as they have equal opportunity to do either and it's a true choice! [Tweet]. Retrieved from https://twitter.com/AmyLord1/status/1117712428530315265

Lorenzo, M., Crouch, C., & Mazur, E. (2006). Reducing the gender gap in the physics classroom. *American Journal of Physics*, *74*(2), 118–122. doi:10.1119/1.2162549

Lovell, K. N. (2018). "Everyone Gets a Blister": Sexism, Gender Empowerment, and Race in the People's Park Movement. *Women's Studies Quarterly*, *46*(3), 103–119. doi:10.1353/wsq.2018.0034

Lundbäck, A, & Trysell, C. (2017). 10 400 läkare skriver under uppropet # utantystnadsplikt, Läkartidningen.se Nov. 30, 2017.

Lundgren, K. (2014). *Barrikaden valde mig. Ada Nilsson. Läkare i kvinnokampen.* Wahlström & Widstrand.

Lyndra, V. (2015). How medical specialties vary by gender. Retrieved from https://www.ama-assn.org/residents-students/specialty-profiles/how-medical-specialties-vary-gender

Lyons, N. B., Bernardi, K., Huang, L., Holihan, J. L., Cherla, D., Martin, A. C., ... Hydo, L. (2019). Gender. disparity in surgery: An evaluation of surgical societies. *Surgical Infections*, *20*(5), 406–410. doi:10.1089ur.2018.220 PMID:30892131

Macaluso, B., Lariviere, V., Sugimoto, T., & Sugimoto, C. (2016). Is Science Built on the Shoulders of Women? A Study of Gender Differences in Contributorship. *Academic Medicine*, *91*(8), 1136–1142. doi:10.1097/ACM.0000000000001261 PMID:27276004

Magee, R. V. (2017). One Field, Different Doors In: Contemplative Higher Education, Transformative Education, and Education for Social Justice. Social Justice, Inner Work & Contemplative Practice, 119.

Magon, A. (2013). Gender, the brain and education: do boys and girls learn differently? [University Library] Retrieved from https://dspace.library.uvic.ca/handle/1828/1411

Mahady, S. E. (2011). Adding flexibility to physician training. *The Medical Journal of Australia*, *194*(9), 460–462. PMID:21534903

Major, D. A., Turner, J. E., & Fletcher, T. D. (2006). Linking proactive personality and the big five to motivation to learn and development activity. *The Journal of Applied Psychology*, *91*(4), 927–935. doi:10.1037/0021-9010.91.4.927 PMID:16834515

Mammen, J. M., Fischer, D. R., Anderson, A., James, L. E., Nussbaum, M. S., Bower, R. H., & Pritts, T. A. (2007). Learning styles vary among general surgery residents: Analysis of 12 years of data. *Journal of Surgical Education*, *64*(6), 386–389. doi:10.1016/j.jsurg.2007.08.005 PMID:18063274

Mangurian, C., Linos, E., Sarkar, U., Rodriguez, C., & Jagsi, R. (2018). What's holding women in medicine back from leadership. *Harvard Business Review*, 24.

Mannberg-Zackari, C. (2015). Män får dyrare sjukvård. Tidningen Curie. Retrieved from https://www.tidningencurie.se/nyheter/2015/08/27/man-far-dyrare-sjukvard/

Manne, K. (2017). Down girl: The logic of misogyny. Oxford, UK: Oxford University Press. doi:10.1093/oso/9780190604981.001.0001

Manne, K. (2016). The logic of misogyny. *Boston Review*, *41*(4), 8–23.

Manner, M. H. (2010). The Impact of CEO Characteristics on Corporate Social Performance. *Journal of Business Ethics. Springer Netherlands*, *93*(S1), 53–72. doi:10.100710551-010-0626-7

Martinez, G., Daniels, K., & Chandra, A. (2012). Fertility of men and women aged 15-44 years in the United States: National survey of family growth, 2006-2010. *National Health Statistics Reports*, *12*, 1–28. PMID:22803225

Martinou, E., Allan, H., & Vig, S. (2014). Personality Differences Among Junior Postgraduate Trainees in the United Kingdom. *The Journal of Surgery*, *72*(1), 122–127. doi:10.1016/j.jsurg.2014.06.014 PMID:25091381

Martin, P., & Barnard, A. (2013). The experience of women in male-dominated occupations: A constructivist grounded theory inquiry. *SA Journal of Industrial Psychology*, *39*(2). doi:10.4102ajip.v39i2.1099

Marx, M. V. (2018). Baby on Board: Managing Occupational Radiation Exposure During Pregnancy. *Techniques in Vascular and Interventional Radiology*, *21*(1), 32–36. doi:10.1053/j.tvir.2017.12.007 PMID:29471998

Mättä, S. (2015). Män kostar mer än kvinnor vid hjärtinfarkt och appendicit [DEYT]. *Lakartidningen*, *2015*, 112.

Mayer, A. P., Blair, J. E., Ko, M. G., Hayes, S. N., Chang, Y. H., Caubet, S. L., & Files, J. A. (2014). Gender distribution of U.S. medical school faculty by academic track type. *Academic Medicine*, *89*(2), 312–317. doi:10.1097/ACM.0000000000000089 PMID:24362384

McClure, E. (2019). Theorizing a Spectrum of Aggression: Microaggressions, Creepiness, and Sexual Assault. *the pluralist*, *14*(1), 91-101.

McCord, J. H., McDonald, R., Sippel, R. S., Leverson, G., Mahvi, D. M., & Weber, S. M. (2009). Surgical career choices: The vital impact of mentoring. *The Journal of Surgical Research*, *155*(1), 136–141. doi:10.1016/j.jss.2008.06.048 PMID:19041099

McCurry, J. (2018). Tokyo medical school admits changing results to exclude women. Retrieved from https://www.theguardian.com/world/2018/aug/08/tokyo-medical-school-admits-changing-results-to-exclude-women

McDonald, R. E., Jeeves, A. E., Vasey, C. E., Wright, D. M., & O'Grady, G. (2013). Supply and demand mismatch for flexible (part-time) surgical training in Australasia. *The Medical Journal of Australia*, *198*(8), 423–425. doi:10.5694/mja12.11685 PMID:23641991

McGregor, L. N., Gee, D. E., & Posey, K. E. (2008). I feel like a fraud and it depresses me: The relation between the imposter phenomenon and depression. *Social Behavior and Personality*, *36*(1), 43–48. doi:10.2224bp.2008.36.1.43

McIntire, M. E. (2015, Sept. 17). Another Research Gender Gap: Men get more start-up money. Retrieved from https://www.chronicle.com/article/Another-Research-Gender-Gap-/233177

McIntosh, P. (1989). *Feeling like a fraud.* Wellesley, MA: Stone Center College.

McKimm, J., Da Silva, A. S., Edwards, S., Greenhill, S., & Taylor, C. (2015), Women and Leadership in Medicine and Medical Education: International Perspectives. In Maria Tsouroufli (Ed.), Gender, Careers and Inequalities in Medicine and Medical Education: International Perspectives (International Perspectives on Equality, Diversity and Inclusion, Volume 2). Emerald Group. doi:10.1108/S2051-233320150000002005

McKinsey & Company. (2017). Women Matter. Retrieved from (https://www.mckinsey.com/~/media/McKinsey/Featured%20Insights/Women%20matter/Women%20Matter%20Ten%20years%20of%20insights%20on%20the%20importance%20of%20gender%20diversity/Women-Matter-Time-to-accelerate-Ten-years-of-insights into gender diversity.ashx)

McKinstry, B. (2008). Are there too many female medical graduates? Yes. [Medical's Women Federation. n.d.]. *BMJ (Clinical Research Ed.)*, *336*(7647), 748. doi:10.1136/bmj.39505.491065.94 PMID:18390524

McManus, I. C., Keeling, A., & Paice, E. (2004) Stress, burnout and doctors' attitudes to work are determined by personality and learning style: A twelve year longitudinal study of UK medical graduates. *BMC Med., 18*(2), 29. Retrieved from http://www.biomedcentral.com/1741-7015/2/29

McManus, I. C., & Sproston, K. A. (2000). Women in hospital medicine in the United Kingdom: Glass ceiling, preference, prejudice or cohort effect? *Journal of Epidemiology and Community Health, 54*(1), 10–16. doi:10.1136/jech.54.1.10 PMID:10692956

McNally, S. (2016) Sexual harassment and bullying in UK surgery: no room for complacency. *BMJ 354.* doi:10.1136/bmj.i4682

McNally, S. (2017). *A woman at a surgical conference: They thought I was the waitress.* Retrieved from https://www.bma.org.uk/connecting-doctors/b/work/posts/a-woman-at-a-surgical-conference-they-thought-i-was-the-waitress

McNally, S. (2018a). How I became a woman in surgery. *Association of Surgeons of Great Britain and Ireland.* Available at www.scarlettmcnally.co.uk

McNally, S. (2018b). Unconscious bias, bullying and behaviour change. *Royal College of Surgeons of Edinburgh event presentations.* Retrieved from https://www.rcsed.ac.uk/professional-support-development-resources/anti-bullying-and-undermining-campaign/resources-to-help-change-the-culture

McNally, S. (2012). Surgical Training: Still Highly Competitive But Still Very Male. *Bulletin Royal College of Surgeons of England, 94*(2), 53–55. doi:10.1308/147363512X13189526438675

McNally, S. (2013). Global population explosion: Economic and health meltdown. *Journal of the Royal Society of Medicine, 106*(2), 38–39. doi:10.1258/jrsm.2012.120246 PMID:23401631

McNally, S., & Huber, J. (2018). Award-winning new doctors' assistants freeing time in acute NHS hospitals *Health Management, 18*(1). Retrieved from https://healthmanagement.org/c/healthmanagement/issuearticle/award-winning-new-doctors-assistants-freeing-time-in-acute-nhs-hospitals

McNally, S., Nunan, D., Dixon, A., Maruthappu, M., Butler, K., & Gray, M. (2017). Focus on physical activity can help avoid unnecessary social care. *BMJ (Clinical Research Ed.), 359*(j4609), 108–110. doi:10.1136/bmj.j4609 PMID:29042359

Medical Licensing Administration at Ministry of Health. (2019). *Physician Statistics*. Kuwait.

Medical Women's Federation [medicalwomenuk]. (2018a, Feb. 16). On average full-time men earned £20,000 more than full-time women when you include bonuses, overtime and awards: £120,890 v £99,833 Even if you look at basic pay, there is a difference of £6,000 for full-time doctors: £87,327 v £81,216 #GenderPayGap [Tweet]. Retrieved from https://twitter.com/medicalwomenuk/status/964410742316220416

Medical Women's Federation. (2018b, May 28). Press Release: Gender Pay Gap Review in Medicine. Retrieved from medicalwomensfederation.org.uk

Medical Women's Federation. (2019, March 29). Press Release: MWF responds to Gender Pay Gap in Medicine Review interim findings. Retrieved from medicalwomensfederation.org.uk

Medscape. (2018). Medscape physician compensation report 2018. Retrieved from https://www.medscape.com/slideshow/2018-compensation-surgeon-6009657

Meghen, K., Sweeney, C., Linehan, C., O'Flynn, S., & Boylan, G. (2013) Women in hospital medicine: facts, figures and personal experiences. [Abstract] *Ir Med J. Feb;106*(2):39-42.

Mehta, S., Burns, K. E. A. A., Machado, F. R., Fox-Robichaud, A. E., Cook, D. J., Calfee, C. S., ... Herridge, M. S. (2017). Gender parity in critical care medicine. *American Journal of Respiratory and Critical Care Medicine, 196*(4), 425–429. doi:10.1164/rccm.201701-0076CP PMID:28240961

Men enjoy five hours more leisure time per week than women. (2018). Men enjoy five hours more leisure time per week than women. Retrieved from ons.gov.uk

Menegatti, M., & Rubini, M. (2017). *Gender bias and sexism in language*. Oxford Research Encyclopaedias. doi:10.1093/acrefore/9780190228613.013.470

Merchant, S., Hameed, M., & Melck, A. (2011). Pregnancy among residents enrolled in general surgery (PREGS): A survey of residents in a single Canadian training program. *Canadian Journal of Surgery, 54*(6), 375–380. doi:10.1503/cjs.015710 PMID:21939607

Mihaila, R., & Botezat, O. (2016). The Gender Construction of Society. *Journal of Research in Gender Studies, 6*(2), 187.

Miller, C. C. (2016, March 18). As Women Take Over a Male-Dominated Field, the Pay Drops. *The New York Times.*

Miller, C. A. (1994). What's a woman doing in a place like this? *Surgical Neurology, 42*, 171–176. doi:10.1016/0090-3019(94)90383-2 PMID:8091297

Miller, J., & Katz, D. (2018). Gender Differences in Perception of Workplace Experience Among Anesthesiology Residents. *The Journal of Education in Perioperative Medicine: JEPM, 20*(1), E618. Retrieved from http://www.ncbi.nlm.nih.gov/pubmed/29928665 PMID:29928665

Miller-Rosser, K., Chapman, Y., Francis, K. (2006). Historical, Cultural, and Contemporary Influences on the Status of Women in Nursing in Saudi Arabia. *The Online Journal of Issues in Nursing*, 2006, 11(3).

Milroy, L. (1980). Language and social networks. Oxford, UK: Basil Blackwell, University Park Press.

Ministry of Health Kuwait. *MOH website history: Historical Overview*. Available at https://www.moh.gov.kw/en/Pages/Aboutus.aspx

Mirkovic, K. R., Perrine, C. G., Scanlon, K. S., & Grummer-Strawn, L. M. (2014). In the United States, a mother's plans for infant feeding are associated with her plans for employment. *Journal of Human Lactation, 30*(3), 292–297. doi:10.1177/0890334414535665 PMID:24868017

Mitchell-Jones, N., Gallos, I., Farren, J., Tobias, A., Bottomley, C., & Bourne, T. (2017). Psychological morbidity associated with hyperemesis gravidarum: A systematic review and meta-analysis. *British Journal of Obstetrics and Gynaecology, 124*(1), 20–30. doi:10.1111/1471-0528.14180 PMID:27418035

Moberly, T. (2018). A fifth of surgeons in England are female. *BMJ (Clinical Research Ed.), k4530*. doi:10.1136/bmj.k4530 PMID:30377150

Moberly, T. (2018). Number of women entering medical school rises after decade of decline. *BMJ (Clinical Research Ed.), 360*, k254. doi:10.1136/bmj.k254

Mohan, H., Ali, O., Gokani, V. J., McGoldrick, C., Smitham, P., Fitzgerald, J. E. F., & Harries, R. L. (in press). Surgical trainees experience of pregnancy, maternity and paternity leave: A cross-sectional study. *Postgraduate Medical Journal.*

Morahan, P., Rosen, S., Richman, R., & Gleason, K. (2011). The Leadership Continuum: A Framework for Organizational and Individual Assessment Relative to the Advancement of Women Physicians and Scientists. *Journal of Women's Health, 20*(3), 387–396. doi:10.1089/jwh.2010.2055 PMID:21351872

Morand, D. A. (1996). What's in a name? An Exploration of the Social Dynamics of Form of Address in Organizations. *Management Communication Quarterly*, *9*(4), 422–451. doi:10.1177/0893318996009004003

More residents building families during training. (2016). [Medical Society Research] Retrieved from https://www.ama-assn.org/residents-students/resident-student-health/more-residents-building-families-during-training

Morgan, E. (2018, March 7). Energy Australia closes gender pay gap overnight, literally. Retrieved from http://www.abc.net.au/news/2018-03-07/energy-australia-closes-gender-pay-gap-overnight/9524770

Morgan, A. U., Chaiyachati, K. H., Weissman, G. E., & Liao, J. M. (2018). Eliminating Gender-Based Bias in Academic Medicine: More than Naming the "Elephant in the Room". *Journal of General Internal Medicine*, 1–3. PMID:29564608

Morgenroth, T., & Ryan, M. K. (2018). Quotas and affirmative action: Understanding group-based outcomes and attitudes. *Social and Personality Psychology Compass*, *12*(3), e12374–e32. doi:10.1111pc3.12374

Morris, M., Chen, H., Heslin, M. J., & Krontiras, H. (2018). A structured compensation plan improves but does not erase the sex pay gap in surgery. *Annals of Surgery*, *268*(3), 442–448. doi:10.1097/SLA.0000000000002928 PMID:29979249

Mouly, F. & Bormes, G. (2017). The New Yorker Cover that's Being Replicated by Women Surgeons Around the World.

Mouly, F., Bormes, G., Wiley, C., Roupenian, K., Berry, P., Cassidy, J., ... (2017). The New Yorker Cover That's Being Replicated by Women Surgeons Across the World. Retrieved from https://www.newyorker.com/culture/culture-desk/the-new-yorker-cover-thats-being-replicated-by-women-surgeons-across-the-world

Murphy, E., & Oesch, D. (2016). The Feminization of Occupations and Change in Wages: A Panel Analysis of Britain, Germany, and Switzerland. *Social Forces*, *94*(3), 1221–1255. doi:10.1093fov099

Nadelson, C. (2006). *A Model for Women's Career Development: An Office for Women's Careers*. Queensland, Australia: Presentation at Griffith University.

Narwan, G. (2019, April 23). Hundreds of errors mar pay gap data. *The Times*.

Natalie, G. (2017). What Happened When A Man And Woman Swapped Names At Work. Retrieved from https://www.refinery29.com/en-gb/2017/03/144692/man-woman-swap-names-workplace-sexism

National Academies of Sciences, Engineering and Medicine. (2018). Sexual Harassment of Women: Climate, Culture and Consequences in Academic Sciences, Engineering, and Medicine.

National Confidential Enquiry into Patient Outcome and Death [NCEPOD]. (1999). *Who operates when?* Retrieved from http://www.ncepod.org.uk/1995_6.html

Nationellt centrum för kvinnofrid. (2018). Kriminalstatistik och våldsutsatthet, Sexualbrott. Retrieved from https://www.nck.uu.se/

Nawrockyi, K. (2016, Nov. 15). Closing the gender pay gap: Stop telling women they just need to negotiate harder. Retrieved from http://www.womanthology.co.uk/pdwti

Neureiter, M., & Traut-Mattausch, E. (2016). An inner barrier to career development: Preconditions of the impostor phenomenon and consequences for career development. *Frontiers in Psychology*, *7*, 53. doi:10.3389/fpsyg.2016.00048 PMID:26869957

Newman, P. (2012). *Releasing Potential: Women Doctors and Clinical Leadership*.

Ng, S. H. (2007). Language-based discrimination: Blatant and subtle forms. *Journal of Language and Social Psychology*, *26*(2), 106–122. doi:10.1177/0261927X07300074

NHS Institute for Innovation and Improvement and Academy of Medical Royal Colleges. (2010). *Medical Leadership Competency Framework* (3rd ed.).

NHS-Digital. (2018) *Analysis of the representation of women across the hospital and community health services workforce.*

NHS-Employers. (2019) *Diversity and Inclusion Partners Programme*. Available at https://www.nhsemployers.org/your-workforce/plan/diversity-and-inclusion/partners-programme

NHS-England. (2013). *A refreshed Equality Delivery System for the NHS*. London, UK: NHS England.

NHS-Leadership-Academy. (2013) *The Healthcare Leadership Model*. Retrieved from https://www.leadershipacademy.nhs.uk/resources/healthcare-leadership-model/

Nietsche, F. (1911). Beyond good and evil (vol. 12 of The complete works. Ed.: O. Levy) Foulis.

NIH Data Book. (2019, April). [Graph illustration the Cumulative Investigator Rate: Research Project Grants, R21, P01, or R01-Equivalents] Retrieved from https://report.nih.gov/nihdatabook/index.aspx

Nilsson, A. (1963). Glimtar ur Mitt liv som läkare. Natur och kultur.

Nine ways to narrow the gender pay gap. (2018, April 5). Nine ways to narrow the gender pay gap. Retrieved from https://www.bbc.com/news/business-43643989

Nomura, K., Yamazaki, Y., Gruppen, L. D., Horie, S., Takeuchi, M., & Illing, J. (2015). The difficulty of professional continuation among female doctors in Japan: A qualitative study of alumnae of 13 medical schools in Japan. *BMJ Open*, *5*(3), e005845. doi:10.1136/bmjopen-2014-005845 PMID:25818268

Nonnemaker, L. (2000). Women physicians in academic medicine: New insights from cohort studies. *The New England Journal of Medicine*, *342*(6), 399–405. doi:10.1056/NEJM200002103420606 PMID:10666431

Norman, H. & Fagan, C. (2017). *Shared parental leave in the UK: is it working? Lessons from other countries.* Retrieved from https://www.workingfamilies.org.uk/workflex-blog/shared-parental-leave-in-the-uk-is-it-working-lessons-from-other-countries/

Noronha, A. (Coord.),& Ferreira, A. P. (Fotogr.) (2016). Mulheres na Ciência. Lisboa: Ciência Viva.

Norström, T. (2009). Män har större chans att få forskningsanslag. *Lakartidningen*, *79*, 1290–1326.

NZ doctor's Hippocratic Oath change passed. (2017). Retrieved from https://www.radionz.co.nz/news/world/341592/nz-doctor-s-hippocratic-oath-change-passed

O'Callaghan, J., Mohan, H. M., & Harries, R. L.Council of the Association of Surgeons in Training. (2017). The non-monetary costs of surgical training. *Annals of the Royal College of Surgeons of England (Suppl)*, *100*(8), 339–344. doi:10.1308/rcsbull.2018.339

O'Hare, E. & O'Donohue, W. (1998). Sexual Harassment: Identifying risk factors. *Archives of Sexual Behaviour; New York, 27*(6), 561 – 80.

O'Neill, T. (2019). *Success and Likability for Women in the Workplace, The Heidi-Howard Study*. Morgan McKinley Go Beyond.

Oaklander, M. (2016, July 11). Women and Black Doctors Still Make Far Less Than White Male Doctors. *Time*. Retrieved from http://time.com/4398888/doctors-gender-wage-gap/

OECD. (2017). The Pursuit of Gender Equality. Retrieved from http://www.oecd.org/gender/the-pursuit-of-gender-equality-9789264281318-en.htm

OECD. (2017). *The Pursuit of Gender Equality: An Uphill Battle*. Paris, France: OECD. doi:10.1787/9789264281318-

OECD. (2019). Retrieved from https://www.catalyst.org/media/companies-more-women-board-directors-experience-higher-financial-performance-according-latest

Office of National Statistics Berlin. (2005). [National Statistics] Retrieved from http://www.rki.de/EN/Content/Health_Monitoring/Health_Reporting/GBEDownloadsT/mittleres_lebensalter.pdf?__blob=publicationFile

Oliveira, D. F. M., Ma, Y., Woodruff, T. K., & Uzzi, B. (2019). Comparison of National Institutes of Health Grant Amounts to First-Time Male and Female Principal Investigators. *Journal of the American Medical Association, 321*(9), 898–900. doi:10.1001/jama.2018.21944 PMID:30835300

Oliver, C. [ChrisOliverNHS]. (2018, March 28). @NHSE_Paul @hcwomenleaders I think the first step is to aknowlege imposter syndrome and realise it is more common than you think! #nhswomen [Tweet]. Retrieved from https://twitter.com/ChrisOliverNHS/status/979074441429872641

Oman medical school. *Homepage*. Available at https://www.squ.edu.om/medicine/About-College/About-CoMHS/History

ONS (Office for National Statistics). (2017). UK Labour Market: Estimates of employment, unemployment, economic inactivity and other employment-related statistics for the UK. Available at https://www.ons.gov.uk/employmentandlabourmarket/peopleinwork/employmentandemployeetypes/bulletins/uklabourmarket/jan2017

Organisation for Economic Co-operation and Development. (2018). *Is the last mile the longest? oecd.org*.

Oriel, K., Plane, M. B., & Mindt, M. (2004, April). Family Medicine Residents and the impostor phenomenon. *Family Medicine*, *36*(4), 248–252. PMID:15057614

Oriel, K., Plane, M. B., & Mundt, M. (2004). Family medicine residents and the impostor phenomenon. *Family Medicine*, *36*(4), 248–252. PMID:15057614

Osika, I. et al. (2005). Tvättsäcksprojektet – genusskillnader in på bara skinnet, Läkartidningen 2846-2851, 40, 2005, 102.

Outlook Magazine. (2019). *Bengal doctors' strike enters day 4*. Healthcare services hit in Delhi, Maharashtra too.

Overcoming gender obstacles in medicine. (2016). [Medical Society Advice] Retrieved from https://www.ama-assn.org/practice-management/physician-diversity/overcoming-gender-obstacles-medicine

Paauw, S. & Kneepkens, E. (2018). #MeToo artsen gaan niet vrijuit. Retrieved from https://www.medischcontact.nl/nieuws/laatste-nieuws/artikel/metoo-artsen-gaan-niet-vrijuit.htm

Paauw, S. & Kneepkens, E. (2018). En hoe zit het eigenlijk met #MeToo bij medici? Retrieved from https://www.medischcontact.nl/arts-in-spe/nieuws/ais-artikel/en-hoe-zit-het-eigenlijk-met-metoo-bij-medici.htm

Palepu, A., Friedman, R. H., Barnett, R. C., Carr, P. L., Ash, A. S., Szalacha, L., & Moskowitz, M. A. (1998). Junior faculty members' mentoring relationships and their professional development in U.S. medical schools. *Academic Medicine, 73*(3), 318-323. Retrieved from https://www.ncbi.nlm.nih.gov/pubmed/9526459

Panagioti, M., Geraghty, K., Johnson, J., Zhou, A., Panagopoulou, E., Chew-Graham, C., ... Esmail, A. (2018). Association Between Physician Burnout and Patient Safety, Professionalism, and Patient Satisfaction. *JAMA Internal Medicine, 178*(10), 1317. doi:10.1001/jamainternmed.2018.3713 PMID:30193239

Park, A. (2019, June 25). NIH Director Francis Collins has a plan to help eliminate "manels". *Time*. Retrieved from https://time.com/5611142/manels-nih-director-francis-collins/?amp=true

Parker, K., Horowitz, J. M., & Rohal, M. (2015). *Women and leadership: Public says women are equally qualified, but barriers persist.* Washington DC: Pew Research Center.

Pasin, L., Nardelli, P., Pintaudi, M., Greco, M., Zambon, M., Cabrini, L., & Zangrillo, A. (2017). Closed-loop Delivery Systems Versus Manually Controlled Administration of Total Iv Anesthesia: A Meta-analysis of Randomized Clinical Trials. *Anesthesia &amp, 124*(2), 456–464. doi:10.1213/ane.0000000000001394

Pastor Gosálbez, M. I., Belzunegui Eraso, A. , & Pontón Merino, P. (2012). Mujeres en sanidad: Entre la igualdad y la desigualdad. *Cuadernos de Relaciones Laborales, 30*(2), 497–518.

Pateman, C. (2018). *The disorder of women: Democracy, feminism and political theory.* John Wiley & Sons.

Patzak, A., Kollmayer, M., & Schober, B. (2017). Buffering impostor feelings with kindness: The mediating role of self-compassion between gender-role orientation and the impostor phenomenon. *Frontiers in Psychology, 8*, 1289. doi:10.3389/fpsyg.2017.01289 PMID:28798714

Pei, K. Y., & Cochran, A. (2019). Workplace Bullying Among Surgeons - the perfect crime. *Annals of Surgery, 269*(1), 43–44. doi:10.1097/SLA.0000000000003018 PMID:30247324

Peters, K., Ryan, M., Haslam, S. A., & Morgenroth, T. (2013). *The psychology and economics of women in leadership.* Retrieved from http://www.europarl.europa.eu/RegData/etudes/workshop/join/2013/474408/IPOL-FEMM_AT(2013)474408_EN.pdf

Peters, K., Ryan, M. K., Haslam, S. A., & Fernandes, H. (2012). To Belong or Not to Belong. Evidence That Women's Occupational Disidentification Is Promoted by Lack of Fit With Masculine Occupational Prototypes. *Journal of Personnel Psychology, 11*(3), 148–158. doi:10.1027/1866-5888/a000067

Pfleiderer, B., Bortul, M., Palmisano, S., Rodde, S., & Hasebrook, J. (2018). Improving female physician's careers in academic medicine: Chances and challenges. *Best Practice & Research. Clinical Anaesthesiology, 32*(1), 15–23. doi:10.1016/j.bpa.2018.04.006 PMID:30049335

Pianosi, K., Bethune, C., & Hurley, K. (2016). Medical student career choice: A qualitative study of fourth-year medical students at Memorial University, Newfoundland. *CMAJ Open, 4*(2), E147–E152. doi:10.9778/cmajo.20150103 PMID:27398357

Piccinato, C., Rodrigues, M., Rocha, L., & Troncon, L. (2017). Characteristics of role models who influenced medical residents to choose surgery as a specialty: Exploratory study. *Sao Paulo Medical Journal, 135*(6), 529–534. doi:10.1590/1516-3180.2017.0053030517 PMID:29116309

Pieri, M., Bonizzoni, M. A., Lembo, R., Dalessandro, V., Alba, A. C., Zangrillo, A., & Landoni, G. (2016, October). Intensive Care and Anesthesia Specialists Would Do More Research If They Could. *Journal of Cardiothoracic and Vascular Anesthesia.* United States. doi:10.1053/j.jvca.2016.04.024

Pletzer, J. L., Nikolova, R., Kedzior, K. K., & Voelpel, S. C. (2015). Does Gender Matter? Female Representation on Corporate Boards and Firm Financial Performance-A Meta-Analysis. *PLoS One, 10*(6). doi:10.1371/journal.pone.0130005 PMID:26086454

Plovnick, M. S. (1975). Primary care career choices and medical student learning styles. *Journal of Medical Education, 50*, 849–855. PMID:1171243

Pohlhaus, J. R., Jiang, H., Wagner, R. M., Schaffer, W. I., & Pinn, V. W. (2011). Sex differences in application success, and funding rates for NIH extramural programs. *Academic Medicine, 86*(6), 759–767. doi:10.1097/ACM.0b013e31821836ff PMID:21512358

Pololi, L. H. & Jones, S. J. (2010). Women faculty: an analysis of their experiences in academic medicine and their coping strategies. *Gender medicine.* Elsevier, 7(5), pp. 438–450.

Poorman, E. (2018). Why does America still have so few female doctors? *The Guardian.* Retrieved from https://www.theguardian.com/commentisfree/2018/jan/14/why-are-there-still-so-few-female-doctors

Pordata, I. N. E. (2018). *Portugal: Mandatos nas eleições para a Assembleia da República deputados do sexo feminino por partido político.* Last update: Nov. 6, 2018. Retrieved from https://www.pordata.pt/

PORDATA, INE. Last update: Aug. 8, 2018.

Pordata. (2018). Graduates in year, in higher education in the area of health: total, by area of education and training and sex. Last update: Sept. 24, 2018. Retrieved from https://www.pordata.pt/</eref>

Pordata. (2018). Retrieved from https://www.pordata.pt/Portugal

Portuguese Medical Association. (2019, January)

Posner, L. (2018, March 13). 4 of the biggest myths about the gender pay gap. Retrieved from https://www.salon.com/2018/03/13/4-of-the-biggest-myths-about-the-gender-pay-gap_partner/

Post, C. & Byron, K. (2015). *Women on Boards and Firm Financial Performance: A Meta-Analysis, Academy of Management Journal, 58, 5.* Thematic Issue on Gender in Management Research.

Post, E. (2015). Professional Titles. *Emily Post Etipedia.* Retrieved from www.emilypost.com/communication-andtechnology/ social-names-and-titles/774-professional-titles

Pottinger, H. [HPottinger]. (2018, March 28). @hcwomenleaders It is can be quite hard to share sometimes when you work in an environment that is fast paced and it can feel like you need to just "get on with it" … it helps to find a trusted [Tweet]. Retrieved from https://twitter.com/HPottinger/status/979078359228604416

Practitioner Health Programme. (2017). Retrieved from https://php.nhs.uk/

Prewitt-Freilino, J. L., Caswell, T. A., & Laakso, E. K. (2012). The gendering of language. A comparison of gender equality in countries with gendered, natural gender, and genderless languages. *Sex Roles*, *66*(3-4), 268–281. doi:10.100711199-011-0083-5

Qatar med school. *Homepage.* Available at http://qatar-weill.cornell.edu/about-us/overview/weill-cornell-medicine-qatar

Quality Worklife Quality Healthcare Collaborative. (2007). *Within Our Grasp: A Healthy Workplace Action Strategy for Success and Sustainability in Canada's Healthcare System.* Ontario, Canada.

Quinn, T. A. (2017). Opening the Doors of Medicine to Women. *The Journal of the American Osteopathic Association*, *117*(3), 149–149. doi:10.7556/jaoa.2017.028 PMID:28241325

Qureshi, M. A., Taj, J., Latif, M. Z., Rafique, S., Ahmed, R., & Chaudhry, M. A. (2017). Imposter syndrome among Pakistani medical students. *Annals of King Edward Medical University*, *23*(2), 1–6. doi:10.21649/akemu.v23i2.1647

Rabinowitz, L. (2018). Recognizing Blind Spots— A Remedy for Gender Bias in Medicine? *The New England Journal of Medicine*, *378*(24), 2253–2255. doi:10.1056/NEJMp1802228 PMID:29897846

Rama-Maceiras, P., Jokinen, J., & Kranke, P. (2015). Stress and burnout in anaesthesia: A real world problem? *Current Opinion in Anaesthesiology*, *28*(2), 151–158. doi:10.1097/ACO.0000000000000169 PMID:25695803

Rangel, E. L., Lyu, H., Haider, A. H., Castillo-Angeles, M., Doherty, G. M., & Smink, D. S. (2018). Factors Associated with Residency and Career Dissatisfaction in Childbearing Surgical Residents. *JAMA Surgery*, *153*(11), 1004–1011. doi:10.1001/jamasurg.2018.2571 PMID:30073246

Rangel, E., Smink, D., Castillo-Angeles, M., Kwakye, G., Changala, M., Haider, A. H., & Doherty, G. M. (2018). Pregnancy and Motherhood During Surgical Training. *JAMA Surgery*, *153*(7), 644–652. doi:10.1001/jamasurg.2018.0153 PMID:29562068

Rassie, K. (2017). The apprenticeship model of clinical medical education: Time for structural change. *The New Zealand Medical Journal*, *130*(1461), 66–72. PMID:28859068

Rayner, C., & Hoel, H. (1997). A summary review of literature relating to workplace bullying. *Journal of Community & Applied Social Psychology*, *7*(3), 181–191. doi:10.1002/(SICI)1099-1298(199706)7:3<181::AID-CASP416>3.0.CO;2-Y

RCP, Royal College of Physicians of London. (2018). *Focus on physicians: 2017–18 census (UK consultants and higher specialty trainees)*. Retrieved from https://www.rcplondon.ac.uk/projects/outputs/focus-physicians-2017-18-census-uk-consultants-and-higher-specialty-trainees

RCSEd (The Royal College of Surgeons in Edinburgh). (2018). Anti-bullying and undermining campaign. Available at https://www.rcsed.ac.uk/professional-support-development-resources/anti-bullying-and-undermining-campaign

Reddy, I. R., Ukrani, J., Indla, V., & Ukrani, V. (2019). Violence against doctors: A viral epidemic? *Indian Journal of Psychiatry*, *61*(10). PMID:31040474

Reed, C. E., Vaporciyan, A. A., Erikson, C., Dill, M. J., Carpenter, A. J., Guleserian, K. J., & Merrill, W. H. (2010). Factors dominating choice of surgical specialty. *Journal of the American College of Surgeons*, *210*(3), 319–324. doi:10.1016/j.jamcollsurg.2009.11.016 PMID:20193895

Reed, V., & Buddeberg-Fischer, B. (2001). Career obstacles for women in medicine: An overview. *Medical Education*, *35*(2), 139–147. doi:10.1046/j.1365-2923.2001.00837.x PMID:11169087

Regitz-Zagrosek, V. (2006). Therapeutic implications of the gender-specific aspects of cardiovascular disease. *Nature Reviews. Drug Discovery*, *5*(5), 425–439. doi:10.1038/nrd2032 PMID:16672926

Regitz-Zagrosek, V. (2012). Sex and gender differences in health. *EMBO Reports*, *13*(7), 596–603. doi:10.1038/embor.2012.87 PMID:22699937

Regitz-Zagrosek, V., Oertelt-Prigione, S., Seeland, U., & Hetzer, R. (2010). Sex and Gender Differences in Myocardial Hypertrophy and Heart Failure. *Circulation Journal*, *74*(7), 1265–1273. doi:10.1253/circj.CJ-10-0196 PMID:20558892

Rego, M. do Céu da Cunha. (2012). *Gender equality policies in the European Union and in Portugal: Influences and inconsistencies*. Ex aequo [online]. 2012, n. 25, pp. 29-44.

Reid-Pharr, R. F. (2019). The Disappearance of Great Men: Or, If You Want to Understand the Wounded Celebrity of Donald Trump, Just Ask Norman Mailer. *Minnesota Review, 2019*(92), 58-72.

Reimann, S., & Alfermann, D. (2018). Female Doctors in Conflict: How Gendering Processes in German Hospitals Influence Female Physicians' Careers. *Gender Issues*, *35*(1), 52–70. doi:10.100712147-017-9186-9

Reynold, E. (2018). Why I want to be a colorectal surgeon: the importance of role models in influencing women to pursue surgery [Abstract]. *Association of Surgeons of Great Britain and Ireland, 53*(Winter): 90-91. Retrieved from http://asgbi.org/Journals/Winter%202018%20JASGBI.pdf

Richardson, A., Mascarenhas, M., & Balen, A. (2019). Is a woman's chronological age or 'ovarian age' more important in determining perinatal outcome after assisted reproductive treatment? *Human Fertility (Cambridge, England)*, 1–7. doi:10.1080/14647273.2019.1597987 PMID:31038011

Riddell, F. [FernRiddell]. (2018a, June 13). My title is Dr Fern Riddell, not Ms or Miss Riddell. I have it because I am an expert, and my life and career consist of being that expert in as many different ways as possible. I worked hard to [Tweet]. Retrieved from https://twitter.com/FernRiddell/status/1006870044331200512

Riddell, F. [FernRiddell]. (2018b, June 16). We need #ImmodestWomen when so many men are unable to accept female expertise. *New Statesman*. Retrieved from https://www.newstatesman.com/politics/feminism/2018/06/we-need-immodestwomen-when-so-many-men-are-unable-accept-female-expertise

Rifkin, G. (2015). Second-generation gender bias. Retrieved from https://www.kornferry.com/institute/second-generation-gender-bias

Rimmer, A. (2017). The gender pay gap: female doctors still earn a third less than male doctors. *BMJ*, j1967. doi:10.1136/bmj.j1967

Rimmer, A. (2014). Why do female doctors earn less money for doing the same job? *BMJ (Clinical Research Ed.)*, *349*, g5604. doi:10.1136/bmj.g5604

Rimmer, A. (2018). Medicine's gender pay gap: Five minutes with . . . Jane Dacre. *BMJ (Clinical Research Ed.)*, *363*, k4559. doi:10.1136/bmj.k4559 PMID:30377157

Risberg, G., Johansson, E., & Hamberg, K. (2009). A theoretical model for analysing gender bias in medicine. *International Journal for Equity in Health*, *8*(1), 28. doi:10.1186/1475-9276-8-28 PMID:19646289

Risberg, G., Johansson, E., Westman, G., & Hamberg, K. (2003). Gender in medicine – an issue for women only? A survey of physician teachers' gender attitudes. *International Journal for Equity in Health*, *2*(1), 10. doi:10.1186/1475-9276-2-10 PMID:14613502

Robertson, J. (2014). Examensarbete, Väntetider på akutmottagningen ur ett jämställdhetsperspektiv, Institutionen för medicin, Sahlgrenska akademin, Göteborgs universitet

Robinson-Walker, C. (2011). The imposter syndrome. *Nurse Leader*, *9*(4), 12–13. doi:10.1016/j.mnl.2011.05.003

Rogers, A. C., Wren, S. M., & McNamara, D. A. (2019). Gender and Specialty Influences on Personal and Professional Life Among Trainees. *Annals of Surgery*, *269*(2), 383–387. doi:10.1097/SLA.0000000000002580 PMID:29099401

Roosevelt, E. (1948). Universal declaration of The human rights, UN.

Rosener, J. B. (2011). Ways women lead. In *Leadership, Gender, and Organization* (pp. 19–29). Springer. doi:10.1007/978-90-481-9014-0_3

Rosenfeld, J., & Denice, P. (2015). The Power of Transparency: Evidence from a British Workplace Survey. *American Sociological Review*, *80*(5), 1045–1068. doi:10.1177/0003122415597019

Ross-Smith, A., & Chesterman, C. (2009). "Girl disease": Women managers' reticence and ambivalence towards organizational advancement. *Journal of Management & Organization*, *15*(5), 582–595. doi:10.1017/S1833367200002431

Rotbart, H., McMillen, D., Taussig, H., Daniels, S., & Md, P. (2012). Assessing Gender Equity in a Large Academic Department of Pediatrics. *Academic Medicine*, *87*(1), 98–104. doi:10.1097/ACM.0b013e31823be028 PMID:22104061

Roter, D. L., & Hall, J. A. (2004). Physician gender and patient-centered communication: A critical review of empirical research. *Annual Review of Public Health*, *25*(1), 497–519. doi:10.1146/annurev.publhealth.25.101802.123134 PMID:15015932

Roter, D. L., Hall, J. A., & Aoki, T. (2002). Physician gender effects in medical communication. *Journal of the American Medical Association*, *288*(6), 7–756. doi:10.1001/jama.288.6.756 PMID:12169083

Royal Australasian College of Surgeons. (2016). *Discrimination, Harassment and Bullying.* Retrieved from www.surgeons.org/respect

Royal College of Surgeons of England. (2015). *National Undergraduate Surgical Curriculum.* Retrieved from www.rcseng.ac.uk/study

Royal College of Surgeons of England. (2016a). *Avoiding unconscious bias: a guide for surgeons.* Retrieved from www.rcseng.ac.uk/avoiding-unconscious-bias

Royal College of Surgeons of England. (2016b). *Learning in operating theatres.* Retrieved from www.rcseng.ac.uk/learning-in-operating-theatres

Royal College of Surgeons of England. (2016c). *Mentoring.* Retrieved from https://www.rcseng.ac.uk/-/media/files/rcs/library-and-publications/non-journal-publications/good-surgical-practice--mentoring.pdf

Royal College of Surgeons of England. (2017). *Improving surgical training.* Retrieved from https://www.rcseng.ac.uk/-/media/files/rcs/careers-in-surgery/improving_surgical_training_text.pdf

Royal College of Surgeons of England. (2019). *Careers.* Retrieved from www.rcseng.ac.uk/career

Royal College of Surgeons of Ireland. (2017) *Promoting gender equity in surgery. Report of a working group.* Retrieved from http://www.rcsi.ie/index.jsp?p=164&n=2790&a=10970

Royal-College-of-Physicians. (2019). *Emerging Women Leaders Programme.* Available at https://www.rcplondon.ac.uk/education-practice/courses/emerging-women-leaders-programme

Royal-College-of-Surgeons. (2019). *Women in Surgery.*

Rue, R. (1967). Employment of married women doctors in hospitals in the Oxford Region. *Lancet*, *1*(7502), 1267–1268. doi:10.1016/S0140-6736(67)92730-4 PMID:4165051

Russell, R. (2017). On overcoming imposter syndrome. *Academic Medicine*, *92*(8), 1070. doi:10.1097/ACM.0000000000001801 PMID:28742562

Rutkow, I. M. (2000). Mary Edwards Walker. *Archives of Surgery (Chicago, Ill.)*, *135*(4), 489–489. doi:10.1001/archsurg.135.4.489 PMID:10768718

Saalwachter, A. R., Freischlag, J. A., Sawyer, R. G., & Sanfey, H. A. (2005). The training needs and priorities of male and female surgeons and their trainees. *Journal of the American College of Surgeons*, *201*(2), 199–205. doi:10.1016/j.jamcollsurg.2005.03.016 PMID:16038816

Saalwachter, A. R., Freischlag, J. A., Sawyer, R. G., & Sanfey, H. A. (2006). Part-time training in general surgery: Results of a web-based survey. *Archives of Surgery*, *141*(10), 977–982. doi:10.1001/archsurg.141.10.977 PMID:17043275

Sadler, G. R., Plovnick, M., & Snope, F. C. (1978). Learning styles and teaching implications. *Journal of Medical Education*, *53*, 847–849. PMID:712775

Sahay, R., Cihák, M., & other IMF staff. (2018). *Women in Finance: A case for closing gaps.* (IMF Staff discussion note, September 2018 SDN/18/5)

Sakulku, J., & Alexander, J. (2011). The impostor phenomenon. *International Journal of Behavioral Science*, *6*(1), 73–92.

Salles, A. (2019). "I Spent my Fertile Years training to be a Surgeon. Now, it might be too late for me to have a Baby". Available at https://time.com/5484506/fertility-egg-freezing/

Salles, A. (2019, Jan. 3). I spent my fertile years training to be a surgeon. Now, it might be too late for me to have a baby. *TIME.* Retrieved from https://time.com/5484506/fertility-egg-freezing/

Salles, A., Mueller, C. M., & Cohen, G. L. (2016). A values affirmation intervention to improve female residents' surgical performance. *Journal of Graduate Medical Education*, *8*(3), 378–383. doi:10.4300/JGME-D-15-00214.1 PMID:27413441

Sambunjak, D., Straus, S. E., & Marušić, A. (2006). Mentoring in academic medicine: A systematic review. *Journal of the American Medical Association*, *296*(9), 1103–1115. doi:10.1001/jama.296.9.1103 PMID:16954490

Samuelson, W. & Zeckhauser, R. (2016, April 26). *Status quo bias in decision making.* doi:10.1007/BF00055564

Sandberg, S. (2011). *Why we have too few women leaders, TED: Ideas Worth Spreading.* Retrieved from http://www.ted.com/talks/sheryl_sandberg_why_we_have_too_few_women_leaders.html

Sandberg, S. (2015). Lean. In *Women, Work, and the Will to Lead.* New York, NY: Knopf.

Sandler, B. J., Tackett, J. J., Longo, W. E., & Yoo, P. S. (2016). Pregnancy and Parenthood among Surgery Residents: Results of the First Nationwide Survey of General Surgery Residency Program Directors. *Journal of the American College of Surgeons*, 1–7. doi:10.1016/j.jamcollsurg.12.004 PMID:26776357

Sandström, U., Wold, A., Jordansson, B., Ohlsson, B., & Smedberg, Å. (2010). Hans Excellens: om miljardsatsningarna på starka forskningsmiljöer. Retrieved from https://www.forskningspolitik.se/files/dokument/Hans_Excellens.pdf

Sanfey, H., Crandall, M., Shaughnessy, E., Stein, S. L., Cochran, A., Parangi, S., & Laronga, C. (2017). Strategies for identifying and closing the gender salary gap in surgery. *Journal of the American College of Surgeons*, *225*(2), 333–338. doi:10.1016/j.jamcollsurg.2017.03.018 PMID:28400299

Sanfey, H., Fromson, J., Mellinger, J., Rakinic, J., Williams, M., & Williams, B. (2015). Surgeons in difficulty: An exploration of differences in assistance between male and female surgeons. *Journal of the American College of Surgeons*, *221*, 621–627. doi:10.1016/j.jamcollsurg.2015.02.015 PMID:25872689

Sanfilippo, F., Noto, A., Foresta, G., Santonocito, C., Palumbo, G. J., & Arcadipane, A., … Maybauer, M. O. (2017). Incidence and Factors Associated with Burnout in Anesthesiology: A Systematic Review. *BioMed Research International.* doi:10.1155/2017/8648925

Sanghani, R. (2017). Feisty, frigid and frump: 25 words we only use to describe women. *The Telegraph.* Retrieved from https://www.telegraph.co.uk/women/life/ambitious-frigid-and-frumpy-25-words-we-only-use-to-describe-wom/

Santana, P. (2013). *Estudo da evolução prospetiva de Médicos no Sistema Nacional de Saúde.* Universidade de Coimbra.

Santos, M., Amâncio, L., & Roux, P. (2015). Numbers do not tell the whole story: Gender and medicine in Portugal. *Women's Studies International Forum*, *53*, 73–82. doi:10.1016/j.wsif.2015.08.005

Sara, B. (2017). In patient satisfaction scores, what role does bias play? [Wedblog] Retrieved from https://www.ama-assn.org/practice-management/physician-diversity/patient-satisfaction-scores-what-role-does-bias-play

Sara, B. (2018). How does gender impact physician burnout? 3 key takeaways. Retrieved from https://www.ama-assn.org/practice-management/physician-health/how-does-gender-impact-physician-burnout-3-key-takeaways

Satyanarayana, M. (2017, April 27). *Female doctors earn less than men, even in the same specialty.* Retrieved from https://www.statnews.com/2017/04/27/gender-pay-gap-specialty-doctor/

Saudi Council for Health Specialties. *SCHS document on Residents statistics.* 2019.

Savage, M. (2018, March 10). Top-paid men outstrip women by 4 to 1, shock figures reveal. *The Guardian.*

Sax, L. (2017). *Why Gender Matters: What Parents and Teachers Need to Know about the Emerging Science of Sex Differences* (2nd ed.). New York, NY: Broadway Books.

Sayres, M., Wyshak, G., Denterlein, G., Apfel, R., Shore, E., & Federman, D. (1986). Pregnancy during residency. *The New England Journal of Medicine, 314*(7), 418–423. doi:10.1056/NEJM198602133140705 PMID:3945268

Schaubnut, N. A., & Thompson, R. A. (2008). *MBTI type tables for occupations.* Mountain View, CA: CPP.

Schieder, J., & Gould, E. (2016). *"Women's work" and the gender pay gap.* Economic Policy Institute.

Schmidt, L. E., Cooper, C. A., & Guo, W. A. (2016). Factors influencing US medical students' decision to pursue surgery. *The Journal of Surgical Research, 203*(1), 64–74. doi:10.1016/j.jss.2016.03.054 PMID:27338536

Schor, N. F. (2018). The Decanal Divide: Women in Decanal Roles at US Medical Schools. *Academic Medicine, 93*(2), 237–240. doi:10.1097/ACM.0000000000001863 PMID:28834842

Schueller-Weidekamm, C., & Kautzky-Willer, A. (2012). Challenges of Work–Life Balance for Women Physicians/Mothers Working in Leadership Positions. *Gender Medicine, 9*(4), 244–250. doi:10.1016/j.genm.2012.04.002 PMID:22626768

Schulte-Rüther, M., Markowitsch, H., Shah, N., Fink, G., & Piefke, M. (2008). Gender differences in brain networks supporting empathy. *NeuroImage, 42*(1), 393–403. doi:10.1016/j.neuroimage.2008.04.180 PMID:18514546

Schuurman, A., Bos, S., de Wit, K., & de Graaf, R. (2018). Een dag het uit het leven van de zaalarts interne geneeskunde. *Nederlands Tijdschrift voor Geneeskunde*, 162.

Schwartz, E. (2015). Läkare kräver genusanalys av sjukvårdens ersättningar. Retrieved from http://www.fria.nu/artikel/117029

Science Guide. (2017). Monitor vrouwen in academie: aantal hougleraren stijgt, aantal bestuurders dealt. Retrieved from https://www.scienceguide.nl/2017/12/monitor-vrouwen-academie/

Sealy, R. (2017). Equal gender representation. *Nursing management, 24*(3), p. 12. doi:10.7748/nm.24.3.12.s15

Sealy, R. (2017). NHS Women on Boards: 50:50 by 2020. Retrieved from nhsemployers.org.

Seebacher, N. (2017). Gender Equity in Medical Specialties. Retrieved from http://levelmedicine.org.au/resources/completed-fellowship-papers/gender-equity-in-medical-specialties/

Seemann, N. M., Webster, F., Holden, H. A., Carol-anne, E. M., Baxter, N., Desjardins, C., & Cil, T. (2016). Women in academic surgery. Why is the playing field still not level? *American Journal of Surgery, 211*(2), 343–349. doi:10.1016/j.amjsurg.2015.08.036 PMID:26723836

Seritan, A. L., & Mehta, M. M. (2016). Thorny laurels: The impostor phenomenon in academic psychiatry. *Academic Psychiatry, 40*(3), 418–421. doi:10.100740596-015-0392-z PMID:26152516

Servicio Madrileño de Salud, Dirección General de Recursos Humanos y Relaciones Laborales. (n.d.). Retrieved from http://www.comunidad.madrid/sites/default/files/doc/sanidad/rrhh/rrhh-portal_estadistico_mes_en_curso_02.pdf

Sexism-in-surgery-females-being-put-off-becoming-surgeons-by-men. (2016). [Online Newspaper] Retrieved from https://wwww.telegraph.co.uk/news/health/11903476/sexism-in-surgery-females-being-put-off-becoming-surgeons-by-men.html%OA

Sexton, K. W., Hocking, K. M., Wise, E., Osgood, M. J., Cheung-Flynn, J., Komalavilas, P., ... Brophy, C. M. (2012). Women in academic surgery: The pipeline is busted. *Journal of Surgical Education*, *69*(1), 84–90. doi:10.1016/j.jsurg.2011.07.008 PMID:22208838

Shah, A., Jalal, S., & Khosa, F. (2018). Influences for Gender Disparity in Dermatology in North America. *International Journal of Dermatology*, *57*(2), 171–176. doi:10.1111/ijd.13875 PMID:29330932

Shalhub, S. (2018). Stop calling me a "female" surgeon. *Op-Med.* Retrieved from https://opmed.doximity.com/articles/stop-calling-me-a-female-surgeon-a2c87f9749f3

Shaw, P. M., Vouyouka, A., & Reed, A. (2012). Time for radiation safety program guidelines for pregnant trainees and vascular surgeons. *Journal of Vascular Surgery*, *55*(3), 862–8.e2. doi:10.1016/j.jvs.2011.11.045 PMID:22277686

Shen, H. (2013). Inequality Quantified: Mind the Gender Gap. *Nature*, *495*(7439), 22–24. doi:10.1038/495022a PMID:23467149

Sikdar, P. (2016). Women surgeons a vanishing tribe. Retrieved from https://timesofindia.indiatimes.com/life-style/health-fitness/health-news/Women-surgeons-a-vanishing-tribe/articleshow/51303079.cms

Silver, J. K. (2016, Oct. 24). Why are female doctors being hidden in plain sight? Retrieved from https://www.statnews.com/2016/10/24/female-doctors-invisible-women/

Silver, J. K., Slocum, C. S., Bank, A. M., Bhatnagar, S., Blauwet, C. A., Poorman, J. A., ... Parangi, S. (2017). Where Are the Women? The Underrepresentation of Women Physicians Among Recognition Award Recipients From Medical Specialty Societies. *PM & R*, *9*(8), 804–815. doi:10.1016/j.pmrj.2017.06.001 PMID:28606837

Simon Gilbody: The importance of being active. (2017). Simon Gilbody: The importance of being active. *BMJ (Clinical Research Ed.)*, *359*, j5371. doi:10.1136/bmj.j5371 PMID:29187359

Simpson, J., & Zeffman, H. (2017). Women prepare for a power grab in church, police and BBC. The Times. Retrieved from https://www.thetimes.co.uk/article/women-prepare-for-a-power-grab-in-church-police-and-bbc-cwgsrwtwm</eref>

Singh, A. (2018). 39.4% of adolescent girls do not attend schools: NCPCR study.

SIR (2019). Swedish Intensive Care Register Jan. 2019.

Skinner, H. (2018). Gender discrimination in leadership roles in surgical specialties in the UK. *Association of Surgeons of Great Britain and Ireland, 53*(Winter): 95. Retrieved from http://asgbi.org/Journals/Winter%202018%20JASGBI.pdf

Skinner, H., Burke, J. R., Young, A. L., Adair, R. A., & Smith, A. M. (2019). Gender representation in leadership roles in UK surgical societies. *International Journal of Surgery*, *67*(1), 32–36. doi:10.1016/j.ijsu.2019.05.007 PMID:31121326

Smirthwaite, G., Lundström, M., & Swahnberg, K. (2017). Doctors doing gender at eye clinics – Gender constructions in relation to waiting times for cataract extractions in Sweden. *NORA*, *25*(2), 107–125. doi:10.1080/08038740.2017.1345006

Smith, C., Galante, J. M., Pierce, J. L., & Scherer, L. A. (2013). The Surgical Residency Baby Boom: Changing Patterns of Childbearing During Residency Over a 30-Year Span. *Journal of Graduate Medical Education*, *5*(4), 625–629. doi:10.4300/JGME-D-12-00334.1 PMID:24455012

Smith, R. (2003). Thoughts for new medical students at a new medical school. *BMJ (Clinical Research Ed.)*, *327*(7429), 1430–1433. doi:10.1136/bmj.327.7429.1430 PMID:14684637

Smith, R. (2006). Medical professionalism: Out with the old and in with the new. *Journal of the Royal Society of Medicine*, *99*(2), 48–50. doi:10.1177/014107680609900202 PMID:16449765

Smith, V., Bethune, C., & Hurley, K. F. (2018). Examining medical student specialty choice through a gender lens: An orientational qualitative study. *Teaching and Learning in Medicine*, *30*(1), 33–44. doi:10.1080/10401334.2017.1306447 PMID:28497985

Socialstyrelsen. (2014). DRG-statistics, Socialstyrelsen.se

Soklaridis, S., Zahn, C., Kuper, A., Gillis, D., Taylor, V. H., & Whitehead, C. (2018). Men's fear of mentoring in the #MeToo era— What's at stake for academic medicine? *The New England Journal of Medicine*, *379*(23), 2270–2274. doi:10.1056/NEJMms1805743 PMID:30281387

Sonnak, C., & Towell, T. (2001). The impostor phenomenon in British university students: Relationships between self-esteem, mental health, parental rearing style and socioeconomic status. *Personality and Individual Differences*, *31*(6), 863–874. doi:10.1016/S0191-8869(00)00184-7

Sorenson, P. S., Hawkins, K., & Sorenson, R. L. (1995). *Gender*. Psychological Type and Conflict Style Preference. doi:10.1136/postgradmedj-2015-133919

Spender, D. (1980). *Man Made Language*. London, UK: Pandora Press.

Spetzler, R. F. (2011). Progress of women in neurosurgery. *Asian Journal of Neurosurgery*, *6*(1), 6–12. doi:10.4103/1793-5482.85627 PMID:22059098

Spraitz, J. (2018). Institutional Sexual Abuse. *Contemporary Issues in Victimology: Identifying Patterns and Trends*, 225.

Statista. (2014). Average age at marriage across rural and urban India in 2013-14, by gender.

Statista. (2019). *Proportion of Female Members of Parliament in the United Kingdom (UK) from 1979 to 2017*. Retrieved from https://www.statista.com

Statistics — Royal College of Surgeons. (2018). [National society Report] Retrieved from https://www.rcseng.ac.uk/careers-in-surgery/women-in-surgery/statistics/

Steinmetz, K. (2019, April 2). Nearly Half of Men Believe the Pay Gap Is "Made Up," Survey Finds. *Time*.

Stephens, E. H., Robich, M. P., Walters, D. M., DeNino, W. F., Aftab, M., Tchantchaleishvili, V., ... Shah, A. A. (2016). Gender and Cardiothoracic Surgery Training: Specialty Interests, Satisfaction, and Career Pathways. *The Annals of Thoracic Surgery*, *102*(1), 200–206. doi:10.1016/j.athoracsur.2016.03.043 PMID:27157051

Stilwell, N., Wallick, M., Thal, S., & Burleson, J. (2000). Myers-Briggs Type and Medical Specialty Choice: A New Look at an Old Question. *Teaching and Learning in Medicine*, *12*(1), 14–20. doi:10.1207/S15328015TLM1201_3 PMID:11228862

Stogdill, R. M. (1974). *Handbook of leadership: A survey of theory and research*. New York, NY: Free Press.

Strang, L. & Broeks, M. RAND Europe report. (n.d.). Maternity Leave Policies. European Commission. Europa EU.

Stratton, T., McLaughlin, M., Witte, F., Fosson, S., & Nora, L. (2005). Does Students?? Exposure to Gender Discrimination and Sexual Harassment in Medical School Affect Specialty Choice and Residency Program Selection? *Academic Medicine*, *80*(4), 400–408. doi:10.1097/00001888-200504000-00020 PMID:15793027

Suddath, C. (2018, March 29). New Numbers Show the Gender Pay Gap Is Real. Retrieved from https://www.bloomberg.com/news/features/2018-03-29/the-gender-pay-gap-is-real-say-new-numbers-from-the-u-k

Sue, D. W., Capodilupo, C. M., Torino, G. C., Bucceri, J. M., Holder, A. M. B., Nadal, K. L., & Esquilin, M. (2007). Racial microaggressions in everyday life: Implications for clinical practice. *The American Psychologist*, *62*(4), 271–286. doi:10.1037/0003-066X.62.4.271 PMID:17516773

Suicides in the UK Statistical bulletins - Office for National Statistics. (2017). Retrieved from https://www.ons.gov.uk/peoplepopulationandcommunity/birthsdeathsandmarriages/deaths/bulletins/suicidesintheunitedkingdom/previousReleases

Sullivan, M. C., Bucholz, E. M., Yeo, H., Roman, S. A., Bell, R. H., & Sosa, J. A. (2012). "Join the Club" Effect of resident and attending social interactions on overall satisfaction among 4390 general surgery residents. *Archives of Surgery*, *147*(5), 408–414. doi:10.1001/archsurg.2012.27 PMID:22785631

Sundaram, V., & Jackson, C. (2018). 'Monstrous men'and 'sex scandals': The myth of exceptional deviance in sexual harassment and violence in education. *Palgrave Communications*, *4*(1), 147. doi:10.105741599-018-0202-9

Supriya, K. E. (2018). Judgment and the Problem of Agency/Accountability: A Postcolonial Critique of Poststructuralist Theory. In Judgment Calls (pp. 42-62). Routledge.

Susan, A. (2012). Why Do So Many Doctors Regret Their Job Choice? Retrieved from https://www.forbes.com/sites/susanadams/2012/04/27/why-do-so-many-doctors-regret-their-job-choice/#e3c420737fae

Sutton, P. A., Mason, J., Vimalachandran, D., & McNally, S. (2014). Attitudes, motivators, and barriers to a career in surgery: A national study of UK undergraduate medical students. *Journal of Surgical Education*, *71*(5), 662–667. doi:10.1016/j.jsurg.2014.03.005 PMID:24776853

Sveriges kommuner och landsting (2017). Öppna jämförelser. Retrieved from https://skl.se/skolakulturfritid/forskola-grundochgymnasieskola/forskolafritidshem/forskola/faktaforskola.3292.html

Sveriges kommuner och landsting. (2018). Vården i siffror. Retrieved from https://vardenisiffror.se/report/view?id=592d2150d4475b02dc29887d

Swanson, J. A., Mara, B., D'Cunha, J., & Maddaus, M. A. (2010). Personality Profiling of the Modern Surgical Trainee: Insights into Generation X. *Journal of Surgical Education*, *67*(6), 417–420. doi:10.1016/j.jsurg.2010.07.017 PMID:21156301

Swanwick, T., & McKimm, J. (2011). What is clinical leadership… and why is it important?. The clinical teacher. *Wiley Online Library*, *8*(1), 22–26. PMID:21324068

Swedish National Agency for University Studies. (2017). Åren1900-2000. Retrieved from http://www.uka.se/fakta-om-hogskolan/den-svenska-hogskolans-historia/aren-1900-2000.html

Tannen, D. (1992). *You Just Don't Understand: Women and Men in Conversation*. London, UK: Virago.

Taylor, E. W. (2017). Transformative learning theory. In *Transformative Learning Meets Bildung* (pp. 17–29). Rotterdam, The Netherlands: SensePublishers. doi:10.1007/978-94-6300-797-9_2

Taylor, K. S., Lambert, T. W., & Goldacre, M. J. (2009). Career progression and destinations, comparing men and women in the NHS: Postal questionnaire surveys. *BMJ (Clinical Research Ed.)*, *338*(jun02 1), b1735. doi:10.1136/bmj.b1735 PMID:19493938

Taylor, T. (2017, Dec. 7). Workplace Flexibility For Millennials: Appealing To A Valuable New Generation. *Forbes*.

Tepper, T. (2015). Amazon's Parental Leave: The New Free Soda? *Money*. http://time.com/money/4098026/amazon-paid-parental-leave-benefits/

Tepper, T. (2015). *The Pros and Cons of Netflix's New Parental Leave Plan.* Retrieved from http://time.com/money/3985632/netflix-unlimited-parental-leave/

Testimonies from #metoo victims. (2018). Confidential mail from victims.

The American College of Obstetricians and Gynecologists Presidential Addresses. (2019, April 15). General format. Retrieved from https://www.acog.org/About-ACOG/ACOG-Departments/Resource-Center/Presidents-and-Their-Inaugural-Addresses?IsMobileSet=false

The American College of Surgeons Archives. (2019). General format. Retrieved from https://www.facs.org/about-acs/archives/acshistory/presidentslist

The British Medical Association. (2018, Dec. 6). Pay scales for consultants in England. Retrieved from https://www.bma.org.uk/advice/employment/pay/consultants-pay-england

'The hijab has no place in NHS hospitals', argues Muslim writer. (2016). [Online Newspaper] Retrieved from https://www.dailymail.co.uk/health/article-3561324/The-hijab-no-place-hospitals-Muslim-writer-says-medicine-free-religion-health-hazard-clothing-banned.html

The Khalil Gibran Chair for Values and Peace. *Dr. Edma Abou Chedid.* Available at https://pioneersandleaders.org/women-pioneers/dr-edma-abou-chedid

The Office for National Statistics. (2016). *The gender pay gap - what is it and what affects it?* The Office for National Statistics. Retrieved from https://www.ons.gov.uk/employmentandlabourmarket/peopleinwork/earningsandworkinghours/articles/thegenderpaygapwhatisitandwhataffectsit/2016-10-26

The state of medical education and practice in the UK. (2018). Retrieved from https://www.gmc-uk.org/about/what-we-do-and-why/data-and-research/the-state-of-medical-education-and-practice-in-the-uk

The Swedish Government. (2017). Sexualbrottslagstiftning. Retrieved from https://www.riksdagen.se/sv/dokument-lagar/arende/betankande/en-ny-sexualbrottslagstiftning-byggd-pa_H501JuU29

The University and College Council. (2018). Statistics regarding universities in Sweden. Retrieved from https://statistik.uhr.se/

The-Academy-of-Medical-Sciences. (2019). *Mentoring.*

Thejournal.ie. (2017). Mothers of premature babies to be given extended paid maternity leave. Available at https://www.thejournal.ie/premature-babies-extended-leave-3627843-Oct2017/

Thibault, G. (2016). Women in Academic Medicine. *Academic Medicine*, *91*(8), 1045–1046. doi:10.1097/ACM.0000000000001273 PMID:27306968

Thiederman, S. (2008). *Making Diversity Work.* New York, NY: Kaplan.

Thompson, A. J. (2014). Linguistic relativity: Can gendered languages present sexist atttitudes? *Linguistics.*

Thompson, T. (2004). Failure-avoidance parenting, the achievement environment of the home and strategies for reduction. *Learning and Instruction*, *14*(1), 3–26. doi:10.1016/j.learninstruc.2003.10.005

Thompson, T., Davidson, J. A., & Barber, J. G. (1995). Self-worth protection in achievement motivation: Performance effects and attribution behavior. *Journal of Educational Psychology*, *87*(4), 598–610. doi:10.1037/0022-0663.87.4.598

Thompson, T., Foreman, P., & Martin, F. (2000). Impostor fears and perfectionistic concern over mistakes. *Personality and Individual Differences*, *29*(4), 629–647. doi:10.1016/S0191-8869(99)00218-4

Thornton International Ltd, G. (2018) *Diversity snapshot – ethnicity, age and gender.*

Thornton, G. (2018). *Women in business: beyond policy to progress.*

Thurber, C., Dugas, L. R., Ocobock, C., Carlson, B., Speakman, J.R., & Pontzer, H. (2019). Extreme events reveal an alimentary limit on sustained maximal human energy expenditure. *Science Advances, 5*(6).

Timeline of women in medicine. (2018). [Museum Information] Retrieved from https://www.ama-assn.org/practice-management/physician-diversity/timeline-women-medicine

Times of India. (2016). More women study medicine, but few practise.

Titjen, F. (2018). *Language and Gender*. Cambridge, UK: Cambridge University Press.

Title VII of the Civil Rights Act of 1964. Retrieved from www.eeoc.gov/laws/statutes/titlevii.cfm

Title XI of the Education Ammendments Act of 1972. Retrieved from http://www.ncaa.org/about/resources/inclusion/title-ix-frequently-asked-questions

Toledo, P., Duce, L., Adams, J., Ross, V. H., Thompson, K. M., & Wong, C. A. (2017). Diversity in the American Society of Anesthesiologists Leadership. *Anesthesia and Analgesia, 124*(5), 1611–1616. doi:10.1213/ANE.0000000000001837 PMID:28277321

Topping, A. & Barr, C. (2018, Feb. 28). What you need to know about gender pay gap reporting. *The Guardian.*

Trades Union Congress. (2016). (pp. 1–8). The Motherhood Pay Penalty.

Triggle, N. (2018, Feb. 16). Top women doctors earn less than men. Retrieved from https://www.bbc.com/news/health-43077465

Trix, F., & Psenka, C. (2003). Exploring the color of glass: Letters of recommendation for female and male medical faculty. *Discourse & Society, 14*(2), 191–220. doi:10.1177/0957926503014002277

Troppmann, K. M., Palis, B. E., Goodnight, J. E. Jr, Ho, H. S., & Troppmann, C. (2009). Women surgeons in the new millennium. *Archives of Surgery, 144*(7), 635–642. doi:10.1001/archsurg.2009.120 PMID:19620543

Tsugawa, Y., Jena, A. B., Figueroa, J. F., Oray, E. J., Blumenthal, D. M., & Jha, A. J. (2017). Comparison of Hospital Mortality and Readmission Rates for Medicare Patients Treated by Male vs Female Physicians. *JAMA Internal Medicine, 177*(2), 206–213. doi:10.1001/jamainternmed.2016.7875 PMID:27992617

Turner, P. L., Lumpkins, K., Gabre, J., Lin, M. J., Liu, X., & Terrin, M. (2012). Pregnancy among women surgeons: Trends over time. *Archives of Surgery, 147*(5), 474–479. doi:10.1001/archsurg.2011.1693 PMID:22351877

Twigg, V., Aldridge, K., McNally, S. A., & Eardley, I. (2018). Does choice of medical school affect a student's likelihood of becoming a surgeon? *Bulletin of Royal College of Surgeons, 100*(2), 90-95. doi:10.1308/rcsbull.2018.90

UAE med school. *Homepage*. Available at https://cmhs.uaeu.ac.ae/en/index.shtml

UN. (n.d.). *Qatar UN goals Qatar: Taking Action for Sustainable Development.* Available at https://www.un.org/sustainabledevelopment/wp-content/uploads/2017/07/Qatar_Govt.pdf

UNDP. (2018). *Human Development Indices and Indicators: 2018 Statistical Update, Kuwait.* Available at http://hdr.undp.org/sites/all/themes/hdr_theme/country-notes/KWT.pdf

UNDP. (2018). *Human Development Indices and Indicators: 2018 Statistical Update*. Available at http://hdr.undp.org/sites/all/themes/hdr_theme/country-notes.pdf

UNDP. (n.d.). *Kingdom of Bahrain. Sustainable Goals. Goal 5: Gender Equality. Bahrain UN goals* Available at http://www.bh.undp.org/content/bahrain/en/home/sustainable-development-goals/goal-5-gender-equality.html

UNDP. (n.d.). *Support Kuwait's implementation of SDG 5.* Available at http://www.kw.undp.org/content/kuwait/en/home/projects/support-kuwait s-implementation-of-sdg-5.html

United Nations. (2002). Committee Experts Praise Portugal's Efforts to Promote Equality of Women [Press release]. Retrieved from https://www.un.org/press/en/2002/WOM1309.doc.htm

Usherwood, T. (1992). Sex bias in the BMJ: an audit. *BMJ,* 304, 880-1. Retrieved from https://www.bmj.com/content/304/6831/880

Uwagba, O. (2019, March 8). *Actually, women do ask for money. They just don't get it.* Retrieved from https://www.thecut.com/2019/03/women-do-ask-money-work-salary-raise.html

Valantine, H., & Sandborg, C. (2013). Changing the Culture of Academic Medicine to Eliminate the Gender Leadership Gap: 50/50 by 2020. *Academic Medicine, 88*(10), 1411–1413. doi:10.1097/ACM.0b013e3182a34952 PMID:23969359

Valsangkar, N., Fecher, A. M., Rozycki, G. S., Blanton, C., Bell, T. M., Freischlag, J., ... Koniaris, L. G. (2016). Understanding the barriers to hiring and promoting women in surgical subspecialties. *Journal of the American College of Surgeons, 223*(2), 387–398. doi:10.1016/j.jamcollsurg.2016.03.042 PMID:27109779

Vaporciyan, A. A., Reed, C. E., Erikson, C., Dill, M. J., Carpenter, A. J., Guleserian, K. J., & Merrill, W. (2009). Factors affecting interest in cardiothoracic surgery: Survey of North American general surgery residents. *The Annals of Thoracic Surgery, 87*(5), 1351–1359. doi:10.1016/j.athoracsur.2009.02.096 PMID:19379863

Velasco, I., Naranjo, S., Lopez-Pedrera, C., Garriga, M. J., Garcıa-Fuentes, E., & Soriguer, F. (2009). Use of povidone-iodine during the first trimester of pregnancy: A correct practice? *BJOG, 116*(3), 452–455. doi:10.1111/j.1471-0528.2008.02059.x PMID:19187379

Vergauwe, J., Wille, B., Feys, M., De Fruyt, F., & Anseel, F. (2014). Fear of being exposed: The trait-relatedness of the impostor phenomenon and its relevance in the work context. *Journal of Business and Psychology, 30*(3), 565–581. doi:10.100710869-014-9382-5

Villwock, J. A., Sobin, L. B., Koester, L. A., & Harris, T. M. (2016). Impostor syndrome and burnout among American medical students: A pilot study. *International Journal of Medical Education, 7,* 364–369. doi:10.5116/ijme.5801.eac4 PMID:27802178

Vinnicombe, S., Doldor, E., & Sealy, R. (2018) *The Female FTSE Board Report 2018: Busy going nowhere with the female executive pipeline.*

Walker, J. J. (2000). Pre-eclampsia. *Lancet, 356*(9237), 1260–1265. doi:10.1016/S0140-6736(00)02800-2 PMID:11072961

Wall, A. (2018, March 30). Pregnancy, new moms, and surgical residency. Association of Academic Surgery. Retrieved from http://www.aasurg.org/blog/pregnancy-new-moms-surgical-residency/

Wallis, C. J., Ravi, B., Coburn, N., Nam, R. K., Detsky, A. S., & Satkunasivam, R. (2017). Comparison of postoperative outcomes among patients treated by male and female surgeons: A population based matched cohort study. *BMJ (Clinical Research Ed.), 2017,* 358. PMID:29018008

Wallis, C., Ravi, B., Coburn, N., Nam, R. K., Detsky, A., & Satkunasivam, R. (2017). Comparison of postoperative outcomes among patients treated by male and female surgeons: A population based matched cohort study. *British Medical Journal, 359,* j4366. doi:10.1136/bmj.j4366 PMID:29018008

Walsh, D. F., Thome, A. P., Mody, K. S., Eltorai, A. E. M., Daniels, A. H., & Mulcahey, M. K. (2019). Radiation safety education as a component of orthopedic training. *Orthopedic Reviews*, *11*(1), 7883. doi:10.4081/or.2019.7883 PMID:30996841

Walton, M. (2015). Sexual equality, discrimination and harassment in medicine: It's time to act. *The Medical Journal of Australia*, *203*(4), 167–169. doi:10.5694/mja15.00379 PMID:26268278

Wänje, A. (2015). Sick leave—A signal of unequal work organizations? *Nordic Journal of Working Life Studies, 5,* 4.

Want, J., & Kleitman, S. (2006). Imposter phenomenon and self-handicapping: Links with parenting styles and self-confidence. *Personality and Individual Differences*, *40*(5), 961–971. doi:10.1016/j.paid.2005.10.005

Warner, A. S., & Lehmann, L. S. (2019). Gender wage disparities in medicine: Time to close the gap. *Journal of General Internal Medicine*, *34*(7), 1334–1336. doi:10.100711606-019-04940-9 PMID:30963441

Watling, C., Driessen, E., van der Vleuten, C. P., & Lingard, L. (2014, July). Learning culture and feedback: An international study of medical athletes and musicians. *Medical Education*, *48*(7), 713–723. doi:10.1111/medu.12407 PMID:24909533

Watling, C., Driessen, E., van der Vleuten, C. P., Vanstone, M., & Lingard, L. (2013, August). Music lessons: Revealing medicine's learning culture through a comparison with that of music. *Medical Education*, *47*(8), 842–850. doi:10.1111/medu.12235 PMID:23837431

Weber, T., Reidel, M., Graf, S., Hinz, U., Keller, M., & Büchler, M. (2005). Careers of women in academic surgery. *Chirurg*, *76*(7), 703–711, discussion 11. doi:10.100700104-005-1017-y PMID:15770490

Webster, F., Rice, K., Christian, J., Seemann, N., Baxter, N., Moulton, C., & Cil, T. (2016). The Erasure of Gender in Academic Surgery: A Qualitative Study. *American Journal of Surgery*, *212*(4), 559–565. doi:10.1016/j.amjsurg.2016.06.006 PMID:27640905

Weir, K. (2013, November). Feel like a fraud? *gradPSYCH Magazine*. doi:10.1002/j.2161-1912.2013.00029.x/abstract

Weiss, A., Lee, K. C., Tapia, V., Chang, D., Freischlag, J., Blair, S. L., & Ramamoorthy, S. (2014). Equity in Surgical Leadership for Women: More Work to Do. *American Journal of Surgery*, *208*(3), 494–498. doi:10.1016/j.amjsurg.2013.11.005 PMID:24933664

Wenger, E. (2000). *Communities of practice: learning, meaning and identity*. Cambridge, UK: Cambridge University Press.

Wennerås, C., & Wold, A. (1997). Nepotism and sexism in peer-review. *Nature*, *387*(6631), 341–343. doi:10.1038/387341a0 PMID:9163412

West, C. & Zimmerman, D. (1987). Doing Gender. *Gender & Society, 1*(2), 125-151. Retrieved from https://www.jstor.org/stable/189945?seq=1#page_scan_tab_contents

West, M., Armit, K., Loewenthal, L., Eckert, R., West, T., & Lee, A. (2015). Leadership and leadership development in healthcare: the evidence base. London, UK: The Kings Fund.

West, M., Dawson, J., Admasachew, L., & Topakas, A. (2011). NHS staff management and health service quality: results from the NHS staff survey and related data. London, UK: Department of Health.

Western, S. (2013). *Leadership: a critical text. Second.* London, UK: Sage.

Whitaker, M. (2018). The surgical personality: Does it exist? *Annals of the Royal College of Surgeons of England, 100*(1), 72–77. doi:10.1308/rcsann.2017.0200 PMID:29260896

White, F. S., McDade, S., Yamagata, H., & Morahan, P. S. (2012). Gender-Related Differences in the Pathway to and Characteristics of U.S. Medical School Deanships. *Academic Medicine*, *87*(8), 1015–1023. doi:10.1097/ACM.0b013e31825d3495 PMID:22722362

White, M. T., & Welch, K. (2012). Does gender predict performance of novices undergoing Fundamentals of Laparoscopic Surgery (FLS) training? *American Journal of Surgery*, *203*(3), 397–400. doi:10.1016/j.amjsurg.2011.09.020 PMID:22364906

Whitman, M. V., & Shanine, K. K. (2012). Research in Occupational Stress and Well-Being: Vol. 10. *Revisiting the impostor phenomenon: how individuals cope with feelings of being in over their heads* (pp. 177–212). doi:10.11081479-3555(2012)0000010009

Wikipedia. Medical Schools List. Available at https://en.wikipedia.org/wiki/List_of_medical_schools_in_the_Middle_East

Wikipedia. Retrieved from https://www.wikipedia.org/

Wilcox, A. R., Trooboff, S. W., Lai, C. S., Turner, P. L., & Wong, S. L. (2019). Trends in gender representation at the American College of Surgeons Clinical Congress and the Academic Surgical Congress: a mixed picture of progress. *J Am Coll Surg*.

Willett, L. L., Halvorsen, A. J., McDonald, F. S., Chaudhry, S. I., & Arora, V. M. (2015). Gender differences in Salary of Internal Medicine Residency Directors: A National Survey. *The American Journal of Medicine*, *128*(6), 659–665. doi:10.1016/j.amjmed.2015.02.002 PMID:25731136

Willett, L. L., Wellons, M. F., Hartig, J. R., Roenigk, L., Panda, M., Dearinger, A. T., ... Houston, T. K. (2010). Do women residents delay childbearing due to perceived career threats? *Academic Medicine*, *85*(4), 640–646. doi:10.1097/ACM.0b013e3181d2cb5b PMID:20354380

Williams, S. (2018). Guiding the higher surgical trainee return to work: a deanery perspective [Abstract]. *Association of Surgeons of Great Britain and Ireland, 53*(Winter), 91-92. Retrieved from http://asgbi.org/Journals/Winter%202018%20 JASGBI.pdf

Winston, B. E., & Patterson, K. (2006). An Integrative Definition of Leadership. *International Journal of Leadership Studies*, *1*(2), 6–66.

Wirtzfeld, D. (2009, August). The History of women in surgery. *Canadian Journal of Surgery*, *52*(4), 317–320. PMID:19680519

Wise, M. R., Shapiro, H., Bodley, J., Pittini, R., McKay, D., Willan, A., & Hannah, M. E. (2004). Factors affecting academic promotion in obstetrics and gynaecology in Canada. *Journal of Obstetrics and Gynaecology Canada*, *26*(2), 127–136. doi:10.1016/S1701-2163(16)30488-1 PMID:14965478

Witz, A. (1992). *Professions and Patriarchy*. London, UK: Routledge. doi:10.4324/9780203167786_chapter_2

Wolfe, L. (2018). *Statistics on the number of women surgeons in the United States. Why is it tough to increase the number of women in surgery?* Retrieved from https://www.thebalancecareers.com/number-of-women-surgeons-in-the-us-3972900

Women in medicine. (n.d.). Retrieved from http://broughttolife.sciencemuseum.org.uk/broughttolife/themes/practising-medicine/women

Women in Surgery. (n.d.). Royal College of Surgeons. Retrieved from https://www.rcseng.ac.uk/careers-in-surgery/women-in-surgery/

Wong, A. V.-K., & Olusanya, O. (2017). Burnout and resilience in anaesthesia and intensive care medicine. *BJA Education, 17*(10), 334–340. doi:10.1093/bjaed/mkx020

Wood, W. & Eagly, A. (2002). A cross-cultural analysis of the behavior of women and men: implications for the origins of sex differences. *Psychological bulletin, 128*(5), 699-727. Retrieved from https://www.ncbi.nlm.nih.gov/pubmed/12206191

Woolston, C. (2016). Psychology: Faking it. *Nature, 529*(7587), 555–557. doi:10.1038/nj7587-555a PMID:26824109

World Health Organization Databases. (2006). Global Atlas of the Health Workforce: Gender Distribution on Selected Health Professions. Geneva.

World Health Organization Databases. (2008). Gender and Workforce statistics.

World Health Organization. (2018). European Health Report. Retrieved from http://www.euro.who.int/en/data-and-evidence/european-health-report/european-health-report-2018

Wright, A. L., Ryan, K., St Germain, P., Schwindt, L., Sager, R., & Reed, K. L. (2007). Compensation in academic medicine: Progress toward gender equity. *Journal of General Internal Medicine, 22*, 1398–1402. doi:10.100711606-007-0329-7 PMID:17694417

Wyatt-Smith, C., Du Plessis, A., Hand, K., Wang, J., Alexander, C., & Colbert, P. (2017). *Why choose teaching? A matter of choice: Evidence from the field. A report prepared for the Queensland College of Teachers.* Brisbane, Australia: Learning Sciences Institute Australia. Retrieved from https://www.qct.edu.au/pdf/WhyChooseTeachingReport.pdf

Wynn-Mackenzie, C. (2016). The Lady Estelle Wolfson Emerging Leaders Fellowships. *Medical Woman, 35*(1), 23.

Wynn, R. (2000). Saints and Sinners: Women and the Practice of Medicine Throughout the Ages. *Journal of the American Medical Association, 283*(5), 668–669. doi:10.1001/jama.283.5.668-JMS0202-4-1 PMID:10665711

Yalom, I. D. (1998). *The Yalom Reader. New York, NY:* Basic Books.

Yedidia, M., & Bickel, J. (2001). Why Aren't There More Women Leaders in Academic Medicine? The Views of Clinical Department Chairs. *Academic Medicine, 76*(5), 453–465. doi:10.1097/00001888-200105000-00017 PMID:11346523

Yeo, H. L., Abelson, J. S., Symer, M. M., Mao, J., Michelassi, F., Bell, R., ... Sosa, J. A. (2018). Association of time to attrition in surgical residency with individual resident and programmatic factors. *JAMA Surgery, 153*(6), 511–517. doi:10.1001/jamasurg.2017.6202 PMID:29466536

Young, V. (n.d.). Impostor Syndrome Quiz. Retrieved from https://impostorsyndrome.com/quiz/

Zalis, S. (2018, Oct. 30). Lessons from the world's most gender-equal countries. *Forbes.*

Zarkov, D. & Davis, K. (2018). Ambiguities and dilemmas around# MeToo:# ForHow Long and# WhereTo?

Zelek, B., & Phillips, S. (2003). Gender and power: Nurses and doctors in Canada. *International Journal for Equity in Health, 2*(1), 1–11. doi:10.1186/1475-9276-2-1 PMID:12605720

Zhuge, Y., Kaufman, J., Simeone, D. M., Chen, H., & Velazquez, O. C. (2011). Is There Still a Glass Ceiling for Women in Academic Surgery? *Annals of Surgery, 253*(4), 637–643. doi:10.1097/SLA.0b013e3182111120 PMID:21475000

Zimmermann, A. (2018). *What can organisations do to close the gender pay gap?* LSE Business Review.

About the Contributors

Maria Irene Bellini is a Transplant Surgeon in Belfast and Social Care Trust. She graduated from the University of Tor Vergata in Rome (IT) in 2007 and very early in her career, she showed an interest in research and transplantation. She trained as a general and transplant surgeon in the same University, achieving a certification of completion of training in 2014 and a research doctorate in 2015. She moved to the UK in 2013, to complete her PhD in Oxford (UK) and undertake further subspecialty training. During this time, she developed an interest in organ perfusion devices and she held the responsibility for the machine perfusion clinical program at Imperial College London (UK) from 2015 until July 2019. She is a Fellow of the European Board of Surgery and an Associate Fellow of the American College of Surgeons. She is also a Board Member of the European Kidney Transplant Section (EKITA) Board member of the Education Committee of the European Society for Organ Transplantation and Lead for the Educational e-platform Transplant Live. She's also the Lead for the ASGBI (Association of Surgeons of Great Britain and Ireland) Women in Surgery section. Maria Irene has broad experience as author and peer-reviewer; she is also involved in editorial board membership of scientific journals as Transplant International and World Journal of Transplantation.

Sharon L. Stein, MD, FACS, FASCRS, is a colorectal surgeon at University Cleveland Medical Center (UH) and Associate Professor, Surgery at Case Western Reserve University (CWRU) School of Medicine. She is also the Surgical Director – Inflammatory Bowel Disease Center at the Digestive Health Institute as well as Director of UH RISES: Research in Surgical Outcomes and Effectiveness Center. She is well accomplished in the world of academic surgery, serving as President elect of the Association of Women Surgeons and on the executive council of the Association of Colon and rectal Surgeons (ASCRS). She was the first women to receive an Honorary Fellowship from the Association of Surgeons of Great Britain and Ireland. As an academician, Dr.Stein has published over 50 articles on a variety of topics from minimally invasive surgery to diversity in surgery. Her programmatic experiences also inform her academic pursuits; she has written about the salary gap in surgery, starting salaries for colon and rectal surgeons, and pregnancy leave internationally, in addition to traditional topics of minimally invasive surgery, rectal cancer and enhanced recovery protocols. She has recently become director of the Director of the University Hospitals Research in Surgical Outcomes & Effectiveness Center (UH RISES). In recognition of her contributions to scholarship, she has been invited to serve as a reviewer for a number of prestigious journalsand to write several book chapters. She has been invited to deliver CME lectures and contribute to scientific publications both nationally and internationally. She was recently chosen by the Society of University Surgeons (SUS) itself along with the Society of Black Academic Surgeons (SBAS), the Society of American Gastrointestinal and Endoscopic Surgeons (SAGES), and the Eastern Association for the Surgery of Trauma (EAST) to participate in 2020 Promising Leaders Program.

* * *

Asmaa Alrashed, General, Bariatric and Metabolic Surgery Senior Specialist in General Surgery Department, Al-Amiri Hospital, Critical Care Senior Specialist in Critical Care and Anesthesia Department, Al-Amiri Hospital, Assistant Program Director of Surgical Foundations, KIMS, Chair of Women Surgeons Committee, KAS.

Helena Alves, specialist on Legal Medicine and Immunohemotherapy, Director of the North Histocompatibility Centre – Oporto, from 2003-2012, created the Public Cord Blood Bank -LusoCord, implemented in the North of Portugal the National Register of Bone Marrow Donors - CEDACE Portugal North, Chief of service working in Immunobiology of Transplantation (1990 - 2012) and coordinator of Histocompatibility Emergency Service to Transplantation in the north of Portugal, Coordinator of Unit of Health Promotion and Chronical Disease Prevention in the National Institute of Health (2012-2019). President of Board of the Medical College of Transfusion Medicine and Immunohemotherapy from the National Medical Association Ordem dos Médicos. Portuguese Delegate to the Biopathology and Laboratory Medicine Section in UEMS U (European Union of Medical Specialists). President of the Scientific Council of Prof Ernesto Morais Foundation. Administrator in the Portuguese Rotary Foundation.

Fátima Carvalho is a Specialist in Pediatric Surgery, Consultant and Assistant Pediatric Surgeon of CHP / CMIN in the paediatrics centre in Oporto, Director of the Pediatric Surgery Service of CHP / CMIN - Oporto Hospitalar Centre. Member of the Board of the College of Competence in Health Services Management of the Medical Association. President of the Northern Disciplinary Council of the National Medical Association Ordem dos Médicos. PhD student at ICBAS at the University of Porto.

Lizzie Chandra is a specialist trainee in Urology rotating in the Yorkshire and Humber region. She has taken the opportunity to complete a Future Leaders Fellowship in addition to surgical training and is actively involved in work focusing on gender equity and less than full time training in surgery.

Stefan De Hert received his medical degree at the University of Antwerp, Belgium in 1984. After his anesthesiology residency training he accepted a faculty position in the Department of Anesthesiology of the Antwerp University Hospital and served as vice chairman of this Department and Professor of Anesthesiology at the University of Antwerp for over 10 years. From 2007 to 2010 he acted as Professor of Cardiothoracic and Vascular Anesthesiology at the University of Amsterdam, The Netherlands, and Director of the Division of Cardiothoracic and Vascular Anesthesiology at the Academic Medical Center in Amsterdam. Presently, he is Professor of Anesthesiology and Director of Research at the Department of Anesthesiology of the University Hospital of Ghent. He has authored and co-authored over 200 articles in peer-reviewed journals and many chapters in different textbooks. He is Associate Editor the Journal of Cardiothoracic and Vascular Anesthesia and acts as regular reviewer for several major anesthesiology, cardiology and surgery journals. Prof. De Hert acted as chair of the ESA Scientific Committee. He is currently President of the European Society of Anesthesiology.

Paul Dent is a Consultant Endocrine and General Surgeon with an interest in Medical Education, surgical training, and unconscious bias in training. Paul was appointed a consultant in 2018 at Croydon University Hospital in South London and is an Honorary Senior Clinical Lecturer at Kings College London. He is currently Educational Supervisor to one of the Improving Surgical Training pilot trainees at Croydon. Paul is a course director for Advanced Trauma Life Support and is the General Surgery representative to the Royal College of Surgeons National Steering Group for ATLS. He graduated in Medical Science at the University of Birmingham in 1999 and then wrote his doctoral thesis on the Neurohumoral control of the kidney in 2002. Paul continued his studies and was in the third intake to study graduate entry medicine at Warwick Medical School, graduating with Honours in Medicine and Surgery in 2006.

Candice Downey is an academic trainee in Yorkshire, United Kingdom. She specialises in General Surgery. Her academic pursuits lie in patient safety, remote monitoring, and risk perception in surgery. She has a strong interest in enhancing the working lives of academic trainees and women in surgery.

Maria Amélia Ferreira, Full Professor at the Faculty of Medicine of the University of Porto (FMUP). She was Dean of FMUP, 2014-2018, and was the first woman - in 190 years of FMUP - to run this prestigious national higher education institution. Amélia Ferreira was responsible for a curricular reform in medical education at FMUP, and she was the forerunner of the strategy of institutional internationalization, through the implementation of mobility programs and international cooperation. She also promoted the intergovernmental cooperation programs in the field of medicine between Portugal and Angola and the implementation of the Medical Education Network in Portuguese Language.

Emma Gans is currently completing her residency in Internal Medicine at a teaching hospital of Leiden University Medical Center. Specific interests are gender medicine and mind-body medicine.

Montserrat González-Estecha, MD, PhD. Specialized in Laboratory Medicine. Vice President of the Federation of European Societies on Trace Elements and Minerals. President of the SEQC_ML Spanish Commission of Trace Elements.

Yitka Graham is an Associate Professor of Health Services Research at the University of Sunderland. She has held a research post within the Bariatric Surgical Unit at Sunderland Royal Hospital for seven years. Her doctorate focused on patient experiences of adjusting to life after bariatric surgery, and she continues her research within bariatric surgery, focusing on patient experience, social support, networks and sexual and reproductive issues in this patient cohort. She was awarded the prestigious award of Fellow of the Obesity Society in 2016. Yitka is the National Research Lead for the British Obesity and Metabolic Surgery Society (BOMSS) and is an Honorary Lifetime Member of the Mexican College of Surgery for Obesity and Metabolic Disorders (CMCOEM). She is a member of the Association of Surgeons of Great Britain and Ireland working party which explores issues affecting women in surgical careers.

Yasmin Grant is a National Institute of Health Research (NIHR) Academic Clinical Fellow (ACF) in General Surgery at Imperial College London. As an undergraduate, she undertook a Bachelor in Science (BSc) in Cancer Studies investigating the clinical and pathological determinants of outcome within the colorectal cancer screening programme in the West of Scotland. She holds an MBChB (Bachelor of Medicine and Bachelor of Surgery) from the University of Glasgow and was awarded the William Hunter and William McEwan Medal for Surgery in her final clinical year. Yasmin commenced her postgraduate career in as Academic Foundation Trainee in Vascular Surgery at Imperial College Healthcare NHS Trust combining clinical work with research. Her research interests include metabonomic profiling of chronic venous disease, behavioural economics in arterial surgery, health economics in general surgery and surgical leadership. Currently, she is undertaking a project investigating the cost implications of margin re-excision in breast conserving surgery. Yasmin is a Member of the Royal College of Surgeons (MRCS) and undertook the Edward Jenner Programme for Leadership at the NHS Leadership Academy. She holds a Postgraduate Certificate in University Learning and Teaching (PGCULT) from Imperial College London and is a Fellow of the Higher Education Academy (FHEA). She is currently undertaking Higher Surgery Registrar Training in North West London.

Rebecca Grossman is a Specialist Registrar in General Surgery in the United Kingdom. She is a regional representative of the Medical Women's Federation, and is on the Royal College of Surgeons of England Women in Surgery Forum.

Rhiannon Harries qualified from Peninsula Medical School in 2007 and completed her higher surgical training in Wales. She is due to start work as a Consultant Colorectal Surgeon at Morriston Hospital, Swansea. Her clinical interests lie in colorectal and hernia surgery and she has published widely with over 50 peer-reviewed papers. She was previously awarded a Royal College of Surgeons Research Fellowship towards her MD awarded by Cardiff University for her research investigating the clinical relevance of Pigment Epithelial Derived Factor in colorectal cancer and wound healing. She is extremely active in collaborative clinical research, currently being a co-investigator for the Hughes Abdominal Repair Trial (HART), a NIHR funded randomised controlled trial comparing suturing techniques for abdominal wall closure in order to prevent incisional hernia formation. Rhiannon has a strong interest in the improvement of surgical education and training and was the 40th President of the Association of Surgeons in Training (ASiT) in 2015-16, representing surgical trainees on numerous meetings including the Royal College of Surgeons Council, Joint Committee on Surgical Training, General Medical Council and the Academy of Medical Royal Colleges Trainee Doctors Group. She was responsible for organising the largest surgical training event to date, with 40 free courses held on one day to celebrate the organisation's 40th anniversary; attended by 570 delegates and representing a total comparable cost saving to trainees of £231,462. The end of her tenure culminated in the ASiT 40th anniversary international conference, which was attended by over 700 attendees. She has convened several educational courses aimed at surgical trainees including ASiT's Foundation Skills in Surgery, Core Laparoscopic Skills, and Introduction to Endoscopy, and has lead on the publications of the accompanying course textbooks. More recently she has co-convened the Welsh FRCS General Surgery Viva Revision Course. Rhiannon has also combined her interest of surgical training with humanitarian surgery, having convened three ASiT Foundation Skills in Surgery training courses to medical students in Rwanda and also teaching surgical skills workshops with the Royal College of Surgeons in Mexico and Guatemala.

Catherine Hayes is Professor of Health Professions Pedagogy and Scholarship in the Faculty of Health Sciences and Wellbeing at the University of Sunderland. She is qualified in podiatry and a Founding Fellow of the Faculty of Podiatric Medicine (Royal College of Physicians and Surgeons, Glasgow) and a Fellow of the College of Podiatry and General Practice (London). She undertakes pedagogic research, evaluation and supervises doctoral and MSc students. She has published widely on qualitative research methodologies and the development of professional practice in health. She has an active interest in transcending disciplinarity between science and arts as signature pedagogies and she is currently working with colleagues on a monograph titled 'Beyond Disciplinarity'. She has been a UK Advisor in Podiatric Medicine for the Royal College of Physicians and Surgeons and was awarded Honorary Membership by

Distinction of the Faculty of Public Health in 2015 and was elected to the Royal Society of Arts in 2016. Catherine was Founder and Convenor of the RAISE Network's Postgraduate and Professional Practice Special Interest Group (SIG). She is a Tenth Anniversary Visiting Professor of Higher Education at the University of Cumbria and Visiting Professor of Higher Education at Liverpool Hope University. She has recently gained Fellowship of both the Chartered Management Institute and Fellowship of the Institute of Leadership and Management following the award of Chartered Manager Status, Principal Fellowship of the Higher Education Academy, a National Teaching Fellowship and Fellowship of the Society for Education and Training, in 2017. Catherine was publicly elected as Secretary to the Executive Board of the Royal College of Physicians and Surgeons (Glasgow) in June 2018. She is also an editorial board member of the College of Podiatry's national journal 'Podiatry Now'.

Christine Heisler matriculated medical school in 2002 at the University of North Dakota School of Medicine and Health Sciences and finished Obstetrics and Gynecology residency in 2006 in Grand Rapids, MI. In 2009, Dr. Heisler completed her 3-year fellowship in Female Pelvic Medicine and Reconstructive Surgery (FPMRS) at the Mayo Clinic in Rochester, MN. She earned her Master's Degree in Biomedical Sciences with studies on quality outcomes related to reconstructive pelvic surgery. Dr. Heisler was among the first within FPMRS to become board certified in 2013. Serving in an educational role at the University of Wisconsin, Dr. Heisler is the FPMRS fellowship program director, Ob/Gyn resident rotation supervisor and Inpatient Advanced Internship course director. She continues to focus on surgical quality improvement with her work on Enhanced Recovery After Surgery (ERAS) within reconstructive surgery.

María Herrera de la Muela is Head of the Breast Cancer Unit. Women's Health Institute. Department of Gynaecology.

Cristina Honorato-Cia graduated in Medicine and Surgery at the University of Navarra in Spain, Trained in Anesthesia and Critical Care in the University Hospital of Navarra. Completed a fellowship in Neurotrauma anesthesia and critical care at the University of Toronto in 2009 and has worked ever since in neuroanesthesia and neurocritical care ever since, obtaining a PhD in this field in 2016. Visiting professor at Washington University, Neuroanesthesia. Representative for Spain at the European Society of Anesthesia since 2017, has been doing work in the field of gender equality and physician wellbeing as a result of her commitment with the ESA.

Ana Jorge, a paediatrician, was Minister of Health between 30 January 2008 and 21 June 2011, in the XVII and XVIII governments. She had previously other positions in the Health Regional Administration. Ana Jorge had coordinated the Sub-region of Health of Lisbon between 1996 and 1997, having transited to the board of Directors of the Regional Health Administration of Lisbon and Tagus Valley, between 1997 and 2000, to which she presided. She was also Director of the Pediatrics service. Ana Jorge was also teacher in the National School of Public Health (specialties of maternal, child, school and Adolescent health) and at the Faculty of Medicine of the University of Lisbon. She was also a member of The Medical College of Paediatrics in the National Medical Association Ordem dos Médicos.

Lap Yan Leung is a Surgical Trainee within the National Health Service (NHS) of England and a Honorary Lecturer of St George's University of London.

Elizabeth Lorraine-Lichtenstein, Swedish Md, specialist and senior consultant in Anesthesiology and Intensive Care, Vice charimn of The Swedish Medical Women´s Association. Coauthor of the book "Läkare, Doktor, Kvinna" that described Women in Medicine in 1997.

Julio Mayol received his MD and PhD from Universidad Complutense in Madrid. After finishing his training in Madrid, he moved to Boston to become research fellow in surgery at Harvard Medical School as part of Prof. Jeffrey B. Matthews' lab at Beth Israel Deaconess Medical Center (1996-1997). Back in Madrid, he became Associate Professor (1998) and Professor (2011) of Surgery and am currently Chief Medical & Innovation Officer at Hospital Clinico in Madrid. He has published on epithelial physiology and minimally invasive surgery. He currently serves as secretary of the BJS company and sit on the editorial boards of the Journal of Gastrointestinal Surgery and World Journal of Gastroenterology.

Maria do Céu Machado is a pediatric physician, President of the INFARMED - National Authority of Medicines and Health Products, I.P. since 2017, has led the Department of Pediatrics of the University Hospital de Santa Maria since May 2011 until 2017. She is also a professor at the University of Lisbon since June 2005. She is member of the National Council of Ethics for the Life Sciences, vice President of the Portuguese Academy of Medicine and vice-President of the Federation of European Medicine Academies. Between February 2013 and September 2014, Maria-Ceu Machado led the direction of the Lisboa Norte University Hospital Center and between 2006 and 2011 was the High Commissioner of Health. She is the author of the essay "Teenagers" and published 172 papers.

Pringl Miller, MD, FACS, is a board-certified General Surgeon and Hospice and Palliative Medicine specialist with additional fellowship training in Clinical Medical Ethics. She received her medical degree from the University of Chicago - Pritzker School of Medicine and completed general surgery training at Santa Barbara Cottage Hospital. After 14 years of general surgery practice she completed fellowships in Hospice and Palliative Medicine and Clinical Medical Ethics both at the University of Chicago. She is an Assistant Professor in the Departments of Surgery and Medicine at Rush University Medical Center. Her clinical and research interests include integrating palliative medicine and clinical medical ethics into the care of high risk surgical patients. Dr. Miller is the guest editor for Surgical Clinics of North America first edition of Practicing Primary Palliative Care in print October 2019. She is a strong advocate for women in surgery as the founder of #WoSurgMeToo and a founding member of TIME'S UP Healthcare. Dr. Miller is the guest editor of the Narrative Inquiry in Bioethics symposium, A Journal of Qualitative Research, entitled #MeToo in Surgery: Narratives by Women Surgeons published by the Johns Hopkins University Press in print and online Winter 2019.

Helen Mohan is a senior colorectal and general surgery SpR in Ireland. She is grateful to be mammy to 3 very special little people, twins and a toddler. She is passionate about improving patient care and surgical training. She has a PhD in pathophysiology of inflammation and cancer. Her academic interests include surgical education, advanced colorectal cancer, molecular biology of colorectal cancer and gender equity in surgical training. She is a past president of the Association of Surgeons in Training. During her time at ASiT she has worked to promote women in surgery and improved conditions for parents in surgery. For example she organised a feeding room and a crèche at the ASiT conference in Belfast. She worked on a survey on pregnancy, maternity and paternity leave with ASiT which has now been accepted for publication in PMJ. During her year as ASiT president she set the conference theme as nurturing excellence emphasising the importance of helping trainees achieve their potential. She is also the assistant editor of the European Journal of Surgical Oncology (EJSO), Vice-Chair of the Irish Surgical Research collaborative and Dukes Club Advanced Colorectal Cancer Representative. She has recently been awarded a scholarship from RCSI and the 30 percent club to pursue a postgraduate diploma in clinical leadership. Other interests include global surgery and she has volunteered with Operation International, most recently in Uganda. She is in her final year of surgical training and plans to pursue further training at fellowship level in advanced colorectal cancer in Australia.

Rebecca Nicholas works as a Plastic & Reconstructive Surgery Specialty Registrar, training in the London Deanery. Alongside her work she is married to Pete for 11 years who is a vicar and she is a mother of two energetic young boys, Oliver (3) and Tobi (1). She is currently training flexibly, and enjoys spending time with her children when she is not at work. She is an elected member on various committees including the PLASTA (PLAstic Surgery Trainees Association) Representative on the ASiT Committee (Association of Surgeons in Training), Trainee Representative on the BSSH Overseas Committee (British Society of Surgery of the Hand), and Vice Chair of the BFIRST Trainees Committee (British Foundation of International Reconstructive Surgery and Training). She has a BSc in International Health and Development, with a particular interests in improving access to surgical training and essential surgery in low- and middle-income countries, and has an MSc in Medical Education, with a particular interest in the use of simulation in surgical training.

Vassilios Papalois is professor of transplantation surgery and consultant transplant and general surgeon at Hammersmith Hospital. He leads a Transplant Centre of Excellence focusing on high risk and extended criteria kidney and pancreas transplantation. Professor Papalois was trained in general and transplant surgery at St Mary's Hospital and in the department of surgery at the University of Minnesota (post-PhD fellowship and clinical fellowship) which is one of the biggest transplant programmes in the world and has led in the field of transplantation for the last 50 years. He has published 200 papers in peer review journals, 20 book chapters and 7 books. His research focuses on pre-transplant assessment and reconditioning of marginal kidney and pancreas grafts, use of stem cells, clinical ethics and health policy. He has been awarded, through competitive processes, more than £2,000,000 in research grants. Professor Papalois is clinical lead for medico-legal issues at Imperial College Healthcare NHS Trust, chairs the Ethics Committee of the Avon and Somerset Constabulary and he is a member of the Research Ethics Committee of the UK Ministry of Defence. He is the Secretary General of the European Union of Medical Specialists (UEMS), the President Elect of the European Society of Organ Transplantation (ESOT), a member of the Executive Board of the Association of Surgeons of Great Britain and Ireland (ASGBI) and a member of the European Society of Surgery (ESS). Professor Papalois organises a series of advanced international courses annually on transplant training, clinical ethics and health policy and has given more than 100 lectures in international forums as an invited speaker. He has been awarded a Bronze National Award for Clinical Excellence by the UK Department of Health, a Senior Clinical Investigator Award by the European Society for Organ Transplantation and a Teaching Excellence Award by Imperial College London. He has also been awarded an Honorary Doctorate from the University of Thessaloniki and he is an Honorary Member of the Spanish Association of Surgeons and the Spanish Transplantation Society.

Monica Sivakumar is a Pathologist at Apollo Gleneagles Hospitals, Kolkata.

Hafdis Svavarsdottir is an Academic Clinical Fellow in General Surgery at the University of Leeds and Core Surgical Trainee in General Surgery at Yorkshire and the Humber Deanery.

Sarah M. Temkin, MD, is a practicing gynecologic oncologist. She is currently the Director for Gynecologic Oncology at the Anne Arundel Medical Center in Annapolis, Maryland. She is widely published on topics including racial disparities in cancer care, screening and prevention, population health as it relates to gynecologic malignancies and clinical trials for women with ovarian, endometrial and cervical cancers.

Maria Theodosopoulou has studied Philosophy, Education, Psychology, has a Master's degree in Career Counselling and a PhD in Lifelong Learning. Currently, she is finishing her second PhD, which focuses on Health Literacy at Imperial College London. She has worked for more than ten years in the fields of lifelong learning and adult education and firmly believes the idea that critical thinking and empowerment skills start in families and schools and stand at the core of learning.

Deborah Verran MBChB, MHSM, FRACS completed medical school in New Zealand in 1981, then worked in hospitals around New Zealand as a junior doctor (unaccredited resident). Undertook accredited General Surgical Training from 1987-1991 (Auckland Regional Scheme), culminating in the FRACS. First consultant position was as a Lecturer in Surgery, 1991-1992 at Auckland Hospital. This was followed by Transplant Surgical Fellowship training in the United States (University of Alabama, Birmingham,1992-1994) and Canada (London, Ontario, 1994-1995). Then commenced my second consultant position as a Transplant Surgeon (Liver & Kidney), in 1995 in Sydney, Australia, which I have held for over 20 years. Undertook and completed an MHSM (Masters in health Service Management) in 2013. Outside interests trekking and hiking. Accomplishments include, over 100 publications, presentations at scientific meetings, committee work at regional and national levels culminating in guideline publication for organ donation and transplantation, medicolegal advisory roles for over 10 years, mentoring of medical students and trainees, membership of International Transplant Societies, clinical Resource Officer for the Australian Organ & Tissue Authority for 6 years – including undertaking Social Media for advocacy purposes for organ donation, ongoing advocacy for gender equity.

Stella Vig is a Consultant Vascular and General Surgeon at Croydon University Hospital, South London. Born in Bangor, North Wales, she trained at the University of Wales College of Medicine. She was appointed as a consultant in 2006. Stella has a strong interest in training and encouraging medical students and foundation years to pursue a career in surgery. She is a champion and advocate for trainees, ensuring their voices are heard. Stella was awarded the NHS Leadership Academy London Mentor of the Year in 2015 and the Silver Scalpel Award as well as the Dr Rose Polge Award in 2018, She was the Foundation Program Director at Croydon University Hospital for 10 years and holds many roles including those of Core Surgery and Higher Surgery Training Programme Director. She has previously completed terms as JCST Chair for Core Surgical Training and General Surgery Surgical Advisory Committee member. She is a member of the Faculty of Surgical Educators. She is one of three Clinical Directors for Croydon and Co-Chairs the London Diabetic Foot Network within the Diabetes Strategic Clinical Network. She was elected to RCS England Council in 2016.

Index

G

H

I

L

M

N

O

P

R

S

T

W

www.ingramcontent.com/pod-product-compliance
Lightning Source LLC
LaVergne TN
LVHW060415300926
849162LV00006B/1430